Peter Manu, MD

The Psychopathology
of Functional
Somatic Syndromes
Neurobiology and Illness Behavior
in Chronic Fatigue Syndrome,
Fibromyalgia, Gulf War Illness,
Irritable Bowel,
and Premenstrual Dysphoria

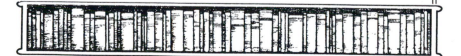

The Psychopathology of Functional Somatic Syndromes

Neurobiology and Illness Behavior in Chronic Fatigue Syndrome, Fibromyalgia, Gulf War Illness, Irritable Bowel, and Premenstrual Dysphoria

THE HAWORTH MEDICAL PRESS®
Haworth Research Series
on Malaise, Fatigue, and Debilitation

Roberto Patarca-Montero, MD, PhD
Senior Editor

The Psychopathology of Functional Somatic Syndromes

Neurobiology and Illness Behavior in Chronic Fatigue Syndrome, Fibromyalgia, Gulf War Illness, Irritable Bowel, and Premenstrual Dysphoria

Peter Manu, MD

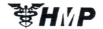

The Haworth Medical Press®
An Imprint of The Haworth Press, Inc.
New York • London • Oxford

Published by

The Haworth Medical Press ®, an imprint of The Haworth Press, Inc., 10 Alice Street, Binghamton, NY 13904-1580.

PUBLISHER'S NOTE
This book has been published solely for educational purposes and is not intended to substitute for the medical advice of a treating physician. Medicine is an ever-changing science. As new research and clinical experience broaden our knowledge, changes in treatment may be required. While many potential treatment options are made herein, some or all of the options may not be applicable to a particular individual. Therefore, the author, editor, and publisher do not accept responsibility in the event of negative consequences incurred as a result of the information presented in this book. We do not claim that this information is necessarily accurate by the rigid scientific and regulatory standards applied for medical treatment. **No warranty, expressed or implied, is furnished with respect to the material contained in this book. The reader is urged to consult with his/her personal physician with respect to the treatment of any medical condition.**

The author has exhaustively researched all available sources to ensure the accuracy and completeness of the information contained in this book. The publisher and author assume no responsibility for errors, inaccuracies, omissions, or any inconsistency herein.

Cover design by Marylouise E. Doyle.

Library of Congress Cataloging-in-Publication Data

Manu, Peter, 1947-
    The psychopathology of functional somatic syndromes : neurobiology and illness behavior in chronic fatigue syndrome, fibromyalgia, Gulf War illness, irritable bowel, and premenstrual dysphoria / Peter Manu.
        p.   cm.
    Includes bibliographical references and index.
    ISBN 0-7890-1259-6 (hard : alk. paper)—ISBN 0-7890-1260-X (pbk. : alk. paper)
    1. Somatoform disorders. I. Title.
    [DNLM: 1. Somatoform Disorders—physiopathology. 2. Colonic Diseases, Functional—physiopathology. 3. Fatigue Syndrome, Chronic—physiopathology. 4. Fibromyalgia—physiopathology. 5. Persian Gulf Syndrome—physiopathology. 6. Premenstrual Syndrome—physiopathology. WM 170 M294p 2004]
RC552.S66M36 2004
616.85′24—dc21

                                                                                                      2003001540

Polonius.
I will be brief. Your noble son is mad.
Mad call I it, for, to define true madness,
What is't but to be nothing else but mad?

Queen.
More matter with less art.

Hamlet, Act 2, Scene 2

ABOUT THE AUTHOR

Peter Manu, MD, is Professor of Clinical Medicine and Professor of Clinical Psychiatry at Albert Einstein College of Medicine at Yeshiva University in New York. He practices and teaches at Long Island Jewish Medical Center, where he is Director of Medical Services at the Zucker Hillside Hospital. Dr. Manu is the author of *The Pharmacotherapy of Common Functional Syndromes: Evidence-Based Guidelines for Primary Care Practice* (Haworth) and editor of *Functional Somatic Syndrome: Etiology, Diagnosis, and Treatment* (Cambridge).

CONTENTS

PART III: THE PSYCHOBIOLOGY OF FUNCTIONAL SOMATIC SYNDROMES

PART IV: ABNORMAL PERSONALITY AND ILLNESS BEHAVIOR IN FUNCTIONAL SOMATIC SYNDROMES

Introduction

Chronic fatigue syndrome, fibromyalgia, irritable bowel syndrome, premenstrual syndrome, and Gulf War illness are common illnesses that lack demonstrable structural or biochemical abnormalities and are characterized by medically unexplained symptoms such as fatigue, myalgias, abdominal pain, difficulty with concentration, mood lability, and sleep disturbance (Manu, 1998).

The way in which these entities have been explained has varied, and some clinicians have interpreted and managed them as physical disorders. However, most physicians have understood them to be mental illnesses (Sharpe and Carson, 2001). This pattern continues, as shown by a recent survey of 400 physicians in the South Thames area of England (Reid et al., 2001). More than half of the respondents (63 percent) thought that the symptoms were best explained by a psychiatric disorder. An even greater proportion of this physician sample (83 percent) believed that patients with medically unexplained symptoms have a personality disorder. Most of the respondents (93 percent) felt that patients with such symptoms are difficult to manage. A solid majority (75 percent) of these physicians rejected the possibility that the symptoms represented evidence of an undiagnosed physical illness. These beliefs were not related to the physicians' training in psychiatry or to the availability of mental health resources in the area they served. Consistent with these beliefs, most of the physicians felt that their main role in managing these patients was to provide reassurance (99 percent of the respondents), act as gatekeepers to prevent inappropriate consultations and laboratory investigations (94 percent), and provide counseling and psychological management (84 percent). The individual comments add support to the strong feelings evoked by these patients in their primary care providers. One physician indicated a frustration possibly felt by many, writing "I would like to have enough courage to tell them that nothing is wrong; you are wasting my time and your time. You must try to learn to live with your symptoms." Another reflected distrust, suggesting that "most of medically unexplained symptoms are related to not wanting to go back to work, and sick benefits usually help to keep away symptoms." The third expressed a degree of annoyance with the fact that "having excluded the impossible as far as one can, the medically unexplained symptom usually has a personality/psychiatric aspect but patients will not be persuaded of this" (Reid et al., 2001, p. 521).

Recent conceptualizations of functional somatic syndromes as mental disorders have proposed four empirical constructs. The first suggested that these syndromes are part of the affective spectrum disorder, together with major depression, bulimia, panic disorder, obsessive-compulsive disorder, and attention deficit disorder with hyperactivity (Hudson and Pope, 1990). The second proposed that patients with functional illnesses are chronic somatizers who present with a large array of complaints, are familiar with the definitions of functional syndromes, have a past history of psychiatric disorders, and tend to embrace poorly documented disease mechanisms such as environmental allergies, overgrowth of *Candida albicans,* and reactivation of dormant herpetic viruses (Stewart, 1990). The third frame of reference encouraged an individualized approach to these syndromes and suggested a variety of explanations such as serotonin deficiency for the pain symptoms in fibromyalgia and physical inactivity for the postexercise malaise of patients with chronic fatigue syndrome (Kellner, 1994). The fourth theory emphasized abnormal illness behavior and focused on these patients' belief that they have a serious problem, their sense that the illness is disabling and catastrophic, and their suspicion of physicians' expertise and motivation (Barsky and Borus, 1999). These constructs have remained largely unproven.

The origin of this book is a cluster of observations made by Tom Lane, Dale Matthews, Victor Hesselbrock, Howard Tennen, Glenn Affleck, Rich Mendola, Javier Escobar, Priscilla Morse, Micha Abeles, Rich Castriotta, the late Bob Watson, and me in a large number of patients with medically unexplainable complaints seen from 1986 through 1993 at the University of Connecticut Health Center, Farmington, Connecticut. From the outset, the structured data collection indicated a high prevalence of major depression (Manu, Matthews, et al., 1989), somatization disorder (Manu, Lane, et al., 1989), and panic disorder (Manu et al., 1991). However, the severity of psychiatric symptoms did not correlate with myalgias and sleep disturbance (Manu et al., 1994). The possibility that the psychiatric syndromes represented reactions to the physical illness appeared unlikely, because their onset preceded the functional complaint in a majority of cases (Lane et al., 1991). Moreover, the depressive symptoms commonly reported by these patients did not influence their disease conviction, disease phobia, and bodily preoccupation (Manu et al., 1996). The findings challenged the view that functional illnesses were manifestations of an affective disorder (Hudson and Pope, 1990), offered only limited support for the chronic somatization hypothesis (Stewart, 1990), and did not confirm the link between depression and hypochondriasis (Barsky and Borus, 1999).

What is the nature of the association between psychopathology and functional illness? Is there a biological gradient between the somatic and psychological features of these syndromes? Do objective findings support a relationship? Are psychiatric symptoms the manifestations of dysfunctional coping? This book attempts to answer these questions by studying the best research work of the past two decades. It starts by describing the modern definitions of chronic fatigue, fibromyalgia, irritable bowel, premenstrual dysphoria, and postcombat ailments and the way in which these entities have evolved into a tightly knit family of self-standing syndromes with a common core of somatic symptoms. The second part presents the frequency of psychiatric disorders in functional syndromes and analyzes the correlation between the burden of psychopathology and the physical features of these illnesses. The third part is a review of advances in the appraisal of the neuroanatomy, neuropsychology, and neurochemistry of functional syndromes and an attempt to determine whether the confirmed abnormalities are similar to those described in psychiatric disorders. The last part of the book focuses on measurable dimensions of personality, coping, and illness behavior and on their correlation with the severity and prognosis of medically unexplainable illness. Throughout the book, the sample selection, methodologies, and findings are described in detail for each of the studies selected. The meta-analytic temptation was resisted: the works were allowed to stand alone and the authors' words permitted to judge the findings.

This book will show that chronic fatigue syndrome, fibromyalgia, irritable bowel syndrome, premenstrual syndrome, and Gulf War illness are overlapping conditions with numerous medically unexplained complaints. The main somatic descriptors of these illnesses are chronic musculoskeletal or abdominal pain, persistent fatigue, sleep disturbance, and cognitive deficits. A past history of mood disorders is common, but only a minority of patients can be diagnosed with current major depression, dysthymia, panic disorder, or post-traumatic stress. Depression and anxiety do not correlate well with the overall severity of functional impairment, but are associated with the features of somatization and poor long-term outcome. The cognitive and neurobiological abnormalities are nonspecific, mild, and variable. No compelling evidence suggests that these syndromes are serotonin-deficient states. The pattern of activation of the hypo-thalamic-pituitary axis distinguishes functional syndromes from melancholic depression and stress-related illnesses. Many patients with functional syndromes have abnormal personality features, a history of sexual and physical abuse, a tendency to attribute their illness to a physical cause, and a catastrophic coping style.

The evidence presented in this book demonstrates that functional syndromes are not atypical manifestations of mood or anxiety disorders. Their psychopathology centers on production of somatic and psychological symptoms as expressions of neuroticism, harm avoidance, sexual victimization, and maladaptive coping. This interpretation of the data accumulated in the past two decades is close to other important themes about the nature of physical symptoms (Katon and Walker, 1998). First, functional illnesses are likely to reflect specific personality traits, prior illness experience, and early family environment. Second, lifetime psychiatric disorders and psychological distress correlate with the number of medically unexplained complaints, a quantitative relationship that highlights the severity of the illness rather than an etiologic relationship. Third, the severity of symptoms increases as the evaluation moves from primary to specialized care settings and creates an unsatisfactory patient-doctor relationship (Katon and Walker, 1998). The central idea generated by this review is the coexistence of somatization with personality abnormalities, an area that has received only scant attention in the research literature. The personality disorders common in patients with somatization disorder are histrionic, passive-dependent, and sensitive-aggressive. The interaction between life situations and personality abnormalities leads to the behavior of complaining, persistence of illness, and resistance to treatment (Stern et al., 1993).

This work was planned during a visiting professorship in the Department of Psychosomatic Medicine, Heinrich-Heine University, Düsseldorf, Germany, made possible by John Kane, Matthias Franz, and Maria Angel. I acknowledge with heartfelt gratitude their support. The writing of the book, as well as my struggle to decipher the complexities of functional disorders, would have been much harder without the clarity brought to this field by Simon Wessely, Michael Sharpe, Steve Straus, Wayne Katon, and Mark Demitrack. I admire and respect the insight, wisdom, and discernment of their work.

PART I:
THE CLINICAL MANIFESTATIONS
OF FUNCTIONAL SYNDROMES

Chapter 1

The Modern Conceptualization
of Unexplained Symptoms

Functional syndromes characterized by malaise, widespread or localized pain, cognitive abnormalities, anxiety, depression, and somatic preoccupation have been identified for more than two centuries. They have received many names and have had many proposed but unproved etiologies (Feinstein, 2001; Sharpe and Carson, 2001). In the past two decades, common illnesses such as chronic fatigue syndrome, fibromyalgia, and irritable bowel have been defined as "medical syndromes" highlighting patterns of somatic distress thought to originate from specific bodily systems (Mayou and Farmer, 2002). The road toward a crisp nosology of functional ailments has been a difficult one, primarily because those involved in the effort have had to abandon traditional demands for appropriate correlation of symptoms and objective abnormalities (Feinstein, 2001).

CHRONIC FATIGUE SYNDROME

Since the early 1980s, a syndrome of persistent fatigue and symptoms resembling those of common viral infections has captured widespread medical and public attention. Initially, the syndrome was etiologically linked to immunological stigmata of Epstein-Barr virus infection (Tobi et al., 1982; Dubois et al., 1984; Jones et al., 1985; Straus et al., 1985) and the illness came to be known as chronic Epstein-Barr virus infection or chronic mononucleosis-like syndrome. However, attempts to confirm the role of Epstein-Barr virus infection in the production of the symptoms refuted a causal relationship (Holmes et al., 1987; Hellinger et al., 1988; Straus et al., 1988). This reality led an interdisciplinary group assembled by the Centers for

Disease Control to name the illness chronic fatigue syndrome and to provide a working case definition (Holmes et al., 1988).

The definition described two major and 14 minor criteria. The first major criterion required a history of new onset of persistent or relapsing, debilitating fatigue or easy fatigability, that did not resolve with bed rest and that was severe enough to reduce daily activities to less than half the premorbid levels for a period of at least six months. The second major criterion mandated that other clinical conditions associated with persistent tiredness be excluded by a thorough clinical and laboratory evaluation. Researchers were also advised to obtain a detailed personal and family psychiatric history. However, a formal psychiatric evaluation was not considered necessary. Patients with psychiatric disorders that preceded the onset of the fatigue-dominated illness were considered ineligible for the diagnosis of chronic fatigue syndrome.

The 14 minor criteria were divided into two groups. The first group included 11 types of subjective complaints: sudden onset, headache, mild fever or chills, sore throat, painful lymph nodes in neck or armpit, muscle weakness, myalgias, migratory arthralgias, postexercise malaise, sleep disturbance, and neuropsychological complaints (i.e., one or more of photophobia, scotomasa, forgetfulness, irritability, confusion, difficulty thinking, inability to concentrate, and depression). The second group included three objective findings: low-grade fever, nonexudative pharyngitis, and palpable or tender lymph nodes in the cervical or axillary areas. The objective findings had to be documented by a physician on at least two occasions, at least one month apart. The diagnosis of chronic fatigue syndrome was to be given to patients with both major criteria and either eight of the 11 subjective complaints or six of the 11 subjective complaints and two of the three objective findings.

Two years later, Australian investigators proposed the second case definition of chronic fatigue syndrome (Lloyd et al., 1990). Compared with the construct adopted in the United States (Holmes et al., 1988), the proposal did not require the presence of physical symptoms, but only a history of chronic, persistent or relapsing fatigue leading to substantial disruption of usual activities; neuropsychiatric dysfunction, including new onset of short-term memory impairment or difficulty with concentration; and postexertional fatigue.

A few months later, a large interdisciplinary group of British investigators produced a new definition for chronic fatigue syndrome (Sharpe et al., 1991). Intended to serve as a guideline for clinical research, the proposal recommended that the diagnosis be given to subjects whose principal symptom of fatigue was definite in onset; whose illness was severe, disabling, and having an effect on physical and cognitive functioning; and in whom the illness had been present at least half the time for at least six months. Patients with psychiatric disorders such as schizophrenia, bipolar mood disorder, substance abuse, and organic brain disorder could not be given this diagnosis. Patients with medical conditions known to produce persistent tiredness were also excluded. Other psychiatric syndromes, including depressive and anxiety disorders, were not considered grounds for exclusion.

A comparison of these case definitions was performed on 805 patients with debilitating fatigue examined at the Brigham and Women's Hospital, Boston, and Harborview Medical Center, Seattle (Bates et al., 1994). Overall, 72 percent of subjects met at least one case definition. Specifically, 61 percent of patients met the American definition (Holmes et al., 1988), 56 percent met the Australian definition (Lloyd et al., 1990), and 55 percent met the British definition of the syndrome (Sharpe et al., 1991). A substantial proportion of patients (41 percent of the total sample) met all three definitions. The authors felt that the multisymptom construct adopted by the American definition was responsible for the preferential inclusion of psychiatric patients and suggested the revision of the current standard with the aim of reducing the number of symptom criteria.

The diagnostic criteria for chronic fatigue syndrome were revised by the International Chronic Fatigue Study Group assembled at the Centers for Disease Control and Prevention in Atlanta, Georgia, in 1993 (Fukuda et al., 1994). The participants included many of the authors of the previous three definitions. The new criteria set required the presence of persistent or relapsing fatigue and at least four of eight specified subjective complaints. The dominant symptom of fatigue had to have a definite onset; had to remain unexplained after clinical evaluation; and had to produce significant reduction in previous levels of occupational and social activities. The eight subjective complaints were substantial impairment in short-term memory and concentration; sore throat; tender cervical or axillary lymph nodes;

muscle pain; joint pains without evidence of acute arthritis; headaches of a new type, pattern, or severity; unrefreshing sleep; and postexertional malaise lasting more than 24 hours. The associated symptoms had to be concurrent with fatigue and had to have persisted or relapsed during at least six consecutive months of illness.

Laboratory tests were to be used only to investigate the presence of other conditions likely to produce the symptoms. The presence of any such condition excluded the diagnosis of chronic fatigue syndrome. The diagnosis was also excluded in individuals with morbid obesity, drug or alcohol abuse within two years prior to the onset of fatigue, and in patients with past or current diagnosis of melancholic or psychotic depression, bipolar affective disorder, schizophrenia, delusional disorder, dementia, and anorexia or bulimia nervosa. The presence of nonmelancholic and nonpsychotic depression, anxiety disorders, and somatoform disorders did not invalidate the diagnosis.

FIBROMYALGIA

The genesis of the current diagnostic criteria for fibromyalgia started with work performed by Canadian investigators from the University of Toronto starting in the 1960s (Smythe and Moldofsky, 1978; Smythe, 1989). In Smythe's (1989) words, the starting position was clear: "If there was no local inflammation, how were the symptoms to be explained? You can imagine the discussion; if there is nothing there, there is nothing there." But to others, "there had to be something there! Psychogenic factors seemed to be important, but there was a reluctance to equate the symptoms with hysteria and malingering. Thus the concept of tension rheumatism evolved, . . . but with a lack of clarity as to whether the symptoms arose peripherally in tense muscles or were manifestations of a psychoneurosis" (p. 4). Smythe's role (Smythe, 1989) was to define the musculoskeletal sites that were very tender in fibrositic patients. A valuable site was to be "unknown to the patient, unknown because it is deep and not central to the area of pain. Because the points were unknown, the tenderness was not susceptible to exaggeration for psychological reasons, conscious or unconscious" (p. 5).

The first set of diagnostic criteria for fibrositis was published by the Canadian clinicians as part of an investigation of sleep disturbance (Moldofsky et al., 1975). The criteria consisted of seven subjective complaints and six clinical observations. The complaints were aching and stiffness for more than three months; chronic fatigue and poor work tolerance; sleep disturbance; morning aching and stiffness; weather effect; temporary relief with heat; and poor appetite. The clinical observations comprised local point tenderness; absence of muscle induration; unrestricted range of musculoskeletal motion; emotional distress (i.e., depression, anxiety, and irritability); dermatographia; and normal findings on radiological and laboratory tests. The number of tender points required for diagnosis was not specified, but the authors provided a list of 13 anatomical locations. A few years later, the same clinicians provided more information on the locations and characteristics of 14 pairs of potentially tender points (Smythe and Moldofsky, 1978) and expressed the opinion that "the existence of exaggerated tenderness at anatomically reproducible locations is central to the acceptance and recognition of the syndrome" (p. 928).

In 1981, investigators from the University of Illinois at Peoria proposed a set of diagnostic criteria for fibromyalgia that was based on a comparison of 50 patients considered to have this condition with 50 healthy control subjects (Yunus et al., 1981). All patients had generalized aching or stiffness and at least four tender points. The authors generated a diagnostic construct that comprised a total of 13 criteria divided into groups of obligatory, major, and minor criteria. The two obligatory criteria were the presence of generalized aches and pains, involving three or more anatomic sites, for at least three months; and the absence of secondary causes (including traumatic, degenerative, endocrinologic, infectious, and malignant disorders) and laboratory abnormalities. The major criterion was defined as the presence of at least five typical and consistent tender points. The ten minor criteria were aggravation of symptoms by anxiety or stress; modulation of symptoms by physical activity; modulation of symptoms by weather; fatigue; poor sleep; anxiety; chronic headache; irritable bowel syndrome; subjective swelling; and numbness.

The diagnosis was to be given to patients who met the two obligatory criteria, the major criterion, and at least three of the ten minor criteria. The criteria set had a specificity of 100 percent and a sensitivity of 96 percent. The authors considered that this definition of fibromyalgia helped to differentiate it from psychogenic rheumatism. In their view, patients with psychogenic rheumatism have bizarre and exaggerated pain symptoms occurring at vague and changing sites, modulated by emotional factors and almost always associated with functional complaints. In contrast, their patients with fibromyalgia complained of aching, pain, or gelling at definite anatomic sites, had symptoms that were modulated by weather, and had few functional complaints.

Five years later, a Boston-based group of investigators used a slightly different set of criteria to define fibromyalgia for clinical research studies (Goldenberg et al., 1986). The definition required three obligatory criteria and three of seven associated clinical features. The obligatory criteria were generalized pain; aches or stiffness involving at least three anatomic sites for three or more months; at least six characteristic and consistent tender points; and the absence of an underlying cause for the illness. The list of associated clinical features included general fatigue; poor sleep; chronic headaches; irritable bowel syndrome; subjective swelling and numbness; anxiety; and modulation of symptoms by stress, anxiety, activity, and weather.

In 1989, the investigators from the University of Illinois College of Medicine, Peoria, published a new set of diagnostic criteria for fibromyalgia (Yunus et al., 1989). The proposed criteria were the result of a study that compared 63 fibromyalgia patients with 63 patients with painful musculoskeletal conditions (32 with mild rheumatoid arthritis and 31 with posttraumatic fibromyalgia) and 30 healthy control subjects. According to their new proposal, the diagnosis of fibromyalgia was to be given to subjects having two obligatory criteria plus either two historical variables and four tender points or three historical variables and three tender points. The obligatory criteria were presence of pain or stiffness at four or more different anatomic sites for at least three months; and absence of a condition that may be responsible for the clinical presentation. The historical variables consisted of a list of six symptoms: hurting all over; pain at more than seven different sites; general fatigue; poor sleep; anxiety or tension; and irritable bowel syndrome. The tender points were to be sought at seven anatomical locations. The definition had a sensitivity of 92 percent and specificity of 94 percent.

The current standard for the definition of fibromyalgia in clinical and research populations was developed by a group of rheumatologists from the United States and Canada on behalf of the American College of Rheumatology (Wolfe et al., 1990). The group included the authors of the Toronto (Moldofsky et al., 1975), Peoria

(Yunus et al., 1981), and Boston (Goldenberg et al., 1986) criteria. The work represented a continuation of an earlier project, which had demonstrated that the tender point count performed better than symptom checklists in separating patients with fibrositis from those with other rheumatological conditions (Wolfe et al., 1985). The criteria set was derived from a study comparing the frequency of symptoms such as widespread pain, fatigue, morning stiffness, and sleep disturbance and the average number of tender musculoskeletal points in 158 patients considered by experts to have primary fibromyalgia and in 135 control subjects with pure musculoskeletal disorders, of whom 42 percent had rheumatoid arthritis, 20 percent had low back pain syndrome, 10 percent had neck pain syndromes, 10 percent had tendinitis, and 18 percent had other rheumatological diagnoses.

Patients with primary fibromyalgia were significantly more likely than rheumatologically ill control subjects to have widespread pain (97 versus 71 percent) and pain at more than 15 different anatomic sites (59 versus 13 percent). They were also much more likely to report fatigue (78 versus 38 percent), sleep disturbance (76 versus 31 percent), paresthesias (67 versus 32 percent), headache (54 versus 30 percent), anxiety (45 versus 22 percent), and irritable bowel (36 versus 13 percent). The most discriminating items were tenderness at 11 of 18 anatomic sites, sleep disturbance, and fatigue.

The criteria set chosen by this group of experts combined the subjective report of widespread pain with tenderness at 11 of 18 (i.e., nine pairs) musculoskeletal sites. The nine pairs of sites at which tenderness must be sought include the suboccipital muscle insertion; the anterior aspect of the intertransverse spaces of the fifth, sixth, and seventh cervical vertebrae; the midpoint of the upper border of the trapezius muscle; the scapula spine near the medial border; the second costochondral junction; 2 cm distal to the ulnar epicondyle; the anterior fold of the gluteal muscle in the upper quadrant of the buttock; the greater trochanter, posterior to its prominence; and the medial fat pad proximal to the joint line of the knee. This construct had a sensitivity of 88 percent and a specificity of 98 percent.

The notion that fibromyalgia is a distinct clinical entity was challenged in a recent analysis of the historical and epidemiological evidence (Wessely and Hotopf, 1999). The authors observed that the diagnosis gained acceptance as a rheumatological disorder only after Smythe and Moldofsky (1978) suggested that reproducible tender points constitute diagnostic proof for the existence of the condition. They also made the point that the efforts made in the 1980s to revise the definition increased its reliability, but did not offer objective findings to support the presence of a discrete disease process. As Wessely and Hotopf (1999) wrote, the origin of this syndrome did not lie in a breakthrough in the interpretation of pathophysiology, but "it was based solely on the clinical intuition of a few rheumatologists" and "on the experiences of examining small number of patients in specialist clinics" (p. 429). The epidemiological case against fibromyalgia is supported by the demonstration of a high prevalence of chronic diffuse musculoskeletal pain in about 10 percent of the general adult population of England and Wales (Croft et al., 1994) and a North American community (Wolfe et al., 1995). Population studies conducted by Wessely's research group (Pawlikowska et al., 1994) have also identified a high frequency of myalgia at rest (14 percent) and after exercise (22 percent). Moreover, the presence of tender points is associated not only with widespread pain, but also with sleep disturbance and fatigue (Croft et al., 1994; Croft et al., 1996). Based on these facts, Wessely and Hotopf (1999) felt that fibromyalgia is a misnomer for a continuum in which patients with more pain have more tender points. From this angle, the tender points could be seen as a nonspecific marker for distress rather than as objective evidence for a unique clinical disorder (Croft et al., 1996; Wolfe, 1997).

PREMENSTRUAL SYNDROME

The modern diagnostic criteria for premenstrual syndrome were published in 1987 in the *Diagnostic and Statistical Manual of Mental Disorders* (American Psychiatric Association, 1987). The condition was named late luteal phase dysphoric disorder, and its diagnosis required that physicians inquire about the presence of ten symptoms or clusters of symptoms: marked affective lability; persistent and marked anger and irritability; marked anxiety and tension; markedly depressed mood, including self-deprecating thoughts or hopelessness; decreased interest in usual activities; easy fatigability; difficulty with concentration; substantial change in appetite, specific food cravings, or overeating; sleep disturbance; and physical symptoms such as headaches, myalgias, arthralgias, bloating, weight gain, and breast tenderness or swelling.

The diagnosis was allowed if at least five symptoms were present during the last seven days of the luteal phase. The symptoms were required to subside within a few days of the onset of menstrual bleeding. At least one of the five symptoms had to indicate a marked change with regard to mood lability, anger or irritability, anxiety or tension, and depression or hopelessness. The luteal phase disturbance had to be severe enough to interfere with occupational, social, or interpersonal activities. The condition had to be distinguished from the premenstrual exacerbation of major depression, dysthymia, panic disorder, and personality pathology. However, the definition stated emphatically that the presence of these conditions did not rule out premenstrual syndrome, as long as "the person experiences characteristic late luteal phase dysphoric disorder symptoms that are markedly different from those they experience as part of the coexisting disorder" (American Psychiatric Association, 1987, p. 368).

The criteria were minimally revised in the 1994 edition of the *Diagnostic and Statistical Manual of Mental Disorders* (American Psychiatric Association, 1994). The number of symptoms or clusters of symptoms was increased from ten to eleven, by adding a complaint of feeling overwhelmed or out of control. The other symptoms were this time named dysphoria; anxiety; affective lability (e.g., feeling suddenly tearful or sad, or having increased sensitivity to rejection); irritability; anhedonia; difficulty with concentration; fatigue; eating disturbance; sleep disturbance; and other physical symptoms. The diagnostic rule was not changed. The manual advised careful consideration of the premenstrual exacerbation of certain medical conditions, such as endometriosis, thyroid gland dysfunction, epilepsy, collagen vascular diseases, and malignancies.

IRRITABLE BOWEL SYNDROME

The modern work toward the definition of irritable bowel syndrome was inaugurated by a study that evaluated 109 unselected patients referred for abdominal pain or change in bowel habit (Manning et al., 1978). All subjects were asked to complete a questionnaire assessing 15 symptoms. The patients' records were reviewed 17 to 26 months later. The audit established the diagnosis of organic gastrointestinal disorder in 33 patients, irritable bowel syndrome in 32 patients, and diverticulosis in 14 patients. Forty patients failed to answer the questionnaire or were lost to follow-up.

Compared with patients with organic disorders, those with irritable bowel syndrome reported a higher frequency of the following four symptoms: abdominal distention, as evidenced by appearance or tight clothing; relief of pain with bowel movement; more frequent stools with the onset of pain; and looser bowel movement with the onset of pain. A feeling of incomplete evacuation and passage of mucus were also common in the irritable bowel group. These six symptoms came to be known as the Manning criteria for the diagnosis of irritable bowel syndrome.

The second set of diagnostic criteria for irritable bowel syndrome were formulated by a multinational group of experts assembled in 1984 (Thompson, 1999). The participants met in Rome in 1988 and published their recommendations in 1989 (Thompson et al., 1989). The criteria were revised by the same group several years later (Thompson et al., 1992). This version was named Rome Criteria I and required the presence of chronic abdominal pain and at least two of five specified symptoms. The abdominal pain or discomfort had to be continuous or recurrent for at least three months; be relieved with defecation; or be associated with a change in the frequency of bowel movements or consistency of stool. The five associated symptoms were abdominal distention; altered stool frequency (more than three bowel movements each day or less than three bowel movements each week); altered stool consistency (hard and lumpy or loose and watery); altered stool passage (urgency to defecate, straining, or a feeling of incomplete evacuation); and passage of mucus. The predominance of constipation or diarrhea was considered significant and researchers were advised to use these variants to stratify subjects enrolled in etiologic and therapeutic studies. The diagnosis could not be given if laboratory studies (i.e., colonoscopy, barium enema, and stool analysis for evidence of infection and malabsorption) indicated evidence of organic pathology (Longstreth, 1998). The diagnosis was not given if the medically unexplained symptoms were better classified as a different functional gastrointestinal disorder, such as functional dyspepsia or functional constipation (Thompson et al., 1992).

The latest definition of irritable bowel syndrome was the result of a consensus-reaching process conducted by the Multinational Working Team to Develop Diagnostic Criteria for Functional Gastrointestinal

Disorders (Thompson et al., 1999). The Rome II definition requires the presence of abdominal discomfort or pain for at least 12 weeks during the preceding year. The pain must have at least two of the following three characteristics: be relieved with defecation; have its onset associated with a change in the appearance of the stool; and have its onset associated with change in the frequency of bowel movements. Other disorders must be ruled out, particularly when the history and physical examination indicate fever, weight loss, or rectal bleeding. A structural examination of the large bowel is recommended in all cases. The type of symptoms and the age of the patient should guide the additional clinical investigations.

Hammer and Talley (1999) summarized the criticisms of the Rome criteria. First, they felt that the current requirement for the duration of abdominal pain and discomfort is arbitrary. Second, symptoms commonly associated with the condition, such as postprandial pain, postprandial urgency or diarrhea, and abdominal bloating were not included in the definition. Third, the criteria were considered more sensitive for the detection of irritable bowel syndrome in women than men.

GULF WAR ILLNESS

In a military conflict triggered by the Iraq's occupation of Kuwait, the United States deployed 697,000 troops to the Persian Gulf starting on August 8, 1990. The armed combat (Operation Desert Storm) began on January 16, 1991, and consisted of a 39-day air war followed by a four-day ground offensive. The United States incurred few combat casualties. The troops were repositioned to bases in Europe and the United States by July 31, 1991. Soon after their return, a substantial number of Gulf War veterans contacted medical clinics of the Department of Defense or Department of Veterans Affairs for a variety of symptoms. By June 1994, 17,000 Gulf War veterans had enrolled for care and 3,000 had a medically unexplained illness that came to be known as Gulf War syndrome (Persian Gulf Veterans Coordinating Board, 1994).

Haley et al. (1997) proposed a definition of the Gulf War illness based on data obtained through surveys of the military personnel deployed for Operation Desert Storm, culled from registries of ill veterans (Persian Gulf Veterans Coordinating Board, 1994) and review of selected cases. The proposal was patterned explicitly after the case definition of chronic fatigue syndrome (Fukuda et al., 1994) and required two major criteria and five of eight clinical features. The first major criterion was documentation of deployment to the theater of operations between August 8, 1990, and July 31, 1991. The second major criterion stipulated the absence of any other physical or psychiatric condition that could cause the illness. The eight clinical features were fatigue; arthralgias or low back pain; headache; intermittent nonbloody diarrhea; sleep disturbance; low-grade fever; weight loss; and neuropsychiatric complaints (i.e., depression, easy irritability, forgetfulness, memory loss, and difficulty with concentration).

A second working case definition for the unexplained Gulf War illness was developed using the Portland, Oregon, component of the Veterans Affairs Persian Gulf War Registry (Bourdette et al., 2001). This definition required the presence of only one of five subjective complaints or clinical findings: unexplained fatigue; musculoskeletal pain; cognitive-psychological changes (i.e., any one of somnolence, mood swings, inability to concentrate, memory loss, and confusion); gastrointestinal complaints; and lesions of the skin or mucous membranes. The symptom had to have its onset during or after deployment to the Persian Gulf; last at least one month; and be present during the three-month period preceding the evaluation. Exclusionary conditions included chronic infections with hepatitis viruses B and C, *Borrelia burgdorferi,* and human immunodeficiency virus (HIV); head injury with loss of consciousness; endocrinologic disorders; autoimmune illnesses; major psychiatric disorders; and other well-defined diseases likely to cause the listed complaints.

The nature and attribution of Gulf War syndrome has been analyzed in the historical frame provided by Great Britain's military involvement in the past century (Jones et al., 2002). The authors reviewed the records of 1,856 veterans randomly selected from among those awarded disability pensions after their service in the Boer War at the turn of the nineteenth century, First and Second World Wars, Malayan and Korean conflicts in the 1950s, and the military campaign in the Persian Gulf in 1991. The ten most common symptoms were difficulty completing tasks; fatigue; shortness of breath; persistent anxiety; weakness; rapid or irregular heartbeat; headaches; difficulty sleeping; tremor or shaking; and dizziness.

The analysis of symptoms revealed three syndromes. The first was a debility syndrome (fatigue, difficulty completing tasks, weakness, and shortness of breath) without cognitive or psychological complaints, which followed participation in military action before the end of the First World War. The second cluster identified a somatic syndrome focused on the heart (rapid heartbeat, shortness of breath, fatigue, and dizziness), which affected mostly veterans of the First World War (49 percent), Second World War (19 percent), and the Persian Gulf campaign (9 percent). The third cluster was a neuropsychiatric syndrome with somatic symptoms (fatigue, depression, anxiety, difficulty sleeping, and headaches) most common (54 percent) among veterans of the Persian Gulf campaign. Cluster membership was easily predicted by war, by contemporary diagnoses, and by the service personnel's attributions of symptoms. The authors felt that "what has changed is not the symptoms themselves but the way in which they have been reported by veterans and interpreted by doctors" and that newly emerging combat syndromes should not be "interpreted as a unique or novel illness but as part of an understandable pattern of normal responses to the physical and psychological stress of war" (Jones et al., 2002, p. 323).

In conclusion, the analysis of these constructs indicates a substantial conceptual and structural overlap between the current definitions of these functional syndromes. First, they all require the presence of multiple medically unexplained symptoms. Second, most focus on establishing the association between four main subjective complaints: chronic pain (musculoskeletal or abdominal); persistent tiredness or easy fatigability; sleep disturbance; and difficulty with concentration or memory. Third, the definitions draw from the same small pool of other symptoms to complete the clinical picture: headache (listed for chronic fatigue syndrome, Gulf War illness, and premenstrual syndrome), abdominal bloating (in irritable bowel syndrome and premenstrual syndrome), nonbloody diarrhea (in Gulf War illness and irritable bowel syndrome), and depression (in premenstrual syndrome and Gulf War illness).

Chapter 2

A Tight-Knit Family of Syndromes

Are functional somatic syndromes specific or are they clinical variants of a single disorder? The conventional clinical wisdom has been shaped by the efforts of research collectives to define these conditions in terms unique to the medical specialties most involved with the care of discrete complaints. Nowadays, gastroenterologists must become comfortable in managing irritable bowel syndrome, rheumatologists diagnose and treat fibromyalgia, virologists are seeing many patients with persistent tiredness, and toxicologists have had to deal with ill veterans of modern warfare. The assumption of specificity has been strongly challenged by keen observers of this reality (Wessely et al., 1999) who have pointed out that substantial overlap exists in the case definitions of these syndromes; that patients with one functional syndrome frequently meet diagnostic criteria for other syndromes; and that patients with different functional syndromes share nonsymptom characteristics such as gender, psychological distress, history of childhood maltreatment, and difficulties in patient-physician relationships.

It is generally acknowledged that Moldofsky and colleagues (1975) were the first writers in the modern era to note that "over the past 100 years the symptom complex of sleep disturbance, musculoskeletal symptoms, fatigue, and mood disturbance in the absence of demonstrable pathology has been given different diagnoses depending on current interests and medical or psychological bias" (p. 347).

The first focused attempt to determine whether functional somatic syndromes represent distinct entities was carried out at the Institute of Community and Family Psychiatry, Sir Mortimer B. Davis–Jewish General Hospital in Montreal, Canada (Robbins et al., 1997). The authors noted that the most common functional illnesses in North America are fibromyalgia, chronic fatigue syndrome, and irritable bowel syndrome. These illnesses are described and managed as separate conditions in clinical practice despite the fact that they have over-lapping symptoms which "raise the question of distinctness and no-sological validity" (p. 606). The study was designed to clarify whether these illnesses are independent of each other, are the clinical presen-tation of an underlying form of somatic distress, or are the somatic manifestation of depression or anxiety.

The sample consisted of 686 consecutive patients receiving care from two hospital-based family medicine clinics in Montreal. The patient group had a mean age of 44 years and a modest preponder-ance of women (58 percent). Data were collected with the Diagnostic Interview Schedule (Robins et al., 1981), a structured instrument that identified the main features of fibromyalgia (e.g., pain in extremities, joint pain, back pain, and headache), chronic fatigue syndrome (e.g., fatigue, weakness, and sleep disturbance), and irritable bowel syn-drome (e.g., bloating, abdominal pain, and diarrhea). In addition, the structured interview recorded the presence of dominant somatic man-ifestations of anxiety (e.g., chest pain, dizziness, palpitations, and shortness of breath) and depression (e.g., loss of appetite, change in weight, restlessness, and slowed thinking). The data were processed by factor analysis to evaluate the validity of the three functional syn-dromes.

The hypothesis that functional somatic syndromes represent enti-ties distinct from each other provided a good fit to the data. However, it was also clear that the syndromes did not occur in isolation. The correlation coefficients between the five latent constructs, i.e., the three functional syndromes and the two forms of psychiatric abnor-malities, were substantial, particularly for the analyses pairing chronic fatigue syndrome with somatic anxiety (coefficient = 0.84), irritable bowel syndrome (0.73), and somatic depression (0.68). The fibro-myalgia construct correlated best with somatic anxiety (coefficient = 0.62) and moderately well with chronic fatigue syndrome (0.57) and irritable bowel syndrome (0.55). The hypothesis that a latent con-struct of somatic distress underlies the three functional illnesses pro-vided only a poor fit to the data because it was dominated by vegeta-tive symptoms of depression.

These data have been recently reevaluated in an editorial discuss-ing the taxonomy of medically unexplained symptoms (Deary, 1999). The author, a psychologist at the University of Edinburgh, Scotland, emphasized that the correlation between the three functional illnesses and features of anxiety and depression was universally significant and positive. The finding suggested that the variance is general and that it cannot be attributed to the individual syndromes. Principal component analysis identified a common factor of the higher order responsible for 69 percent of the variance. This variable, or general latent trait, correlated very highly with all of the constructs evaluated by Robbins et al. (1997), the coefficients being 0.93 for chronic fatigue syndrome, 0.92 for somatic anxiety, 0.85 for irritable bowel syndrome, 0.72 for somatic depression, and 0.70 for fibromyalgia. In the author's view, the strength of these associations challenged the specificity of these syndromes.

In a small study conducted at the University of Washington, Seattle (Aaron et al., 2000), the investigators explored the presence of overlapping conditions in 25 patients with chronic fatigue syndrome, 22 patients with fibromyalgia, and 25 patients with temporomandibular disorder recruited from specialty hospital-based clinics. The patient groups were similar with respect to gender, duration of illness, and educational level. Most patients were females (range for groups 73 to 96 percent). A sample of 22 individuals seen in the dermatology clinic formed the control group. The participants received a complete physical examination and completed a 138-item symptom checklist designed to identify the three index syndromes and seven additional functional illnesses (irritable bowel syndrome, chronic tension-type headache, interstitial cystitis, postconcussive syndrome, multiple chemical sensitivities, chronic low back pain, and chronic pelvic pain).

Patients with chronic fatigue syndrome had numerous overlapping functional syndromes, including fibromyalgia (80 percent), irritable bowel syndrome (36 percent), chronic low back pain (32 percent), interstitial cystitis (8 percent), chronic pelvic pain (8 percent), and postconcussive syndrome (8 percent). The comorbid functional illnesses of patients with fibromyalgia were chronic low back pain (67 percent), irritable bowel syndrome (59 percent), temporomandibular disorder (24 percent), chronic tension-type headache (23 percent), chronic pelvic pain (18 percent), multiple chemical sensitivities (18 percent), and chronic fatigue syndrome (28 percent). The temporomandibular disorder overlapped only with other chronic pain illnesses, e.g., chronic tension-type headache (36 percent) and chronic low back pain (16 percent), but not with chronic fatigue syndrome or multiple chemical sensitivities. Among the subjects in the control group, the evaluation uncovered four cases of low back pain and three of temporomandibular disorder. The analysis of individual symptoms showed that four functional syndromes overlapped consistently in all patient groups (chronic fatigue syndrome, fibromyalgia, irritable bowel syndrome, and chronic tension-type headache). For instance, the diagnostic criteria for irritable bowel syndrome were present in 92 percent of patients with chronic fatigue syndrome, 77 percent of those with fibromyalgia, and 64 percent of temporomandibular disorder patients.

The analysis of individual symptoms disclosed a number of clusters. First, there were symptoms common to patients in all of the three groups. This cluster included myalgias, sleep disturbances, cognitive difficulties, abdominal pain relieved by bowel movements, and abnormal stool consistency. Second, symptoms such as fatigue, muscle weakness, and arthralgias were common among patients with fibromyalgia and chronic fatigue syndrome, but were unusual in the temporomandibular disorder group. Third, sore throat and mild fever were specific for chronic fatigue syndrome, while pain made better by heat and worse by sitting or standing was a characteristic feature of the fibromyalgia group. Therefore, it would appear that functional illnesses overlap because they share "generalized pain sensitivity, sleep and concentration difficulties, and bowel complaints" (Aaron et al., 2000, p. 225).

The overlap between functional somatic syndromes was also explored in a prospective study by investigators from Guy's, King's, and St. Thomas' School of Medicine and Institute of Psychiatry in London (Nimnuan et al., 2001). A total of 550 individuals referred by their general practitioner to outpatient clinics operated by two hospitals in southeast London agreed to participate. Data collection relied on questionnaires addressing the presence of 11 groups of symptoms corresponding to 13 recognized functional somatic syndromes. The most common syndromes identified in this group were premenstrual syndrome (25 percent), tension headache (18 percent), noncardiac chest pain (17 percent), and fibromyalgia (14 percent). Chronic fatigue syndrome was diagnosed in 8 percent of the sample. As expected, the point prevalence of these syndromes was higher among patients referred for care to clinics specializing in the evaluation of their main symptoms. For instance, the prevalence of irritable bowel syndrome ranged from 4 percent in the neurology clinic to 25 percent among those seen in the gastroenterology clinic. Similarly, fibromyalgia was identified in 25 percent of individuals seen by rheumatologists, noncardiac chest pain in 39 percent of those evaluated by respiratory medicine physicians, and premenstrual syndrome in 34 percent of women seeking care in the gynecology clinic. Overall, 56 percent of subjects had evidence of a functional illness, and the majority (53 percent of the total) had at least two functional somatic syndromes. The overall frequencies of functional illnesses varied relatively little with the clinical site, as it ranged from a low of 49 percent in the dental clinic to a high of 60 percent in the gastroenterology clinic.

Data analyses indicated considerable overlap between the syndromes. For example, a patient with irritable bowel syndrome was also quite likely to have nonulcer dyspepsia (28 percent), tension headache (22 percent), fibromyalgia (21 percent), and chronic pelvic pain (19 percent). Chronic fatigue syndrome overlapped with tension headache (18 percent), irritable bowel syndrome (17 percent), fibromyalgia (15 percent), and nonulcer dyspepsia (10 percent). Premenstrual syndrome was associated with hyperventilation syndrome (23 percent), tension headache (14 percent), fibromyalgia (13 percent), and nonulcer dyspepsia (13 percent). Two groups of symptoms, dominated by sleep disturbance and mood changes, were each responsible for 9 percent of variance and explained a substantial portion of the overlap.

The overlap between the unexplained Gulf War illness and other functional somatic syndromes was studied by investigators from the Veterans Affairs Medical Center, Portland, Oregon (Bourdette et al., 2001). The regional component of the Persian Gulf War Registry allowed the recruitment of 244 veterans who had at least one of the five unexplained symptoms or signs: persistent tiredness; musculoskeletal pain; cognitive/psychological disturbance; gastrointestinal complaints; and skin or mucosal lesions. The subjects (204 males and 40 women) had a mean age of 26 years and had served an average of 4.3 months in the theater of military operations. The authors conducted interviews and physical examinations to establish the prevalence of fibromyalgia, chronic fatigue syndrome, and multiple chemical sensitivity. The last condition was diagnosed in subjects who reported sensitivity to substances contained in household cleaning supplies, garden sprays, paints, and perfumes.

Fifty veterans (21 percent) met diagnostic criteria for fibromyalgia. This diagnostic overlap was gender-sensitive, as shown by the fact that almost half (43 percent) of the female veterans with unexplained Gulf War illness had fibromyalgia. Among male veterans, fibromyalgia was diagnosed in 16 percent of the cases. Forty-four veterans (18 percent of the total sample) had chronic fatigue syndrome. All of these veterans belonged to a subsample ($N = 103$) of cases with the chief complaint of persistent tiredness. The frequency of chronic fatigue syndrome in this particular subsample was 43 percent. Multiple chemical sensitivity was reported by 16 percent of the study group. Among the 44 veterans with Gulf War illness who had chronic fatigue syndrome, 41 percent had fibromyalgia and 32 percent multiple chemical sensitivity. Similarly, of the 50 ill Gulf War veterans with fibromyalgia, 46 percent had both chronic fatigue syndrome and multiple chemical sensitivity.

Investigators from the University of Washington, Seattle, and University of Illinois, Chicago, further expanded the body of evidence for the overlap between medically unexplained somatic syndromes in a co-twin control study that controlled the data for genetic and environmental factors (Aaron et al., 2001). The participating twins had been recruited for the CFS Twin Registry established in 1993 at the Harborview Medical Center in Seattle, Washington. Of the 632 inquiries, 454 twins returned the screening questionnaires, and 233 pairs of twins were found to have at least one member with a history of chronic fatigue. Data were collected with questionnaires designed to assess the presence of ten conditions: fibromyalgia, irritable bowel syndrome, multiple chemical sensitivity, temporomandibular disorder, interstitial cystitis, tension headache, postconcussion syndrome, chronic low back pain, chronic nonbacterial prostatitis (in males), and chronic pelvic pain (in females). A structured psychiatric interview, the Diagnostic Interview Schedule (Robins and Helzer, 1985) was administered by telephone to establish the lifetime presence of somatization disorder, major depression, dysthymia, generalized anxiety, panic, agoraphobia, post-traumatic stress disorder, mania, bipolar disorders, schizophrenia, substance use disorders, and eating disorders. Twins with a complaint of persistent tiredness were further subdivided into subsamples of twin pairs discordant for idiopathic chronic fatigue (127 pairs), chronic fatigue syndrome (22 pairs), and presumptive chronic fatigue syndrome (80 pairs) diagnosed according to standard criteria (Fukuda et al., 1994). Statistical analyses determined the prevalence of functional illnesses in twins with and without these types of chronic fatigue, and regression models were used to control for sociodemographic characteristics and nonexclusionary psychiatric morbidity (i.e., nonpsychotic and nonmelancholic major depression, dysthymia, generalized anxiety and panic disorder, somatization disorder, and post-traumatic stress disorder).

The groups were similar with regard to ethnicity (99 percent white), mean years of education (range 14 to 15), proportion married (range 59 to 63 percent), and number of children. Twins with chronic fatigue syndrome were on average four years younger than the subjects included in the other two groups. Female-female monozygotic pairs predominated in the chronic fatigue syndrome group (91 percent) and formed a slim majority (54 percent) of the remaining subjects.

Fibromyalgia was present in 77 percent of the subjects with chronic fatigue syndrome and in none of their nonfatigued twins. Similar differences were observed in the group of subjects with presumptive chronic fatigue syndrome (75 versus 4 percent) and idiopathic chronic fatigue (72 versus 7 percent). Irritable bowel syndrome was present in 59 percent of fatigued subjects, but in only 14 percent of their nonfatigued twins. Overall, 76 percent of subjects with definite chronic fatigue syndrome and 69 percent of those with presumptive chronic fatigue syndrome had at least three other functional somatic syndromes, a fact noted for only 9 percent of their nonfatigued twins. The odd ratios for chronic fatigue and comorbid functional somatic syndromes were very impressive and were dependent on the clinical classification and presence of nonexclusionary psychiatric disorders. For example, twins with presumptive chronic fatigue syndrome were 29 times more likely to have an associated functional illness than their siblings.

A further attempt to evaluate the associations of functional somatic syndromes was a systematic review of the comorbidity of irritable bowel performed by investigators from the University of North Carolina at Chapel Hill (Whitehead et al., 2002). The authors searched all scientific papers published since 1966 to assess the comorbidity of irritable bowel with nongastrointestinal somatic disorders, other functional gastrointestinal disorders, and mental illnesses. The work aimed to test the hypothesis that the extent of comorbidity challenges the understanding of irritable bowel syndrome as a distinct entity. For each comorbid condition, the investigators established the prevalence in the general population, its frequency in patients with irritable bowel syndrome, and the incidence of irritable bowel syndrome in subjects with the comorbid condition.

The best-documented associations were found to exist between irritable bowel syndrome and fibromyalgia, chronic fatigue syndrome, chronic pelvic pain, and temporomandibular disorder. For instance, the published record indicated that a majority of patients with chronic fatigue syndrome (median, 51 percent; range 35 to 92 percent) have irritable bowel syndrome. The frequency of chronic fatigue syndrome among patients with irritable bowel syndrome was more than 30 times greater than the prevalence of chronic fatigue syndrome in the community. The review established that an average of 48 percent of patients with fibromyalgia have irritable bowel syndrome (range, 32 to 77 percent). Fibromyalgia was diagnosed in 32 percent of patients with irritable bowel syndrome (range, 28 to 65 percent). The average is 16 times greater than the estimated prevalence of fibromyalgia in the general population. Other conditions commonly found in patients with irritable bowel syndrome included chronic pelvic pain (35 percent), premenstrual syndrome (18 percent), and temporomandibular joint disorder (16 percent). Irritable bowel syndrome was strongly associated with other functional gastrointestinal disorders such as functional dyspepsia and noncardiac chest pain syndrome. The authors also concluded that most patients with irritable bowel (range, 54 to 94 percent) have at least one current psychiatric illness, the most common being major depression, generalized anxiety disorder, panic disorder, and somatization disorder.

The authors' interpretation of the data was based on the postulate that the comorbid functional somatic syndromes are relatively independent of each other and are not manifestations of a defined psychiatric disorder such as anxiety, somatization, or depression. The data indicated a degree of overlap that was much greater than expected by chance, suggesting a common mechanism or factor relevant for the production of the clinical manifestations of these disorders. The nature of the common mechanism(s) appeared to be psychological and included selective attention to and vigilance for somatic sensations; a tendency to amplify bodily complaints; and an increased reactivity to stress. The interaction between these mechanisms was thought to center on increased pain perception; on stress leading to enhanced physiological arousal and increased autonomic activity; and on the somatization trait as a nonspecific amplifier of bodily sensations. The review emphasized the quantitative aspect of psychiatric comorbidity, by pointing out that patients with more than one functional somatic disorder were more depressed and anxious than those with only one type of functional illness. The authors felt that the comorbid associations between functional somatic syndromes were not due to diagnostic ambiguity (Barsky and Borus, 1999), medical subspecialization (Wessely et al., 1999), affective spectrum disorder (Hudson and Pope, 1990), or neuroendocrine abnormalities (Tache et al., 1999; Mayer, 2000).

In summary, a substantial overlap exists between chronic fatigue syndrome, fibromyalgia, irritable bowel syndrome, and Gulf War illness, and between irritable bowel and premenstrual syndrome. The evidence indicates that a common core of clinical dimensions explains the phenomenon. This core includes increased sensitivity to pain, sleep disturbance, difficulty with concentration, and depressed or labile mood. Patients with these syndromes also share a high degree of somatic anxiety, expressed as hypervigilance, somatic amplification of bodily complaints, and increased reactivity to stress. In the absence of a common physical cause, the common denominator of these functional somatic illnesses may be found in their association with psychiatric disorders, in neurobiological abnormalities, or in personality traits leading to maladaptive coping and abnormal illness behavior.

PART II:
PSYCHIATRIC MORBIDITY
IN FUNCTIONAL SOMATIC ILLNESS

Chapter 3

Depression and Somatization in Chronic Fatigue Syndrome

Chronic fatigue syndrome is characterized by persistent tiredness, a variety of other physical complaints, cognitive dysfunction, and symptoms commonly associated with mood and anxiety disorders (Garralda and Rangel, 2002). The presence of cognitive dysfunction and the high prevalence of depression have complicated the study of chronic fatigue syndrome and have contributed to the continuing debate about the nature of the illness. However, recent analyses have postulated a qualitative difference between the symptoms of depression experienced by patients with mood disorders and those with somatic illnesses (Valentine and Meyers, 2001). Moreover, there is no evidence that the cognitive dysfunction reported by patients with chronic fatigue syndrome correlates with the severity of depression and anxiety (Michiels and Cluydts, 2001). In this chapter the best available evidence linking chronic fatigue syndrome and psychiatric morbidity is evaluated in an attempt to determine whether this functional somatic illness is a clinical variant of traditional mood or somatization disorders.

MOOD DISORDERS AND CHRONIC FATIGUE SYNDROME

The first controlled investigation of the prevalence and characteristics of mood disorders in chronic fatigue syndrome was carried out at The National Hospital for Nervous Diseases in London, England (Wessely and Powell, 1989). The study group comprised 47 adult patients referred by the neurological staff for a chief complaint of medically unexplained fatigue lasting six or more months. The control group included 33 patients with neuromuscular disorders (17 with myasthenia gravis, eight with myopathies, three with Guillain-Barré syndrome, and five with other disorders), and 26 inpatients with major depression. Data regarding psychiatric diagnoses were collected with a structured interview schedule (Spitzer and Endicott, 1978). The presence of fatigue was not taken into account in establishing psychiatric diagnoses for which fatigue is a diagnostic criterion.

Patients with chronic fatigue syndrome and neuromuscular disorders were similar with respect to age and duration of illness. Patients with major depression were older and had a longer duration of illness than the other two groups. All patients described themselves as markedly fatigued, but the severity of fatigue was rated much higher by the chronic fatigue syndrome and major depression patients. Patients from these two groups felt that their illness was primarily a mental impairment (e.g., problems with concentration, clear thinking, and memory). In contrast, the fatigue symptom of patients with neuromuscular disorders had mainly physical features (e.g., lacking energy, having less muscle strength, and feeling weak).

The prevalence of current psychiatric disorders was much greater in the chronic fatigue syndrome group than among fatigued patients with neuromuscular conditions (72 versus 36 percent, $p < 0.001$). A past psychiatric history was identified in 43 percent of patients with chronic fatigue syndrome, 64 percent of subjects from the major depression group, and 30 percent of the neuromuscular patients. The most common psychiatric diagnosis in the chronic fatigue syndrome group was major depression (47 percent). The authors interpreted their findings to suggest that the same pattern of mental or central fatigue exists in both chronic fatigue syndrome and major depression. However, given the fact that only about half of patients with chronic fatigue syndrome met criteria for major depression, "depression is not the sole explanation" for the syndrome (Wessely and Powell, 1989, p. 946).

The prevalence of mood disorders among patients with chronic fatigue syndrome was also evaluated by researchers from the University of Connecticut School of Medicine (Lane et al., 1991). The inception cohort comprised 200 patients with a chief complaint of chronic fatigue. Sixty patients were found to meet all the requirements of the working case definition for chronic fatigue syndrome (Holmes et al., 1988). Each patient was matched for gender and age (within five years) to a control subject selected at random from the remaining 140 chronic fatigue subjects. Organic disorders were excluded in the entire group by a comprehensive physical and laboratory evaluation. The main data collection instrument was the Diagnostic Interview Schedule (Robins and Helzer, 1985), which was used to discover past and present symptoms of major depression, dysthymia, and bipolar disorder. The psychiatric diagnoses were made according to the definitions included in the contemporary version of the *Diagnostic and Statistical Manual of Mental Disorders* (American Psychiatric Association, 1987).

The mean age of patients in both groups was 37 years, and 70 percent of the patients were female. The groups were similar with respect to average duration of fatigue (4.6 versus 7 years), its self-rated severity on a 10-point scale (7.8 versus 7.6), and the number of physicians consulted for the condition (4.6 versus 3.1). Patients with chronic fatigue syndrome indicated a greater degree of functional impairment and were more likely to be currently employed.

Using the entire life as time frame, mood disorders were diagnosed in 45 patients (75 percent) with chronic fatigue syndrome and 46 fatigue control subjects (77 percent). Major depression with recurrent episodes was the most common psychiatric disorder in this cohort, being identified in 26 of the chronic fatigue syndrome patients (43 percent) and 32 members of the control group (53 percent). The prevalence of a single episode of major depression was 28 percent among the chronic fatigue syndrome patients and 17 percent in the control group. Dysthymia was less common, being diagnosed as the primary mood disorder in one patient with chronic fatigue syndrome and three control subjects. Finally, bipolar disorder with depressed mood was identified once in each group.

Thirty chronic fatigue syndrome patients (50 percent) were in the midst of a major nonpsychotic depressive episode at the time of examination. Seventeen of these cases had a history of recurrent episodes of depression. The remaining 13 patients were experiencing the first depressive episode of their lives. The prevalence of current major depression in the control group was 45 percent; 19 patients were suffering a recurrent episode of major depression and 8 had the symptoms of the first depressive illness of their lives.

A subset analysis focused on the subjects diagnosed with major depression indicated that the prevalence of the individual depressive symptoms among chronic fatigue syndrome patients was similar to that of the fatigue controls. The symptoms reported by the patients with chronic fatigue syndrome and the corresponding frequencies in the control group were anhedonia (100 versus 100 percent), poor concentration (89 versus 87 percent), insomnia (82 versus 73 percent), slow thinking (75 versus 65 percent), hypersomnia (73 versus 54 percent), worthlessness or guilt (64 versus 52 percent), psychomotor retardation (60 versus 48 percent), and suicidal ideation (55 versus 50 percent). Episodes of major depression led to suicide attempts in 20 percent of patients with chronic fatigue syndrome and 7 percent of control subjects; the difference did not reach statistical significance.

The major depressive disorder had preceded the onset of the fatigue illness by at least one year in 51 percent of the patients with chronic fatigue syndrome meeting diagnostic criteria for a mood disorder. This subset comprised a large majority (81 percent) of patients given the diagnosis of major depression with recurrent episodes. Among the fatigue control subjects, the major depressive disorder predated the onset of their new illness in 50 percent of cases. Taken together, the data indicated that a chief complaint of fatigue is associated with depressive symptomatology. The presence of the other symptoms of chronic fatigue syndrome did not change the frequency and quality of this association or the severity of depressive features.

The prevalence of mood disorders among chronic fatigue patients was also evaluated in a controlled study performed by an interdisciplinary team from the University of Wales College of Medicine and the University of Bristol, United Kingdom (Farmer et al., 1995). The 100 South Wales patients from the study group had been referred for evaluation of chronic fatigue of at least six month's duration. All subjects had negative results on a standardized battery of laboratory tests that included extensive immunologic, virologic, and bacteriologic assays. The participants met the requirements of the current diagnostic standard (Fukuda et al., 1994). The control group consisted of 50 healthy age and gender-matched subjects who responded to a newspaper advertisement.

The main data-collecting instrument was the Schedule for Clinical Assessment of Neuropsychiatry (Wing et al., 1990), a highly structured psychiatric interview and computer algorithm developed by the World Health Organization to generate diagnoses according to current criteria (American Psychiatric Association, 1987). Data were collected from all participants at the start of the study. Seventy-five patients with chronic fatigue syndrome were reinterviewed an average of 11 months later to determine the stability of the diagnostic classification over time.

The chronic fatigue syndrome sufferers had an average age of 40 years and a mean duration of illness of five years. The fatigue illness was described as developing rapidly after a viral infection in 69 percent of cases. None of the chronic fatigue patients had any significant physical or laboratory abnormalities. The subjects from the physically healthy control group had a mean age of 45 years.

Twenty-seven percent of patients with chronic fatigue syndrome and 4 percent of the age- and gender-matched healthy control group were diagnosed with a current depressive disorder. The prevalence of depressive disorders in remission was similar in the two groups (4 versus 8 percent). Data generated by reinterviewing 75 chronic fatigue syndrome patients one year after the initial evaluation indicated a significant shift toward improvement of major depression.

A high lifetime prevalence of mood disorders was also identified in a carefully controlled study performed by investigators from the Free University of Brussels, Belgium (Fischler et al., 1997). The patient sample consisted of 53 subjects consecutively evaluated in the fatigue clinic of an academic hospital. A medical control group was assembled by randomly selecting 50 patients from among individuals receiving care in the ear, nose, and throat and dermatology clinics. The operating assumption here was that these patients reflected the normative baseline regarding psychopathology; their somatic symptoms, level of disability, and duration of illness were not factored into the selection process. These subjects were 17 to 55 years of age and carried diagnoses such as chronic sinusitis ($N = 11$), chronic rhinitis ($N = 6$), benign skin tumors ($N = 7$), and benign pigmented lesions ($N = 6$).

The main data collection instrument was the Structured Clinical Interview (Spitzer et al., 1990) a clinician-administered tool enabling the formulation of psychiatric diagnoses according to standardized criteria (American Psychiatric Association, 1987). The diagnostic investigation was carried out in all cases by one of the authors, a psychiatrist who used his clinical judgment to limit minimization or outright denial of psychopathology. Validated psychometric scales were used to determine the severity of depression and depressogenic thought processes.

The groups comprised a majority of women (74 percent among chronic fatigue syndrome and 64 percent of medical control patients) and had a mean age of 37 years. The mean duration of the fatigue illness was 6.5 years. The lower and middle socioeconomic classes were more prevalent in the chronic fatigue syndrome group, but the significance of the difference was confounded by the fact that more of these patients were unemployed or were classified as permanently disabled. One of the patients from the medical control group was diagnosed with chronic fatigue syndrome; two others had chronic fatigue. Current major depression was diagnosed in 15 percent of the patients with chronic fatigue syndrome and 10 percent of the medical control group, while dysthymia was identified in 17 percent and 6 percent, respectively. At least one previous episode of major depression was recorded for 45 percent of chronic fatigue patients and 22 percent of the control subjects. Overall, the lifetime prevalence of a clinically significant mood disorder reached 77 percent in the chronic fatigue syndrome group, but only 38 percent among the outpatient control subjects, a highly significant difference. The difference in the rates of current mood disorders (30 versus 10 percent) was just short of statistical significance.

The role of depression in the production of pain and other medically unexplained symptoms associated with chronic fatigue syndrome was evaluated in a carefully controlled study performed by an interdisciplinary group from the University of Manchester in the United Kingdom (Morriss et al., 1999). The initial cohort was selected from among 227 consecutive patients presenting with a chief complaint of chronic fatigue. The British criteria for the diagnosis of chronic fatigue syndrome (Sharpe et al., 1991) identified the condition in 165 individuals. Of these 165 patients, 119 agreed to participate in the study. Structured psychiatric interviews diagnosed current mood disorders in 42 of the participants (25 percent); 29 had dysthymia or mood disorder not otherwise specified and 13 had major depression. Six patients from this group also had an anxiety disorder. Among the 77 chronic fatigue syndrome patients without a mood disorder, 68 had no psychiatric illness, seven had an anxiety disorder, and two were diagnosed with somatization disorder. The control group included 26 patients with depressive disorders. Twenty-four of these patients had major depression, and two were diagnosed with dysthymia. The three groups, i.e., chronic fatigue syndrome without comorbid depression ($N = 77$), chronic fatigue syndrome with depression ($N = 42$), and depression without chronic fatigue ($N = 26$), were statistically similar with regard to gender, age, employment, and marital status. The depressed chronic fatigue syndrome group had a significantly lower severity of depressive symptoms than the depressed patients without chronic fatigue.

All of the participants underwent a semistructured clinical interview designed to establish the number of lifetime medically unexplained symptoms, and the number of symptoms for which medical care was sought and treatment prescribed. Self-rating questionnaires measured the severity of current pain, fatigue, depression, and anxiety, and perceived disability and general health.

The most important findings of the study were those elucidating the prevalence of widespread bodily pain and unexplained physical symptoms. Both groups of patients with chronic fatigue syndrome reported a high frequency of widespread body pain (65 and 64 versus 15 percent) and felt more impaired by pain in activities of daily living. The presence of depression did not seem to correlate with the number of medically unexplained symptoms; depressed and nondepressed chronic fatigue patients had an average of seven such symptoms during their lifetime, while the patients with depressive disorder had experienced an average of one unexplainable symptom. The data were interpreted to suggest that the presence of depression is unlikely to explain the totality of clinical features of chronic fatigue syndrome.

Investigators from the Center for Community Research, DePaul University in Chicago, Illinois, completed a study comparing the physical symptoms of 32 subjects with chronic fatigue syndrome, 16 individuals with chronic fatigue who were diagnosed with melancholic depression, and 47 control subjects without a history of persistent tiredness (Jason et al., 2002). Data were collected with a detailed questionnaire that assessed the presence of physical and neuropsychiatric symptoms, including the features of chronic fatigue syndrome (Fukuda et al., 1994).

The examination of the data showed that most of the symptoms defining chronic fatigue syndrome were relatively common in patients with melancholic depression. The finding applied not only to the overlapping features of chronic fatigue syndrome and depression, such as unrefreshing sleep (91 percent in chronic fatigue syndrome versus 84 percent in melancholic depression) and difficulty with memory and concentration (87 versus 63 percent), but also with regard to postexertional malaise (69 versus 47 percent), new onset headache (75 versus 68 percent), muscle pain (84 versus 53 percent), and sore throat (62 versus 42 percent). The spread was somewhat larger with regard to joint pain (56 versus 26 percent) and painful lymph nodes (41 versus 21 percent). None of these differences were statistically significant. The only significant differences between the patient groups were recorded for shortness of breath (which was reported by 66 percent of the chronic fatigue syndrome patients, 26 percent of melancholic depression patients, and 23 percent of nonfatigued subjects) and decreased sexual interest (50 versus 16 versus 7 percent). Both patient groups had high frequencies of depressed mood (56 percent in the chronic fatigue syndrome group, 74 percent in the melancholic depression group, and 14 percent in nonfatigued subjects), irritability (50 versus 42 versus 11 percent), and general muscle weakness (75 versus 47 versus 18 percent). Other symptoms common in both patient groups were bloating (40 percent in the chronic fatigue syndrome group and 26 percent in the melancholic depression group), impairment of sexual functioning (50 versus 37 percent), nocturia (44 versus 32 percent), orthostatic dizziness (47 versus 21 percent), chest pains (41 versus 10 percent), morning stiffness (56 versus 37 percent), and puffy face (41 versus 21 percent). Twenty-two percent of chronic fatigue syndrome patients and 16 percent of patients with melancholic depression reported recurrent fever or chills. The value of the study is the identification of a similar symptom core in chronic fatigue syndrome and melancholic depression. This core included postexertional malaise, cognitive difficulties, and unrefreshing sleep and distinguished both groups of patients from nonfatigued control individuals. Nonetheless, the overlap appears to expand the meaning of the chief complaint, rather than to suggest an etiologic relationship between the two conditions.

SOMATIZATION DISORDER
AND CHRONIC FATIGUE SYNDROME

Wessely and Powell (1989) performed the first systematic evaluation of somatization disorder in chronic fatigue syndrome in a study that compared patients having idiopathic fatigue with subjects having neuromuscular disorders and major depression. Fifteen percent of chronic fatigue syndrome patients had somatization disorder. As a group, the patients with chronic fatigue syndrome endorsed an average of 15 different somatic symptoms. The average number of somatic symptoms reported by patients with neuromuscular disorders (eight per patient) and major depression (12 per patient) was significantly lower ($p < 0.002$). The authors pointed out that the prevalence of symptoms considered specific for chronic fatigue syndrome, such as postexercise myalgia, was similar in chronic fatigue syndrome and major depression groups (83 versus 67 percent). Most patients with chronic fatigue syndrome attributed their symptoms to a physical cause.

The results of this study overlap substantially with the findings reported by a group of investigators from the University of Connecticut School of Medicine (Lane et al., 1991). The authors identified somatization disorder in 28 percent of 60 patients with chronic fatigue syndrome, but in only 5 percent of a gender- and age-matched control group with a chief complaint of tiredness and without symptomatic evidence of chronic fatigue syndrome. The exclusion of symptoms defining chronic fatigue syndrome reduced the frequency of somatization disorder to 12 percent in the study group and 2 percent in the fatigue control group, but the difference remained statistically significant. A number of unexplainable symptoms were much more common among the chronic fatigue patients: heavy menstrual bleeding (71 versus 11 percent), abdominal pain (47 versus 21 percent), diarrhea (45 versus 27 percent), irregular menstrual periods (36 versus 14 percent), and back pain (27 versus 12 percent). Close to 90 percent of patients with chronic fatigue syndrome diagnosed with somatization disorder experienced medically unexplained symptoms before the onset of their fatigue illness.

A study devoted exclusively to the examination of the rate of somatization disorder in chronic fatigue syndrome was conducted by researchers from the New Jersey Medical School and Kessler Institute for Rehabilitation, West Orange, New Jersey (Johnson et al., 1996). The authors studied 42 patients with chronic fatigue syndrome and compared them with 18 patients with "mild" multiple sclerosis, 21 patients with either major depression or dysthymia, and 33 healthy individuals. Subjects with a history of schizophrenia, substance abuse, eating disorders, and bipolar mood disorder were screened out. The patients with chronic fatigue syndrome were diagnosed according to standard criteria (Holmes et al., 1988) and had an illness duration of less than four years. The subjects were included only if their symptoms produced significant problems in their lives during the month preceding the evaluation. Control patients with multiple sclerosis had no other organic diagnoses, were mostly asymptomatic, and showed no major neurological deficits. Chronic fatigue syndrome and multiple sclerosis patients with mood or anxiety disorders during the five years prior to the onset of the illness were not allowed into the study.

The principal measures of the study were the computerized version of the Diagnostic Interview Schedule (Robins et al., 1991) and the pencil-and-paper version of its somatization disorder section, administered by a psychologist or a neuropsychology technician trained in their use. The answers were scored according to four different criteria sets. The first set had a psychogenic conceptualization, that is, the symptoms were coded as psychiatric when the explanation given them by a health professional was anxiety, depression, stress, "nerves," or mental illness. The same coding was used for chronic fatigue syndrome, Epstein-Barr virus infection or candidiasis, fibromyalgia or fibrositis, premenstrual syndrome, migraines, irritable bowel syndrome, vague food allergies, mitral valve prolapse, and hypoglycemia. The psychiatric coding was also used to classify symptoms for which no explanation had been provided, as well as those for which the subject had not contacted a health professional, but were treated with medications or impaired activities of daily living. The second set classified the symptoms of chronic fatigue syndrome, i.e., headaches, arthralgias, myalgias, and muscle weakness, as a reflection of physical rather than psychiatric disorder. In the third set, the physical conceptualization was extended to include all symptoms that had occurred since the onset of chronic fatigue syndrome or were considered by the patient to be related to the fatigue illness. Finally, the fourth set considered the diagnosis of somatization disorder only among patients whose chronic fatigue syndrome had its onset before age 30; as in the previous two sets, the symptoms of chronic fatigue syndrome were coded as physical.

The chronic fatigue syndrome group included 37 women and five men, with a mean age of 34 years and a mean of 15 years of education. Gender distribution, age, and level of education were similar to those recorded for the control groups of patients with depressive disorders and multiple sclerosis and for the healthy sedentary subjects.

The prevalence of somatization disorder in the study group was 12 percent when the symptoms of chronic fatigue syndrome were coded as physical and 54 percent when they were coded as psychiatric. In the control groups, the corresponding frequencies were 8 percent and 46 percent among patients with depressive disorders, 0 percent and 15 percent in the multiple sclerosis sample, and 0 percent and 3 percent among the healthy sedentary subjects. The psychogenic conceptualization differentiated chronic fatigue syndrome from all of the control groups. The physical conceptualization confirmed the higher prevalence of somatization disorder among chronic fatigue syndrome patients as compared with healthy subjects, but not for those diagnosed with a depressive disorder or multiple sclerosis. Somatization disorder could not be diagnosed in any of the groups included in the study when all of the symptoms thought by the patients to be related to their fatigue illness were given a physical explanation. The requirement that chronic fatigue syndrome start before the age of 30 coupled with the physical conceptualization of its symptoms identified only one patient (2 percent) with somatization disorder.

A number of symptoms of somatization disorder were clearly more frequent among patients with chronic fatigue syndrome. Unexplained shortness of breath was reported by 55 percent of these patients, as compared to 19 percent of patients with depressive disorders, 5 percent of those with multiple sclerosis, and none of the healthy subjects. The sensation of "lump in the throat" had been experienced by 38 percent of patients with chronic fatigue syndrome, 28 percent of the depressed control group, 16 percent of patients with multiple sclerosis, and 3 percent of the healthy control group. Similarly, blurred vision was among the unexplained symptoms of 36 percent of chronic fatigue patients, but none of the multiple sclerosis or healthy control groups. Overall, the pattern of individual symptom reporting was similar for the chronic fatigue syndrome and depressive disorders groups. The presence of a comorbid association between chronic fatigue syndrome and other psychiatric disorders was not associated with a higher number of somatization disorder symptoms.

The largest study assessing the association between psychological and somatic symptoms in subjects with chronic fatigue was conducted by researchers from the medical faculties of the King's College, Charing Cross and Westminster, and Royal Free Hospital in London (Wessely et al., 1996). The study group consisted of 185 subjects with fatigue persistent for at least six months. Thirty-six subjects fulfilled standard criteria for the diagnosis of chronic fatigue syndrome, while the others ($N = 149$) were classified as having idiopathic chronic fatigue (Fukuda et al., 1994). The control group was composed of 193 age- and gender-matched subjects without complaints of tiredness. All participants were recruited from among 2,376 individuals evaluated for acute viral ($N = 1,199$) or nonviral ($N = 1,177$) illnesses by general practitioners located in the southern part of England. The subjects from the viral and nonviral cohorts were paired for age and time of evaluation. Psychiatric diagnoses were established with the Revised Clinical Interview Schedule, a structured instrument with confirmed validity in primary care settings (Lewis et al., 1992). The instrument was modified to exclude fatigue from the list of symptoms required for any psychiatric diagnosis. Current depressive and anxiety disorders were also assessed with the Hospital Anxiety and Depression Scale (Zigmond and Snaith, 1983). Symptoms of psychological distress were detected with the General Health Questionnaire (Goldberg and Williams, 1988). Somatic symptomatology was recorded on a 32-item checklist. Clinical interviews and reviews of medical records were used to collect data regarding past psychiatric disorders and use of psychotropic medications.

Current psychiatric disorders were identified with the Revised Clinical Interview Schedule in 111 patients (60 percent) with chronic fatigue. The prevalence was somewhat higher among the chronic fatigue syndrome patients (75 percent) than in the idiopathic chronic fatigue group (57 percent). In contrast, only 19 percent of the subjects without complaints of tiredness had a current psychiatric disorder ($p < 0.001$). The Hospital Anxiety and Depression Scale identified a probable depressive disorder in 81 percent of patients and a probable anxiety disorder in 67 percent of patients with chronic fatigue syndrome. The exclusion of fatigue as a contributing symptom reduced the proportion of depressive disorders to 44 percent of the chronic fatigue syndrome group. More than two-thirds of chronic fatigue syndrome patients (68 percent) had been previously diagnosed with a psychiatric disorder, and 43 percent of them had received prescriptions for psychotropic drugs prior to entering the study. The corresponding frequencies among the control subjects were 32 percent for past psychiatric illnesses and 14 percent for previous psychotropic treatment ($p < 0.01$). As expected, these variables were also strong predictors for the presence of current psychiatric morbidity. The previous use of psychotropic medications showed a significant correlation with the severity of psychological distress.

Somatic symptoms were significantly more prevalent among patients with chronic fatigue syndrome. The observation retained its validity for symptoms not part of the syndrome's definition. For instance, compared with subjects without fatigue, patients with chronic fatigue syndrome were more likely to endorse nausea (69 versus 21 percent), stomach pain (50 versus 25 percent), palpitations (44 versus 15 percent), frequency of urination (44 versus 12 percent), eye pain (42 versus 13 percent), shortness of breath (33 versus 4 percent), and tremor (25 versus 12 versus 6 percent [chronic fatigue syndrome, idiopathic fatigue, and control group, respectively]). Of the eight symptoms used as diagnostic criteria, the study found that only post-exertion malaise (63 versus 23 percent), muscle weakness (94 versus 63 percent), and myalgia (89 versus 50 percent) produced significant differences between chronic fatigue syndrome and idiopathic chronic fatigue. The number of somatic symptoms correlated with the depression and anxiety scores as well as with the burden of psychopathology uncovered by the structured psychiatric interview ($p < 0.001$).

A high rate of somatization disorder was identified by researchers from Brussels, Belgium (Fischler et al., 1997). In a controlled study already described in this chapter, the authors diagnosed somatization disorder in 11 of 53 patients with chronic fatigue syndrome (21 percent), but in none of 50 subjects from a medical control group ($p = 0.002$). All of these patients were female. The subgroups with and without somatization disorder were statistically similar in age, but differed substantially with respect to the mean duration of illness, which was 8.3 years longer for patients with somatization disorder (13.3 versus 5 years; $p < 0.001$). The number of comorbid lifetime psychiatric disorders was significantly higher among patients with somatization disorder (3.6 versus 1.9 disorders).

PSYCHOPATHOLOGY AND CHRONIC FATIGUE: ENVIRONMENTAL OR GENETIC COVARIATION?

The genetic and environmental determinants of the association between prolonged fatigue and affective distress were first studied by investigators from the University of South Wales, Sydney, and Queensland Institute of Medical Research, Brisbane, Australia (Hickie et al., 1999). The authors' hypothesis postulated that chronic fatigue is strongly heritable and has unique genetic determinants. The hypothesis was tested in a cohort of 2,281 pairs of twins enrolled with a national registry. The data-collecting instrument assessed the presence and severity of fatigue, psychological distress, anxiety, and depression. Zygosity was determined with standard questions about physical similarity. Data were divided into genetic influences, common environmental influences, and unique environmental determinants. Data analysis was carried out using structural equation modeling.

A total of 1,004 twin pairs (533 monozygotic and 471 dizygotic) returned usable data. The survey identified prolonged fatigue in 9 percent, psychological distress in 13 percent, anxiety in 14 percent, and depression in 7 percent of the sample. The monozygotic correlations were significantly higher than dizygotic ones for fatigue, anxiety, and psychological distress, indicating a genetic determination of the observed familial aggregation. In contrast, the monozygotic and dizygotic correlations for depression were essentially the same, suggestive of a role for the shared common environment. The correlation between fatigue and psychological distress (0.38) was substantially weaker than the correlation between psychological distress and anxiety (0.67) and depression (0.79). The final model identified a unique genetic contribution responsible for 44 percent of the variance in fatigue, which was not shared with the markers of psychological distress. The contribution of environmental factors to fatigue variance was minimal (less than 6 percent). Gender did not influence the magnitude of the genetic contribution. The authors felt that "prolonged fatigue states are etiologically distinct from the other common presentations of psychological distress" and that "a specific, independent genetic factor contributes to fatigue" (Hickie et al., 1991, p. 266). In later work, the same group of investigators expanded the scope of their inquiry from prolonged fatigue to somatic distress, and found it to be explained in a large measure (33 percent of variance) by a specific genetic influence that was unrelated to depression or anxiety (Gillespie et al., 2000).

The second contribution to the understanding of psychopathology in patients with unexplained chronic fatigue was made in a unique co-twin study carried out at the University of Washington, Seattle (Roy-Byrne et al., 2002). The aim of the work was to determine whether the psychological distress experienced by 100 fatigue-discordant white female twin pairs was due to genetic covariation or environmental factors. The majority of these pairs (69 percent) were monozygotic. The affected twin had moderately severe fatigue for an average of six years. Data were collected with structured instruments assessing psychiatric morbidity, general psychological distress, and self-reported health conditions. The findings were analyzed according to zygosity and clinical type of fatigue (i.e., chronic fatigue, chronic fatigue not explained by medical exclusions, and chronic fatigue not explained by medical and psychiatric exclusions).

Chronically fatigued monozygotic twins were more depressed and socially dysfunctional than their sisters ($p < 0.001$). Monozygotic and dizygotic twins with chronic fatigue indicated substantially more anxiety and somatic preoccupation than their nonfatigued twins ($p < 0.01$). Monozygotic and dizygotic twins appeared to be similar in a direct comparison of the four principal components of psychological distress (anxiety, depression, insomnia, and social dysfunction). The severity of psychological distress did not correlate with the clinical type of fatigue. The authors interpreted their findings to show that "prolonged fatigue is the critical symptom in the association between chronic fatigue-related disorders and psychological distress" (Hickie et al., 1991, p. 32).

In conclusion, a past history of major depression and a large number of medically unexplained bodily complaints have been identified in a substantial proportion of patients with chronic fatigue syndrome. Current mood disorders were present in less than half of the patients with this functional disorder, and the severity of depressive symptomatology was clearly milder than that observed in control populations of patients with major depression. On the other hand, the severity of depression and anxiety showed a robust association with the number of medically unexplained symptoms, somatic preoccupation, and frequency of somatization disorder. Taken together, the evidence reviewed in this chapter pleads against interpretations of chronic fatigue syndrome as a form of affective disorder. The magnitude of somatization phenomena identified throughout the life of many patients with chronic fatigue syndrome is the most consistent research finding of the past two decades.

Chapter 4

Somatization and Depression in Fibromyalgia

Fibromyalgia is a chronic illness characterized by musculoskeletal pain, fatigue, sleep disturbance, and psychological distress with a prevalence of 2 percent in the general population and 20 percent among rheumatology outpatients (Cathebras et al., 1998). Recent interpretations of the pathogenic mechanisms of fibromyalgia have emphasized a primary disturbance thought to originate in the central nervous system (Neeck, 2002). Depressive, anxiety, and somatoform disorders are commonly diagnosed in both male and female fibromyalgia patients (Yunus, 2001) and are associated with the onset and maintenance of the syndrome (McBeth and Silman, 2001). In this chapter we explore the best work on the clinical dimensions of the relationship between fibromyalgia and psychiatric morbidity. The aim of this analysis is to identify a direct link between the presence and severity of fibromyalgia and the burden of psychopathology.

The pioneering body of research that has attempted to determine the psychiatric disorders associated with fibromyalgia consists of five studies that used structured interviews and control groups of patients with rheumatoid arthritis (Hudson et al., 1985; Kirmayer et al., 1988; Ahles et al., 1991; Krag et al., 1994; Walker et al., 1997).

In the first of these studies, investigators from Harvard Medical School and Boston University (Hudson et al., 1985) recruited 31 consecutive fibromyalgia patients referred for rheumatological evaluation. The diagnosis was established according to the Yunus criteria (Yunus et al., 1981), which require the continuous presence of diffuse musculoskeletal pain for at least three months; at least six tender points; and absence of trauma or arthritis. Three control groups were also assembled. The first included 14 subjects with rheumatoid arthritis referred to the same rheumatologist. Their diagnosis was established according to criteria endorsed by the American Rheumato-logical Association (Ropes et al., 1958). The second control group comprised 41 individuals who were first-degree relatives of 17 patients with schizophrenia. This group was assumed to reflect the prevalence of affective disorders in the general population. The third control group included 24 female outpatients diagnosed with major depression. The main data collecting instrument was the Diagnostic Interview Schedule of the National Institute for Mental Health (Robins et al., 1980), an extensively validated method for establishing current and past psychiatric diagnoses as defined by the American Psychiatric Association (1980). A second researcher interviewed the groups of patients with fibromyalgia, rheumatoid arthritis, and major depression in order to detect the psychiatric morbidity of their first-degree relatives. Experienced psychiatrists who were not aware of the subjects' rheumatological diagnosis administered the interviews. The blind condition of the study could not be maintained for three control subjects with rheumatoid arthritis on account of their prominent joint deformities.

Demographic and clinical data were provided only for the groups with fibromyalgia and rheumatoid arthritis. The fibromyalgia group had 27 women and four men, a mean age of 45 years, and a mean duration of illness of 5.3 years. The patients with rheumatoid arthritis (10 women and four men) had a mean age of 49 years and had been diagnosed an average of 8.5 years prior to entry into this study.

Current major depression was identified in eight of the 31 fibromyalgia patients (26 percent). In contrast, none of the 14 patients with rheumatoid arthritis was in the midst of a major depressive episode. The lifetime prevalence of major affective disorders was 71 percent in the fibromyalgia group, but only 13 percent among patients with rheumatoid arthritis. The differences in these proportions were statistically significant. The lifetime prevalence of mood disorders among the 41 healthy control participants was 12 percent. The onset of major depression preceded the first symptoms of fibromyalgia in 64 percent of cases.

The prevalence of lifetime anxiety disorders was 26 percent in the fibromyalgia group. The disorders identified were panic disorder and/or agoraphobia (23 percent) and obsessive-compulsive disorder (5 percent). There were no cases of anxiety disorder among the rheumatoid arthritis patients. Other psychiatric disorders identified only among patients with fibromyalgia were somatization disorder (6 percent), bulimia nervosa (3 percent), and antisocial personality disorder (1 percent).

The assessment of major mood disorders among first-degree relatives found that 54 percent of patients with major depression, 47 percent of patients with fibromyalgia, and 14 percent of patients with rheumatoid arthritis had a family history of major affective disorder. These data translated into a 22 percent prevalence of depression among the family members of patients with fibromyalgia, which was similar to the rate of 15 percent predicted for the relatives of the control group of subjects with major depression. In contrast, only 3 percent of the first-degree relatives of rheumatoid arthritis patients were expected to have major depression. The authors felt that their method was unlikely to exaggerate the prevalence of affective disorders in the families of patients with fibromyalgia, but acknowledged the fact that the absence of contact with family members limited the accuracy of this portion of their data.

The second scientific investigation comparing the psychiatric morbidity of patients with fibromyalgia with those afflicted by rheumatoid arthritis took place at the Sir Mortimer B. Davis–Jewish General Hospital and McGill University, Montreal, Canada (Kirmayer et al., 1988). The authors recruited 20 patients with fibromyalgia and 23 patients with rheumatoid arthritis from the practice of one local rheumatologist. Care was taken to exclude fibromyalgia patients involved in litigation or receiving monetary support for their disability. The diagnostic criteria for the two conditions were identical to those used by Hudson et al. (1985). Likewise, psychiatric diagnoses (restricted to major depression and somatization disorder) were made by using the same version of the Diagnostic Interview Schedule. An experienced psychiatrist reviewed the interview findings to adjudicate the physical or psychogenic attribution of the somatic symptoms. One year after the initial interview, the subjects were contacted by telephone, and follow-up data regarding the presence of depressed mood were obtained by a research assistant.

The fibromyalgia and rheumatoid arthritis groups had a female preponderance (95 versus 74 percent) and were similar in age (57 versus 59 years) and level of education (11 versus 12 years in school). Thirty percent of fibromyalgia patients and 43 percent of patients with rheumatoid arthritis were not working at the time of the study.

The lifetime prevalence of major depression was 20 percent in the fibromyalgia group and 9 percent in the rheumatoid arthritis group; the difference did not reach statistical significance. The interview identified dysthymia in three patients (13 percent) with rheumatoid arthritis but in none of those with fibromyalgia. Only one patient in the entire sample fulfilled the authors' definition of somatization disorder. At follow-up, 50 percent of fibromyalgia patients and 22 percent of the rheumatoid arthritis group reported having had a two-week period of depressed mood during the previous year, a statistically insignificant difference. The groups were also similar with regard to the prevalence of the vegetative symptoms of depression, i.e., change in appetite or weight, insomnia or hypersomnia, psychomotor agitation or retardation, anhedonia, and fatigue.

The arbitration of the contradictory results of the Boston and Montreal studies was attempted by investigators from the University of Illinois College of Medicine at Peoria (Ahles et al., 1991), who recruited 35 patients with fibromyalgia, 33 patients with rheumatoid arthritis, and 31 healthy control subjects without pain symptoms. The patients in the first two groups were diagnosed according to the same criteria as those used by Hudson et al. (1985) and Kirmayer et al. (1988). The healthy control subjects were selected from among the friends and neighbors of the patients with fibromyalgia in an effort to obtain socioeconomic comparability.

The principal instrument of the study was the Psychiatric Diagnostic Interview (Othmer et al., 1983), a criterion-referenced, highly structured method for establishing psychiatric diagnoses as defined by the American Psychiatric Association (1980). In the authors' opinion, the instrument was expected to perform better than the Diagnostic Interview Schedule (Robins et al., 1980) with regard to the ability to distinguish psychiatric and medical populations. However, the evidence supporting this assumption (Powell et al., 1985; Weller et al., 1985) had been provided only by the authors of the instrument and to our knowledge has not been independently confirmed.

The interviews were conducted in conditions designed to minimize the possibility that the physical appearance could unblind the investigators to the presence of rheumatoid arthritis. The patients were instructed to avoid making any mention of their diagnosis, and care was taken to conceal gait abnormalities and hand deformities. All interactions were audiotaped and the data scored independently by the interviewer and a second investigator. The two raters disagreed in the cases of three patients with fibromyalgia, three with rheumatoid arthritis, and one pain-free control subject. In these situations, both raters audited the tape and reached a consensus regarding the final diagnosis. To evaluate the presence and severity of pain, all participants were given a schematic drawing of the body and asked to rate the intensity of aches and pains in 25 areas.

In the fibromyalgia group, there were five men and 30 women with a mean age of 43 years and mean duration of illness of 9.5 years. The rheumatoid arthritis group consisted of one man and 30 women, with a mean age of 47 years. These patients had been ill for an average of six years. In the pain-free control group there were fewer than 30 women, with a mean age of 45 years. The two clinical groups were similar with regard to pain frequency and severity.

The frequency of major depression at any point during lifetime was 43 percent in the fibromyalgia group, 39 percent among patients with rheumatoid arthritis, and 26 percent in the group of pain-free subjects. The combined frequency of panic disorder and obsessive-compulsive disorders reached 20 percent in the fibromyalgia group, 9 percent in patients with rheumatoid arthritis, and 3 percent in the pain-free control group. Somatization disorder was identified in 14 percent of patients with fibromyalgia and 6 percent of those with rheumatoid arthritis. None of the intergroup differences reached statistical significance. There were no gender differences in the distribution of psychiatric diagnoses.

Subsequent work performed in Denmark suggested that the burden of psychopathology is greater in fibromyalgia than in equally painful rheumatological conditions (Krag et al., 1994). Working at Frederiksberg Hospital in Copenhagen, the investigators reviewed the files of patients evaluated in the rheumatology clinic and identified 60 patients with fibromyalgia, 40 with rheumatoid arthritis, and 24 with lumbar disk herniation. The intention was to enroll patients experiencing pain on a daily basis. A letter to determine eligibility and willingness to participate was sent to each patient, and 49 patients with fibromyalgia, 25 with rheumatoid arthritis, and eight with lumbar disk herniation were included in the study cohort. The data collected included the clinical features of illness; the severity of pain experienced in the past week and in the past 24 hours; and functional capacity as measured by walking distance. The psychometric measurements relied on four structured interviews with some overlapping features: a melancholia scale with 11 items evaluating motor, verbal, and intellectual activity, suicidal ideation, lowered mood, self-reproach and guilt, reduced interest in work and leisure activities, fatigue, and sleep disturbance (Bech and Rafaelsen, 1980); a ten-item atypical depression scale assessing symptoms such as suicidal ideation, tension, impatience, emotional dependence, increased appetite, hypersomnia, and intellectual retardation (Larsen et al., 1991); a scale designed to discriminate between endogenous and reactive depression and between somatic illness and depression (Carney et al., 1965); and a scale measuring symptoms of anxiety (Hamilton, 1959). The data were appropriately analyzed both with and without the exclusion of the items that are common in somatic and psychological disorders, i.e., sleep disturbance, fatigue, and pain.

The fibromyalgia and control groups were similar in age (53 versus 56 years), proportion of females (92 versus 85 percent), duration of illness (ten versus nine years), and proportion of patients who had received inpatient (16 versus 6 percent) or outpatient (29 versus 15 percent) psychiatric care. The severity of current pain was only marginally higher among fibromyalgia patients, and the groups were similar with respect to consumption of nonnarcotic and opiate analgesics.

Patients with fibromyalgia had a higher burden of affective psychopathology, as demonstrated by significantly higher scores on the scales measuring melancholia, atypical depression, and anxiety. The exclusion of the items identifying the severity of sleep disturbance, fatigue, and pain did not change the magnitude of the observed differences. In both groups, the severity of current pain correlated with the severity of changes recorded on the melancholia and anxiety scales. However, for the same pain level, patients with fibromyalgia were significantly more depressed and anxious than the subjects from the control group.

Investigators from the University of Washington Medical School in Seattle provided support for the higher prevalence of psychiatric disorders in fibromyalgia patients as compared with rheumatoid arthritis patients (Walker et al., 1997). The project was designed as an attempt to correct the methodological shortcomings of previous studies (Hudson et al., 1985; Kirmayer et al., 1988; Ahles et al., 1991) by selecting homogenous samples and using a broad array of instruments to assess the presence and impact of psychopathology. The subjects were recruited from among patients referred for evaluation to rheumatology clinics in a continuous, sequential manner that identified 41 individuals with rheumatoid arthritis and 49 with fibromyalgia. Thirty-six fibromyalgia patients and 33 rheumatoid arthritis patients agreed to participate and were administered the Diagnostic Interview Schedule (Robins et al., 1980) and a battery of self-rated questionnaires assessing functional disability, appraisal of illness, pain, and sleep disturbance as well as data regarding past and current illnesses and treatments. The interviewers were not blinded to the principal diagnosis.

Patients with fibromyalgia were significantly younger than those with rheumatoid arthritis (47 versus 54 years) and more likely to be single (70 versus 44 percent). The groups were similar with respect to education and comorbid physical disorders. At least one lifetime psychiatric disorder was identified in 90 percent of patients with fibromyalgia and 49 percent of those with rheumatoid arthritis. The most striking intergroup differences were observed for the prevalence of somatization disorder (70 percent in the fibromyalgia group versus 3 percent in the rheumatoid arthritis group, for an odds ratio of 73), dysthymia (53 versus 6 percent, odds ratio 17), lifetime depression (86 versus 31 percent, odds ratio 14), and current panic disorder (25 versus 3 percent, odds ratio 11). Other common diagnoses were lifetime panic (47 versus 12 percent) and agoraphobia (42 versus 12 percent). All of these differences were statistically significant. The prevalence of current depression was 14 percent in the fibromyalgia group and 6 percent among rheumatoid arthritis patients (odds ratio 2.5), a difference that did not reach statistical significance.

Overall, the fibromyalgia group had significantly more psychiatric diagnoses per patient than the rheumatoid arthritis group (3.6 versus 0.8, $p < 0.001$) and more medically unexplained physical symptoms (15 versus 5, $p < 0.001$). Fibromyalgia patients had higher levels of pain and more sleep disturbances. They also had more impairment in coping than patients with rheumatoid arthritis. Self-ratings of functional impairment indicated that patients with fibromyalgia felt substantially more affected in their occupational, social, and emotional activities. The scores for physical disability were similar in the two groups. A logistic regression analysis of all the variables for which intergroup differences were observed indicated that the best predictor of group membership was the number of medically unexplained symptoms ($p < 0.0001$). The authors noted that the lifetime prevalence of psychiatric disorders in the rheumatoid arthritis group was similar to that found in the general population (Kessler et al., 1994). In contrast, fibromyalgia patients had a significantly higher burden of psychopathology and "taken together, these findings suggest that the psychological distress and psychiatric disorders found in this patient group are unlikely to be secondary to the rheumatological symptoms" (Walker et al., 1997, p. 570).

An important contribution to the understanding of the association between mood disorders and fibromyalgia was made in a general population study conducted by investigators from the Arthritis and Rheumatism Council Epidemiology Research Unit, University of Manchester, England (Croft et al., 1994). The participants were recruited from among people living in the catchment area of two general practices in the north of England. Using mailed questionnaires and follow-up clinical evaluations, the authors identified individuals with chronic widespread pain ($N = 74$), regional pain ($N = 67$), and no pain ($N = 36$). The mean age of the group was 53 years, and 120 of the 177 participants were female. A nurse unaware of the subject's pain complaints visited the subject at home and performed an examination of the 18 anatomical sites recommended by the American College of Rheumatology for the detection of tender points (Wolfe et al., 1990). Subjects also filled out questionnaires designed to assess depressive symptomatology, sleep disturbance, and severity of fatigue. Data were analyzed by comparing subgroups of participants with no tender points, one to four tender points, five to ten tender points, and with at least 11 tender points.

Thirty-eight (21 percent) of the 177 participants had at least 11 tender points, 50 (28 percent) had five to ten tender points, 65 (36 percent) had one to four tender points, and 26 (15 percent) had no tender points. The female subjects had an average of six tender points, while the males had an average of only three tender points. The proportion of females increased in parallel with the number of tender points, from 34 percent in the subgroup without tender points to 89 percent in the subgroup with at least 11 tender points. Most participants with four or fewer tender points had no pain complaints. In contrast, 80 percent of those with five to ten tender points and 95 percent of those with at least 11 tender points complained of widespread or regional pain. Of the latter group, 18 participants had widespread pain, thus fulfilling positive diagnostic criteria for fibromyalgia.

The number of tender points had a positive correlation with the severity of depression ($p < 0.001$). The scores on the instrument used to assess depressive symptomatology, the General Health Questionnaire (Goldberg and Williams, 1988), a 12-item instrument with the highest score 48, averaged 20 for subjects with no tender points and 28 for those with at least 11 tender points. The subjective experience of pain as widespread or localized, the age, and the gender did not influence this association. The severity of sleep disturbance and fatigue were shown to correlate with the tender point counts. The data support the authors' conclusion that "depression scores rise with tender point count irrespective of the pain status" and with their suggestion that "depression and fatigue may play a part in the genesis of the tender points" (Croft et al., 1994, p. 699).

These findings were supported by an investigation of pain thresholds and fibromyalgia symptoms in the general population performed in Wichita, Kansas (Wolfe, Ross, Anderson, and Russell, 1995), which indicated that the severity of depressive symptomatology had a stronger correlation with the tender point count than with the pain threshold. A second report of this epidemiological study provided further clarification of the association between psychological factors and fibromyalgia (Wolfe, Ross, Anderson, Russell, and Herbert, 1995). The authors contacted 3,006 randomly selected households and obtained rates of 11 percent for chronic widespread pain, 20 percent for chronic regional pain, and 5 percent for transient musculoskeletal pain. The individuals with widespread pain were given a clinical examination and were administered two questionnaires aimed at detecting psychological abnormalities, the Symptom Checklist 90 (Derogatis, 1983) and the anxiety and depression scales of the Arthritis Impact Multidimensional Scale (Meenan et al., 1980). The statistical processing used logistic regression to calculate the prevalence of fibromyalgia and its correlation with the level of severity of the psychological disturbance. The analysis included control procedures for age and gender.

Of the 319 respondents with chronic widespread pain identified in the survey, 36 (19 percent) met the American College of Rheumatology criteria (Wolfe et al., 1990) for fibromyalgia. Fibromyalgia was significantly more common among subjects who described their health status as poor and who were very dissatisfied with their health. Fibromyalgia was also much more likely among women, subjects with the most severe perception of pain, individuals who had applied for disability benefits, divorced subjects, and those who had completed only nine to 11 years of education. Of the psychometric variables, fibromyalgia was strongly associated with somatization, anxiety, past or current depression, and family history of depression. The total burden of psychopathology was a significant predictor of fibromyalgia, as reflected by the number of positive items and global severity of psychological distress. The authors noted that the level of psychological distress of the individuals with fibromyalgia identified in this epidemiological study of the general population was similar to that of patients with the same diagnosis referred for specialty consultation. As indicated by the investigators, the inference drawn from this comparison was that the psychological distress is not correlated with the care-seeking behavior, severity of pain, advancing age, or female gender, but is an intrinsic dimension of fibromyalgia.

The relationship between pain and depression in patients with fibromyalgia was also studied by researchers from the Department of Rheumatology, University Hospital, Basel, Switzerland, and the Max Planck Institute of Psychiatry, Munich, Germany (Fassbender et al., 1997). The study group included 30 consecutive patients (24 women and six men; mean age 50 years) found by the Swiss investigators to meet standard criteria required for the diagnosis of fibromyalgia (Wolfe et al., 1990). The control group consisted of 26 patients (14 women and 12 men; mean age 45 years) diagnosed by the German co-authors of the report to have major depression (American Psychiatric Association, 1987).

The main measurements included the evaluation of tenderness at the 18 musculoskeletal sites in the manner recommended by the American College of Rheumatology for the assessment of fibromyalgia (Wolfe et al., 1990); the self-rated grievousness of depressive symptoms (Zung, 1965); and the presence and severity of 14 functional symptoms (e.g., dry mouth, cold hands or feet, lump in the throat, headache, dizziness, and tremor).

Patients with fibromyalgia had tenderness at an average of 16.5 musculoskeletal locations. In contrast, the average numbers of tender points in the major depression group was 1.3. The majority (62 percent) of patients with major depression had no tender points and only one patient (4 percent) had the 11 tender points required for a diagnosis of fibromyalgia. Four patients (15 percent) with major depression were found to have generalized pain; two of these patients had no tender points. Patients with fibromyalgia had significantly more frequent and more severe functional symptoms than patients with major depression.

Six patients (20 percent) from the fibromyalgia group were moderately depressed (self-rated score greater than 48), and 14 patients (46 percent) were mildly depressed (score greater than 41 and less than 49). The self-rated severity of depression was higher among the patients with major depression (scores 58 versus 42, $p < 0.001$), and the difference retained significance when comparisons were carried out separately for men and women. The correlation between the number of tender points and the severity of depressive symptomatology was weak and statistically insignificant in both groups. The study suffers from an important methodological shortcoming, because the investigators were not blinded to the primary diagnosis. With this caveat, the findings suggest that the threshold for pain is lower in fibromyalgia than in mood disorders and it is not influenced by the severity of depression.

The most recent evaluation of the psychiatric morbidity in fibromyalgia was conducted from 1994 to 1995 on 73 subjects enrolled at four study sites located in Washington, DC; Long Island, New York; Charleston, South Carolina; and San Diego, California (Epstein et al., 1999). Patients were recruited by calling previously diagnosed fibromyalgia patients and through advertisements placed in the local print media. Lifetime and current psychiatric diagnoses were established with the mood and anxiety disorders modules of the well-validated Structured Clinical Interview for DSM-III-R (Spitzer et al., 1990). The instrument's somatoform disorder module was not administered because the research team "did not believe that a distinction between FMS [fibromyalgia syndrome] with somatization and FMS without somatization could be made reliably" (Epstein et al., 1999, p. 58). The validity of this assumption was not fully documented and appeared to be based on only one study, which has been described in Chapter 3 (Johnson et al., 1996). Psychometric assessments used instruments measuring depression, state anxiety, functional impairment, personality traits, somatosensory amplification, and hypochondriasis.

Most of the patients were white (96 percent), middle-aged (mean 46 years), well-educated (mean 16 years in school) women (94 percent) with an average duration of illness of six years. The lifetime prevalence of major depression was 69 percent. Approximately one in every four patients (23 percent) was in the midst of an episode of major depression at the time of the evaluation. The lifetime prevalence of panic disorder was 17 percent and current panic disorder was identified in 9 percent of patients. After adding the prevalence of social and simple phobia to the above frequencies, the authors concluded that 48 percent of their fibromyalgia patients had a current psychiatric disorder.

Compared with patients who were depression-free ($N = 57$), those with current major depression ($N = 16$) rated themselves as significantly more impaired with regard to their physical functioning. The correlation was linked to the presence of the mood disorder, because the self-assessed severities of pain and fatigue were statistically similar in the two groups. While current anxiety disorders were not associated with a change in physical health scales, the severity of the anxiety state, as determined by psychometric self-assessment, correlated significantly with a decrease in physical functioning. A comparison of patients with or without a lifetime history of mood and anxiety disorders detected no differences in any of the dimensions of physical health measured by the study.

An important addition to this body of data is research focusing on the prevalence of post-traumatic stress disorder and its impact on patients with fibromyalgia (Sherman et al., 2000). The subjects were 93 patients consecutively referred to the fibromyalgia syndrome program at the University of Washington School of Medicine's interdisciplinary pain treatment center in Seattle. All patients had been diagnosed according to the standard criteria of the American College of Rheumatology (Wolfe et al., 1990). Most of the participants were middle-aged (mean 46 years), well-educated (90 percent high school graduates; 30 percent college graduates), white (91 percent) women (98 percent). The average duration of fibromyalgia symptoms averaged 9.5 years.

The diagnosis of post-traumatic stress disorder was established with an empirically derived 28-item scale that was known to have high sensitivity, specificity, and internal consistency (Arata et al., 1991). A widely used multidimensional pain inventory (Kerns et al.,

1985) was employed to measure the severity of pain and the patient's affective and cognitive responses to it; the patient's perception of how significant others had reacted to the pain complaints; and the general activity level. Additional measurements included assessments of the presence and severity of depressive symptomatology and measures of disability and functional impairment.

Fifty-two patients (56 percent) were diagnosed with high levels of post-traumatic stress disorder symptoms and were compared with the 41 patients who did not. The two groups were similar with regard to age (47 versus 45), gender distribution, and marital status. The percentage of patients who completed a high school education was smaller in the posttraumatic stress subgroup (84 versus 97 percent). The onset of fibromyalgia coincided with an accident or injury in 42 percent of patients with posttraumatic stress symptoms and 30 percent in the subgroup without such symptoms, but the difference did not reach statistical significance. The duration of the chronic pain illness (120 versus 112 months), the prevalence of current depressive disorders (69 versus 51 percent), and the proportion of patients in active litigation related to their pain syndrome (22 versus 15 percent) were statistically similar in the two subgroups.

The severity of pain experienced by the fibromyalgia patients with posttraumatic stress symptoms was significantly greater than that of patients without such symptoms ($p = 0.001$). Significant differences between the subgroups were also observed with regard to the degree to which pain interfered with life activities. Patients with posttraumatic stress symptoms also reported significantly more depressive symptoms and higher levels of affective distress. Finally, only 15 percent of the patients with posttraumatic stress symptoms were considered to show adaptive coping to their illness, as compared with 48 percent of those without such symptoms. The features of adaptive coping included reporting low levels of pain, distress, and disability; satisfactory control over life's demands; and minimal functional impairment. In contrast, dysfunctional coping characterized 37 percent of fibromyalgia patients with posttraumatic stress symptoms, but only 19 percent of the other fibromyalgia patients. Patients with this type of maladaptive coping style felt helpless and pessimistic about their chronic pain illness and reported much more distress and disability than subjects with adaptive coping. The patients with this coping style reported frequent negative responses from significant others and perceived the social support for their pain, distress, and disability to be inadequate.

The data reviewed in this chapter indicate that a past history of mood and anxiety disorders is reported by a majority of patients with fibromyalgia. However, active psychiatric illnesses are present only in a minority of subjects with this chronic pain illness. The evidence presented in this chapter does not support a direct correlation between depression and pain in fibromyalgia. The best predictor for the severity of illness is the magnitude of somatization, expressed as the number of medically unexplainable somatic complaints.

Chapter 5

The Spectrum of Mood Disorders Associated with Premenstrual Dysphoria

Reproductive-related hormonal changes are considered an important factor for the well-established increase in the prevalence of major depression and other mood disorders in women from early adolescence until a few years after the cessation of menses (Burt and Stein, 2002). With a prevalence of 5 to 10 percent, premenstrual syndrome is probably the most common functional illness of fertile women and is characterized by affective abnormalities that manifest themselves as depressed mood, lability, tension, and irritability (Eriksson et al., 2002). The relationship between premenstrual syndrome and psychopathology is quite complex. The majority of patients have a past history of depressive symptoms and show premenstrual exacerbation of established mental illnesses (e.g., schizophrenia, obsessive-compulsive disorder, and alcohol abuse), but only a distinct minority is thought to have disabling major depression (Limosin and Ades, 2001). In this chapter we evaluate recent studies of psychiatric morbidity in premenstrual syndrome in an attempt to determine whether this illness is an independent entity or the manifestation of another major mood disorder.

The first controlled data regarding the prevalence of psychiatric disorders in women with late luteal phase dysphoric disorder were collected by experienced investigators from the Columbia University College of Physicians and Surgeons and the New York Psychiatric Institute (Harrison et al., 1989). The participants were recruited through advertisements in the print and broadcast media or were referred by health care professionals for a therapeutic trial of premenstrual symptoms. Of the 350 individuals considered eligible for the study after a brief screening interview, 195 completed and returned questionnaires regarding their symptoms (i.e., daily ratings for at least one month), medical history, psychiatric diagnoses and treatment, and family history of mental illnesses. The final cohort included 140 subjects. Fifty-five women were considered ineligible: 33 had unequivocal evidence of current affective or other psychiatric disorders and 22 had significant medical illnesses, gave a history of regular treatment with hormone-based drugs, or failed to meet the severity criteria for late luteal phase dysphoric disorder (American Psychiatric Association, 1987). The 140 participants were administered instruments assessing the presence of luteal phase dysphoria and a structured psychiatric evaluation. The procedure identified a group of 86 women with definite late luteal phase dysphoric disorder but without any current psychiatric illness. The authors also assembled a control group of 45 women who were assessed with the same instruments and were shown to be free of premenstrual dysphoria and current psychiatric disorders.

The patients and control subjects were similar with regard to age (mean 32 versus 33 years), ethnic background (82 versus 90 percent white), years of education (15 versus 17), and marital status (42 versus 32 percent married and 16 versus 12 percent separated or divorced). Compared with control subjects, the participants with premenstrual syndrome were more likely to describe their marriage as unhappy (39 versus 3 percent). Eighty percent of women with premenstrual syndrome and 67 percent of control subjects confirmed a history of prior use of oral contraceptive agents. The frequencies of mood symptoms (38 versus 16 percent) and physical symptoms (42 versus 11 percent) leading to the discontinuation of oral contraceptives were significantly greater in the premenstrual syndrome group.

The most important data collected in the study were those addressing the history of personal and family mental illness. In the premenstrual syndrome group, 70 percent of subjects had a history of major depressive disorder lasting for at least four weeks. The corresponding frequency among the control subjects was significantly lower at 41 percent. The premenstrual syndrome patients reported prior treatment with psychotropic medications significantly more often than control subjects (27 versus 2 percent). The frequencies of suicide attempts (12 versus 7 percent), postpartum depression (7 versus 0 percent), panic disorder (16 versus 5 percent), and alcohol or drug abuse (16 versus 11 percent) were statistically similar. The groups were also similar with regard to the frequency of history of depression in at least one parent (38 versus 28 percent) or at least one sibling (24 versus 19 percent). However, women with late luteal dysphoric disorder syndrome were significantly more likely to have a family member experiencing premenstrual symptoms.

The evaluation of the psychiatric morbidity of women with prospectively confirmed premenstrual syndrome was continued by investigators from the Healthsource Premenstrual Syndrome Program, Magee-Women's Hospital, and the University of Pittsburgh (Pearlstein et al., 1990). The 97 subjects had been referred for diagnostic evaluation and treatment of premenstrual discomfort. They were asked to rate their symptoms prospectively on a daily basis for three months and were diagnosed with late luteal phase dysphoric disorder according to the accepted standard (American Psychiatric Association, 1987). The authors were careful to include only patients who reported more than 30 percent premenstrual increase in the majority of their complaints and no detectable postmenstrual distress.

Psychiatric disorders were diagnosed with the Schedule for Affective Disorders and Schizophrenia, a semistructured interview providing a detailed description of current and past psychopathological changes (Endicott and Spitzer, 1978). To avoid potential confusion between long episodes of late luteal phase dysphoric disorder and short episodes of depression, the authors decided to diagnose mood disorders only when the duration of the episode was greater than one month.

Past or current psychiatric disorders were identified in 80 (82 percent) of these 97 patients with premenstrual syndrome. Nineteen women (20 percent) were found to have a current psychiatric disorder, specifically depressive disorders (12 patients), anxiety disorders (six patients), schizophrenia or schizoaffective disorder (two patients), and drug or alcohol abuse (two patients). A history of one or more past psychiatric disorders was present in 61 (63 percent) of the cases. The most common remitted disorders were major depression (37 percent of the entire group) and other depressive disorders (19 percent). Of the 51 women with children included in this sample, 15 (29 percent) had suffered from postpartum depression. Other remitted syndromes included anxiety disorders (10 percent) and alcohol or drug abuse (9 percent). Personality disorders were diagnosed in 8 percent of subjects and consisted of avoidant personality disorder in five patients, paranoid personality disorder in two, and compulsive personality disorder in one.

The power of premenstrual dysphoria as a predictor of future major depressive episodes was prospectively evaluated by investigators from the New York State Psychiatric Institute and Columbia University, New York (Graze et al., 1990). The issue is important, because most patients with premenstrual syndrome have a past personal history or a family history of major depressive illness. Both variables are, of course, strong predictors of subsequent affective disorder and may confound clinical features specific to this syndrome.

The subjects were recruited in 1981-1982 from among women responding to notices calling for paid volunteers for a study of biological and mood characteristics of the menstrual cycle. The inclusion criteria required the absence of current medical or psychiatric illnesses. Thirty-six subjects were reevaluated in 1984-1985 as part of the current study.

The presence of premenstrual dysphoric changes was assessed with an instrument scoring the severity of nine items: feeling depressed; having suicidal ideation; feeling guilty; feeling "empty"; feeling sad or blue; feeling lonely; having a decrease in self-esteem; wanting to be alone; and having a pessimistic outlook. The temporal pattern of mood changes was demonstrated by premenstrual worsening of depression, mood swings, anxiety, irritability, and social withdrawal. The initial interviews determined the presence of a family history of major affective disorders and the duration of the longest previous episode of depression experienced by the subject. The follow-up interview ascertained whether the subject had experienced symptoms enabling the diagnosis of major depression after enrollment. The interviewer was unaware of the diagnoses established at the onset of the study.

Thirteen patients (36 percent) had at least one episode of major depression during the follow-up interval, which ranged from 2.7 to 4.4 years (mean 3.6 years). The follow-up interval was identical for the subgroups of patients with and without a new major depression episode. The mean age of the two subgroups was similar (33 versus 36 years). Univariate comparisons between subgroups indicated similar frequencies of prior major depressive disorder (77 versus 78 percent) and positive family history (54 versus 65 percent). The index of severity of premenstrual dysphoria, as measured at entry into the study, was twice as high in the patients who developed an episode of major depression later on. Bivariate analyses indicated that the severity of premenstrual dysphoria at the initial assessment correlated strongly with the development of depression during the follow-up period. In contrast, neither prior depressive episodes nor a family history of depression correlated significantly with the target outcome. The hierarchical multiple regression analysis confirmed these data and established a significance level of 0.01 for the significance of the contribution of premenstrual dysphoria to the onset of a major depressive epidode during the next several years. The correlation appears specific for the premenstrual "depressive" symptoms, because symptoms such as anxiety, irritability, and erratic mood throughout the menstrual cycle did not separate those with and without new episodes of major depression.

Investigators from Massachusetts General Hospital, Boston (Bailey and Cohen, 1999), also assessed the prevalence of active mood and anxiety disorders among women with premenstrual symptoms. The subjects were 206 women recruited for a clinical trial of antidepressant therapy through media advertisements or fliers posted at fitness centers, health centers, and hospitals. A screening interview followed by daily symptom ratings established the diagnosis of premenstrual dysphoric disorder. The psychiatric morbidity was assessed with a structured instrument that included modules for mood (major depression, dysthymia, and bipolar disorder) and anxiety disorders (generalized anxiety disorder, panic disorder, and obsessive-compulsive disorder).

As a group, active mood disorders were identified in 23 percent and anxiety disorders in 7 percent of patients. An additional 8 percent of the sample suffered from both mood and anxiety disorders. The three most common individual diagnoses were dysthymia (13 percent), major depression (12 percent), and panic disorder (9 percent). Forty-eight (60 percent) of the 80 patients with an active mood and/or anxiety disorder had not been previously diagnosed.

The prevalence of seasonal affective disorder among patients with premenstrual dysphoric disorder was studied at the University of British Columbia, Vancouver (Maskall et al., 1997). Clinical evaluations were carried out on 154 women referred by their family physicians for consultation to a premenstrual syndrome outpatient clinic, and 100 of them were found to have high or moderate likelihood of premenstrual dysphoric disorder. The diagnosis was based on unstructured interviews, chart reviews, and, when available, prospective symptom diaries. A nonclinical control group included 50 female medical students and hospital employees. The individuals with premenstrual dysphoria were significantly older (36 versus 28 years) and weighed more (140 versus 126 lb) than the control subjects. The two groups were similar with respect to the time of residence in Vancouver's climatic area (21 versus 20 years). All participants completed the Seasonal Pattern Assessment Questionnaire (Rosenthal et al., 1987), an instrument assessing seasonal changes in sleep, appetite, level of energy, mood, and social activities. The instrument allowed the classification of the subjects as cases or noncases of seasonal affective disorder according to established criteria (Kasper et al., 1989).

The point prevalence of seasonal affective disorder was much higher among women with premenstrual dysphoria than nonclinical control subjects (38 versus 8 percent, $p < 0.001$). In most of these cases (34 of 38), the seasonal disorder had a winter pattern, characterized by hypersomnia and weight gain. The analysis of the individual items indicated a greater seasonal worsening of mood lability, fatigue, and hyperphagia in the women with premenstrual symptoms. A majority (59 percent) of patients with late luteal phase dysphoria indicated seasonal changes in their premenstrual symptoms, and almost half of the subjects in this subsample felt that these changes were marked or severe. The authors thought that the essential link between late luteal phase dysphoric disorder and seasonal affective illness is the previously demonstrated summer-to-winter variation in serotonin availability (Brewerton et al., 1988; Sarrias et al., 1989).

Work carried out by investigators from the University of Vienna, Austria, confirmed the high prevalence of premenstrual dysphoric disorder among women with seasonal affective disorder (Praschak-Rieder et al., 2001). The sample recruited for the study included 46 women attending a seasonal affective disorder outpatient clinic and 46 premenopausal healthy women recruited through advertisements in local newspapers. Exclusion criteria were the presence of major medical, gynecological, or psychiatric disorder (other than seasonal affective disorder) and irregular menstrual cycles. Psychiatric morbidity was assessed with semistructured interviews, and the seasonal pattern confirmed with validated questionnaires (Rosenthal et al., 1987).

The patients with seasonal affective disorder were older than the control subjects (33 versus 24 years). They had been suffering from a mood disorder for an average of ten years and had had an average of eight previous depressive episodes. Twenty-one women (46 percent) with seasonal affective disorder and one healthy control subject (2 percent) met criteria for premenstrual dysphoric disorder ($p < 0.001$). The age of the patients did not correlate with the prevalence of premenstrual dysphoria in this sample.

The same group of Austrian investigators published evidence establishing a role for the serotonin transporter promoter gene in the association between premenstrual syndrome and seasonal affective disorder (Praschak-Rieder et al., 2002). The polymorphism of this gene region has been identified as a risk factor for seasonality of abnormalities in mood (Rosenthal et al., 1998), as well as for neuroticism and depression (Lesch et al., 1996). The study tested the hypothesis that the risk of premenstrual syndrome in patients with seasonal affective disorder has a positive correlation with a family history of depression and with the serotonin transporter promoter repeat length polymorphism (5-HTTLPR). A group of 89 patients with seasonal affective disorders and no other current psychiatric diagnoses participated in the study. Forty-eight patients fulfilled criteria for premenstrual dysphoric disorder (American Psychiatric Association, 1994). Patients with and without premenstrual dysphoria were similar with regard to age, number of pregnancies, mood polarity, and global seasonal variation of their symptoms. Family members were assessed with a structured interview. Biological data were obtained with polymerase chain reaction amplification of genomic material isolated from nucleated blood cells.

A family history of affective disorders significantly increased the likelihood of premenstrual syndrome in patients with seasonal affective disorder (odds ratio 3.6; $p < 0.003$). The presence of the heterozygous state for the short allele of 5-HTTLPR doubled the likelihood of premenstrual syndrome (odds ratio 2.7; $p < 0.04$). The specific polymorphism of the specified genetic region, i.e., the presence of the short allele, did not correlate with a family history of mood disorders. The data were correctly interpreted to suggest that a family history of mood disorders indicates a higher genetic vulnerability for premenstrual syndrome and that the condition most likely follows a polygenic inheritance pattern.

Finally, in a long-term prospective study of the relationship between premenstrual dysphoria and major depressive disorders, investigators from Rush–Presbyterian–St. Luke's Medical Center and Rush Medical College in Chicago, Illinois, followed for two years eight patients with premenstrual syndrome and a randomly selected healthy control group (Hartlage et al., 2001). The groups were similar in age, ethnic background, employment status, and income level. Data were collected with structured psychiatric interviews at baseline and repeatedly during the following two years. To avoid overlap with premenstrual depression, the diagnosis of major depression was made only for episodes lasting one month or more, rather than the usual two-week period.

Four of the eight women with premenstrual dysphoria and two of the seven control subjects had a history of major depression. However, the only current diagnosis at baseline was phobic disorder, identified in one of the patients with premenstrual syndrome. By the end of the two-year follow-up period, seven patients (88 percent) and three control subjects (33 percent) had had at least one episode of major depression ($p < 0.05$). A past history of major depression was present in five of the ten participants with current depressive episodes (three premenstrual syndrome patients and two control subjects). The authors' calculations indicated that women with premenstrual syndrome are 14 times more likely to develop a major depressive disorder, as compared with the entire control group, and six times more likely than control subjects with a past history of major depression. Conversely, women with major depression were three times more likely to have the symptoms of premenstrual syndrome than nondepressed individuals. The data were interpreted to indicate that "the effect of premenstrual dysphoric disorder on the development of major depressive disorder appears to be independent and relevant" (Hartlage et al., 2001, p. 1575) and that premenstrual syndrome is either a risk factor for or a prodromal form of major depression.

In conclusion, the majority of patients with moderate or severe premenstrual syndrome do not have a current mood disorder. Prospective research carried out in the last decade has produced robust evidence that women with premenstrual syndrome have a family history of seasonal affective disorder or major depression and that severe premenstrual dysphoria predicts a high frequency of subsequent episodes of depression.

Chapter 6

Anxiety, Depression, and Somatization in Irritable Bowel Syndrome

More than half of the patients with irritable bowel symptoms have psychiatric disorders, including major depression, panic disorder, generalized anxiety disorder, social phobia, and post-traumatic stress disorder (Lydiard, 2001). Psychiatric disorders are particularly frequent among patients presenting with comorbid associations between irritable bowel and other functional somatic syndromes, such as fibromyalgia, chronic fatigue syndrome, temporomandibular joint syndrome, and chronic pelvic pain (Whitehead et al., 2002). Moreover, the severity of somatic manifestations of irritable bowel syndrome and their response to treatment are also thought to correlate with the presence of psychiatric morbidity (Creed, 1999). In this chapter, we evaluate in depth the best evidence exploring the link between irritable bowel syndrome and psychosocial variables and attempt to determine whether the presence of depression and anxiety is linked with the clinical manifestations of this common functional illness.

The association between irritable bowel syndrome and psychiatric illness has been assessed in a carefully controlled study performed by investigators from the University of Washington School of Medicine, Seattle (Walker et al., 1990). The authors recruited a sequential sample of 63 patients diagnosed with irritable bowel syndrome by a clinic-based or private practice gastroenterologist according to the prevailing standard (Thompson et al., 1989). Twenty-eight patients agreed to participate in the study. For the control group, the authors had access to a group of 24 patients with inflammatory bowel disease, of whom 19 gave their consent for the study. Thirteen patients from the control group suffered from Crohn's disease; the other six carried a diagnosis of ulcerative colitis. The irritable bowel syndrome and inflammatory bowel disease groups were comparable with respect to age (mean 37 versus 35 years), gender (proportion of females 79 versus 53 percent), marital status, and social class.

The psychiatric morbidity was assessed with the Diagnostic Interview Schedule of the National Institute for Mental Health (Robins et al., 1981) and the diagnoses established according to standard criteria (American Psychiatric Association, 1987). The severity of current symptomatology and the somatic and autonomic perceptions were measured with the Hopkins Symptom Checklist-90 (Derogatis et al., 1973), the Beck Depression Inventory (Beck, 1978), and the Modified Somatic Perceptions Questionnaire (Main, 1983).

The prevalence of psychiatric disorder at any time during life was significantly higher among patients with irritable bowel syndrome (93 versus 21 percent). The finding applied to depressive disorders (61 versus 16 percent), generalized anxiety disorder (54 versus 11 percent), panic disorder (29 versus 0 percent), and somatization disorder (32 versus 0 percent). Intragroup comparisons showed no difference between patients with Crohn's disease and ulcerative colitis. The prevalence of lifetime simple phobia, social phobia, and alcohol abuse or dependence was statistically similar in the two groups. The proportions of patients diagnosed with current depression (21 versus 5 percent), current generalized anxiety disorder (11 versus 5 percent), and current panic disorder (7 versus 0 percent) were statistically similar among patients with irritable bowel syndrome and inflammatory bowel conditions. A majority of patients (82 percent) with irritable bowel syndrome, but only a couple of patients (7 percent) with inflammatory bowel disease had developed a psychiatric disorder prior to the onset of their gastrointestinal illness.

Secondary analyses focused on the number of medically unexplained symptoms and indicated that patients with irritable bowel syndrome had a significantly higher number of these symptoms (mean 10.6 versus 2.5, $p < 0.0001$). The difference retained its significance after the exclusion of gastrointestinal symptoms of abdominal pain, diarrhea, constipation, nausea, and vomiting (mean of remaining unexplained symptoms 6.1 versus 1.7, $p < 0.0001$). To evaluate the role of generalized anxiety disorder in the production of medically unexplained symptoms, the authors recalculated the number of these symptoms after the exclusion of palpitations and dyspnea; the difference remained significant (5.5 versus 1.6, $p < 0.0001$).

The psychometric data indicated that the severity of current depressive symptomatology was similar in the two groups (mean score on Beck Depression Inventory 7.3 versus 4.2). On the other hand, patients with irritable bowel syndrome had significantly higher scores on somatic perceptions and somatization, anxiety, interpersonal sensitivity, paranoia, and psychoticism, leading to a substantial difference in the global severity of their psychological distress ($p < 0.005$). The authors felt that patients with irritable bowel show evidence of psychological distress with negative affectivity and multiple medically unexplained symptoms occurring on the background of past psychiatric illness. The hypothesis that their symptoms were the somatic manifestations of a current psychiatric condition was not confirmed.

Structured psychiatric interviews were used to assess the prevalence of psychiatric disorders in patients with irritable bowel syndrome by investigators from the Institute of Psychiatry, Medical University of South Carolina, Charleston (Lydiard et al., 1993). A sample of convenience comprising 35 subjects was recruited by one of the co-authors from his private practice of gastroenterology. All participants met standard diagnostic criteria for irritable bowel syndrome (Thompson et al., 1989). The study group included 30 females and five males whose age ranged from 19 to 82 years (mean 45 years). The symptoms of irritable bowel syndrome had been present for an average of 18 years and were at least moderately severe in all cases. Data regarding lifetime and current psychiatric morbidity were collected with the Structured Clinical Interview (Spitzer et al., 1990).

Criteria for at least one psychiatric diagnosis were met by 94 percent of the sample. The most common lifetime psychiatric disorder was major depression (46 percent), followed by generalized anxiety disorder (34 percent), panic disorder (31 percent), social phobia (29 percent), somatization disorder (26 percent), bipolar or cyclothymic disorder (15 percent), dysthymic disorder (14 percent), obsessive-compulsive disorder (9 percent), and hypochondriasis (6 percent). Current anxiety disorders were identified in 65 percent and current mood disorders in 37 percent of this group of patients with irritable bowel syndrome. The current anxiety disorder group was dominated by panic disorder (26 percent of patients), generalized anxiety disorder (26 percent), and social phobia (26 percent). Six of the nine patients with current panic disorder suffered from agoraphobia and described fear of losing bowel control while outside the home. The dominant symptoms of social phobia diagnosed in this group centered on interpersonal sensitivity unrelated to the gastrointestinal illness. The current mood disorders diagnosed in this sample were major depression (23 percent), bipolar or cyclothymic disorder (15 percent), and dysthymia (9 percent). The prevalence of somatization disorder was 17 percent. The analysis of the temporal relationship between the psychiatric illness and the onset of irritable bowel syndrome showed that in 43 percent of patients the psychiatric illness preceded the onset of the irritable bowel. In 34 percent of patients the onset of the two conditions occurred at the same time. The study confirmed the magnitude of the somatization phenomenon and the fact that only a minority of patients with irritable bowel syndrome suffer from currently active depressive or anxiety disorders.

A significant advance in understanding the relationship between irritable bowel syndrome and psychiatric illness was achieved by a family study performed by investigators from the University of Iowa, Iowa City, and the University of Kentucky, Louisville (Woodman et al., 1998). The authors hypothesized that the demonstration of increased rates of psychiatric illness among relatives of patients with irritable bowel syndrome would increase the likelihood of a causal association between the two clinical entities.

A consecutive sample of 128 patients who had been newly diagnosed with irritable bowel syndrome was identified as potential participants. Sixty-two of them were randomly selected for interviews, 27 agreed to participate, and 20 were found to be eligible for the study. The diagnosis used an acceptable set of criteria (Manning et al., 1978). Eligibility required the absence of poorly controlled medical conditions, psychosis, dementia, or mental retardation. A review of medical records confirmed that none of the participants had organic gastrointestinal pathology or a history of abuse of antidiarrheal or laxative medications. The control group comprised 20 age- and gender-matched subjects who had undergone laparoscopic cholecystectomy. The control subjects were required to have no biliary tract symptoms or evidence of irritable bowel syndrome.

The investigators identified 99 first-degree relatives of patients with irritable bowel syndrome and collected complete data on 46 (47 percent). They were also able to contact 112 first-degree relatives of the control subjects and obtained the cooperation of 75 (67 percent).

A researcher blinded to the proband status interviewed the relatives. Data regarding lifetime psychiatric morbidity were collected with the Structured Clinical Interview (Spitzer et al., 1990). Psychological and somatic symptoms were recorded with the 53-item Brief Symptom Inventory (Derogatis and Melisaratos, 1983), and hypochondriasis was measured with the 14-item Whiteley Index (Pilowski, 1967). The family history of psychiatric disorders and gastrointestinal symptoms was assessed with questionnaires developed for this study.

Patients with irritable bowel syndrome and postcholecystectomy control subjects were similar with regard to age (41 versus 43 years), proportion of females (80 percent), and marital, educational, and occupational status. The frequency of lifetime psychiatric diagnoses was substantially higher among patients with irritable bowel syndrome (90 versus 40 percent, $p < 0.005$). The difference reflected the higher rate of major depression (70 versus 25 percent), somatoform disorders (35 versus 0 percent), and substance use disorders (35 versus 0 percent) in the irritable bowel group. The frequencies of social phobia (30 versus 10 percent), generalized anxiety disorder (20 versus 10 percent), and panic disorder (15 versus 5 percent) were statistically similar in the two groups. Overall, probands with irritable bowel syndrome had an average of 2.8 lifetime psychiatric disorders, compared with an average of only 0.6 psychiatric disorder in the postcholecystectomy group.

The two groups of first-degree relatives were similar in age, gender, marital status, and occupational class. Relatives of patients with irritable bowel syndrome had achieved a lower educational level compared to the relatives of the control subjects. The prevalence of irritable bowel syndrome among relatives of patients with irritable bowel was 2.1 percent, statistically similar to the prevalence of 1.3 percent recorded among the relatives of the postcholecystectomy control subjects. Functional upper or lower gastrointestinal disorders, including subthreshold irritable bowel, functional constipation or diarrhea, abdominal pain, globus, rumination, functional chest pain, heartburn, and aerophagia were identified in 47 percent of the irritable bowel syndrome group's relatives and in 32 percent of the control group's relatives.

A past or current psychiatric disorder was identified in 72 percent of the first-degree relatives with a functional gastrointestinal disorder, but in only 32 percent of relatives without such conditions. The prevalence of depressive disorders was significantly higher among relatives of patients with irritable bowel syndrome (33 versus 17 percent, $p < 0.05$). An even greater difference was noted for the prevalence of anxiety disorders (42 versus 19 percent, $p < 0.005$). The difference between the two groups of relatives was attributable mainly to major depression (32 versus 17 percent, $p < 0.05$) and generalized anxiety disorder (15 versus 5 percent, $p < 0.05$). The frequencies of somatoform and substance use disorders were similar in the two groups of relatives. Psychometric data confirmed the fact that the severity of symptoms of depression and anxiety was higher among the first-degree relatives of patients with irritable bowel syndrome. In contrast, the two groups of relatives had similar scores on measures of extroversion, neuroticism, hostility, interpersonal sensitivity, and hypochondriasis. Given the strong association between functional gastrointestinal disorders and psychiatric illnesses dominated by depression and anxiety in both probands and first-degree relatives, the authors postulated that "they [these disorders] may be transmitted together and may represent features of a single disturbance" (Woodman et al., 1998, p. 52). However, a causal explanation of the association between psychiatric morbidity and irritable bowel syndrome was not provided and is very difficult to conceptualize given the very low frequency of the syndrome among first-degree relatives.

The link between irritable bowel syndrome and psychiatric disorders was studied in a large community by researchers from the University of Sydney, Australia (Talley et al., 2001). The investigators were able to access the participants in the Dunedin Multidisciplinary Health and Development Study, a complete one-year birth cohort ($N = 1,037$) of individuals born in 1972-1973 in Dunedin, New Zealand. Ninety-three percent of the participants were of European descent, and 52 percent were males. The cohort was assessed at age 18 and age 21 with a structured psychiatric interview and diagnoses made according to standard U.S. criteria (American Psychiatric Association, 1987). Data were coded to indicate no psychiatric morbidity, episodic psychiatric morbidity, and chronic psychiatric disorder. At age 26 the participants completed a bowel symptom questionnaire that allowed the diagnosis of irritable bowel syndrome.

Irritable bowel syndrome was diagnosed according to the Manning criteria (Manning et al., 1978) in 12.7 percent of the sample, or 10.8

percent of males and 14.6 percent of females. The more restrictive Rome criteria (Thompson et al., 1989) diagnosed the syndrome in 4.3 percent of the participants (3.3 percent of males and 5.3 percent of females). The structured interviews identified psychiatric disorders at the age of 18 and/or 21 in 54 percent of the sample. The most common disorders were anxiety disorders (33 percent), depression (30 percent), and substance dependence (21 percent).

The presence of irritable bowel syndrome did not identify a group with a higher prevalence of psychiatric disorders in this community sample. The prevalence of any psychiatric disorder at age 18 or 21 was 31 percent among subjects without irritable bowel syndrome, 21 percent in the group diagnosed by the Rome criteria, and 35 percent in those who met the Manning criteria. The prevalence for anxiety disorders was 21 percent among those without bowel symptoms and 16 percent and 26 percent in those diagnosed by the Rome and Manning criteria, respectively. The frequency of the diagnosis of depression was also similar in these three groups (22 percent, 24 percent, and 28 percent). Intergroup similarities were also observed for the prevalence of substance dependence (15 percent, 13 percent, and 12 percent).

Another study assessing psychiatric morbidity of patients with irritable bowel syndrome was an exploration of the prevalence of somatization disorder carried out by researchers from Washington University, St. Louis, Missouri (Miller et al., 2001). The study was justified by the considerable theoretical and practical overlap between two conditions characterized by multiple unexplainable physical symptoms. The participants were recruited from among patients referred for evaluation to gastroenterology clinics with the diagnosis of irritable bowel syndrome ($N = 24$) and ulcerative colitis ($N = 26$). All irritable bowel syndrome patients met the revised Rome diagnostic criteria (Thompson et al., 1999). The participants were evaluated by psychiatrists who used the highly structured Diagnostic Interview Schedule (Robins et al., 1995) to establish the presence of mental disorders according to the most recent standard (American Psychiatric Association, 1994). The diagnosis of somatization disorder was made in patients who had at least four out of ten medically unexplained symptoms. Three of the ten symptoms (i.e., abdominal pain, abdominal distention, and diarrhea) overlap with the diagnostic criteria and the clinical manifestations of irritable bowel syndrome and are common also in patients with ulcerative colitis. In addition to making the diagnosis of definite somatization disorder, the authors also established the diagnosis of probable somatization disorder when three out of ten symptom criteria were present. The interviewers were blinded to the group membership of their subjects. The researchers also reviewed the participants' clinic charts in order to increase the accuracy of the assessment of somatization disorder. Illness behavior was measured with self-administered questionnaires.

The irritable bowel syndrome and ulcerative colitis groups were similar with regard to age (42 versus 43 years), proportion of females (75 versus 54 percent), duration of illness (nine versus 11 years), and average number of visits to the clinic in the previous year (2.6 versus 2.5). Slightly more patients with irritable bowel syndrome were symptomatic at the time of referral (92 versus 69 percent).

Ten female patients with irritable bowel syndrome (42 percent of the sample) were classified as having somatization disorder. Six patients (25 percent) had definite somatization disorder, and four patients (17 percent) were diagnosed with probable somatization disorder. In contrast, none of the patients with ulcerative colitis met criteria for somatization disorder. The subgroup of patients with irritable bowel syndrome and somatization disorder had an average of 7.4 of the ten possible symptoms required for the diagnosis of this psychiatric disorder. In contrast, the average number of somatization symptoms was 3.4 in the remaining patients with irritable bowel syndrome, reflecting the overlap in the definition of these conditions. Patients with ulcerative colitis had an average of 2.2 somatization symptoms. Major depression was diagnosed in 58 percent of patients with irritable bowel syndrome and 31 percent of the ulcerative colitis group, a difference that did not reach statistical significance. The prevalence of depression among patients with somatization disorder was 80 percent.

The overall burden of psychopathology was clearly increased only in patients with somatization disorder, as reflected by larger symptom counts for generalized anxiety disorder, posttraumatic stress, schizophrenia, eating disorders, and attention deficit hyperactivity disorder. The excess of somatization and depressive symptoms was particularly prevalent in women with irritable bowel syndrome. Global assessments of illness behavior did not reveal significant differences between groups. However, the subgroup of patients with irritable bowel syndrome and somatization disorder scored significantly higher on all three dimensions tested, i.e., denial ($p < 0.04$), affective disturbance ($p < 0.04$), and disease conviction ($p < 0.05$). Gender did not influence illness behavior. The authors interpreted the evidence to imply that a substantial proportion of patients with irritable bowel syndrome "may meet IBS [irritable bowel syndrome] criteria as part of multisystem medical complaints, in the gastrointestinal system as well as elsewhere" (Miller et al., 2001, p. 29).

These data show that the vast majority of patients with irritable bowel syndrome and their first-degree relatives have a past history of depressive and anxiety syndromes, but only one in four patients suffers from an active mood disorder. Moreover, the severity of functional gastrointestinal disorder does not correlate with the presence of depression or anxiety, but is linked to the magnitude of the somatization phenomena expressed by these patients. In turn, the severity of somatization predicts the burden of psychopathology and the overall psychological distress experienced in irritable bowel syndrome.

Chapter 7

Somatization and Posttraumatic Stress in Gulf War Illness

The assessment of psychiatric morbidity in veterans of the Persian Gulf conflict has been hampered by imprecise definition of their illnesses, the overlap with chronic fatigue syndromes, and by controversy regarding the role of stress in the causation of the syndrome (Tournier et al., 2002). The issue is further complicated by the many interpretations of illnesses reported by soldiers involved in modern warfare and peace-keeping missions, including a psychotrauma start model, a somatic start model, a premorbidity model, and a complaints-not-related-to-war model (de Vries et al., 1999). However, a consensus is emerging that cultural and psychological factors are major contributors to the genesis and maintenance of Gulf War illness (Sartin, 2000).

A careful cross-sectional study authored by researchers from the Medical University of South Carolina, Charleston, Uniformed Services University of Health Sciences, Bethesda, Maryland, and the Walter Reed Army Medical Center, Washington, DC, focused on veterans who returned from the Gulf area and sought medical attention for illnesses related to their service experiences (Labbate et al., 1998). The aim of the study was to investigate the frequency of psychiatric syndromes and somatic symptoms, as well as their relationship with traumatic events such as combat experience, combat injury, and handling dead bodies.

The study used the patient population accrued through the Walter Reed Army Medical Center's participation in the Comprehensive Clinical Evaluation Program of the Department of Defense, a clinical initiative designed to serve veterans self-referred for symptoms thought to be connected to their tour of duty to the Persian Gulf. The boundaries of the catchment area were the Atlantic seaboard to the east and the states of Virginia to the south, West Virginia and Pennsylvania to the west, and Maine to the north. The symptomatic veterans were first evaluated in a military community hospital. If the presenting symptoms could not be diagnosed or treated, the veterans' care was transferred to a regional medical center for in-depth specialty evaluations. The study sample included the 131 veterans referred consecutively for this comprehensive evaluation in 1994 and 1995.

Psychiatric diagnoses were made with the Structured Clinical Interview (Spitzer et al., 1990) and the Clinical Assessment of Post-traumatic Syndrome Scale (Blake et al., 1995). Issues related to physical or psychiatric attribution of the symptoms were resolved by consensus after the data were collected. Trauma questionnaires enabled assessments of five Gulf War experiences (chemical alarms, rocket alarms, witnessed casualties, direct combat, and wounded in action) as well as past combat experience and injury, handling of dead bodies, and previous psychological trauma.

The symptomatic Gulf-deployed veterans were mostly male (86 percent) and had a mean age of 36 years. The majority (69 percent) were noncommissioned officers. Moderate or severe past trauma was reported by 41 percent of veterans. Only a minority of these troops had been exposed to live fire combat (15 percent), had been injured in combat (6 percent), or had handled dead bodies (19 percent).

Mood disorders were diagnosed in 35 percent of these veterans (major depression in 28 percent and dysthymia in 7 percent). Anxiety disorders were identified in 32 percent of the sample (post-traumatic stress disorder in 18 percent, panic disorder in 7 percent, generalized anxiety disorder in 5 percent, and social phobia in 2 percent). Undifferentiated somatoform disorder was the diagnosis given to 26 percent of this patient population. Finally, 8 percent of the symptomatic Gulf veterans suffered from alcohol abuse or dependence.

Younger age was a strong predictor for all psychiatric diagnoses other than post-traumatic stress disorder. The latter illness was correlated significantly with combat injury or exposure to one of the Gulf-specific combat experiences. Handling dead bodies was a strong predictor for both post-traumatic stress disorder and undifferentiated somatoform disorder. The possibility of a causal relationship between medically unexplained somatic symptoms of these veterans and their psychiatric morbidity was not explored.

The study of psychiatric morbidity of individuals diagnosed with Gulf War syndrome has been substantially helped by investigators from Boston University and Tulane University in work designed at the National Center for Posttraumatic Stress Disorder, Boston Veterans' Administration Medical Center (White et al., 2001). In this carefully controlled investigation conducted from 1994 to 1996, the authors attempted to establish not only the psychiatric morbidity of Gulf War veterans, but also the relationship between psychiatric disorders, particularly major depression and post-traumatic stress disorder, and the number and pattern of somatic complaints in this population. The deployed veteran sample consisted of 2,949 Army troops from New England deployed to the Gulf War zone from Fort Devens and 928 Louisiana troops from all military branches who departed from New Orleans. An appropriately complex sampling strategy was used to select 353 subjects from Fort Devens and 194 from New Orleans. This sample was thought to represent well the gender distribution and the prevalence of somatic complainers in the initial cohort. Complete data were provided by 148 veterans from Fort Devens and 73 from New Orleans. The control group was recruited from among the members of an air ambulance company called for duty at the same time as the study subjects, but sent to Germany for the duration of the Persian Gulf conflict. These troops did not see military action in the Persian Gulf, but assisted with transport missions and German civilian evacuations. Of the 95 members of the unit, 48 agreed to complete all the measures of the study.

The main data collection instrument was the Structured Clinical Interview (Spitzer et al., 1990), designed to identify current and lifetime psychiatric diagnoses. The diagnosis of post-traumatic stress disorder was made with a clinical rating scale (Blake et al., 1995). The presence of 49 somatic symptoms during the most recent 30-day period was assessed with a standardized questionnaire. Twenty-four of these 49 symptoms were used to calculate a separate score indicating distress into one of nine different body systems. Finally, combat exposure was assessed with a standardized instrument that included traditional military experiences, such as being surrounded by the enemy, as well as items specific for the Persian Gulf conflict, such as being on alert for attacks with biological weaponry.

The two groups of Gulf War veterans and the control troops were remarkably similar with respect to age (range of means 36 to 41 years), educational status (range of means 13 to 14 years in school), and previous combat exposure. The group of deployed Louisiana veterans comprised significantly more women (21 versus 8 percent in the Fort Devens group and 12 percent in the control group) and nonwhite troops (44 versus 4 percent and 0 percent). The two deployed groups had significantly fewer officers and personnel with prior service or combat experience in Vietnam than the control group.

The troops deployed to the Persian Gulf reported an average of three symptoms, while the control group reported an average of only 0.2 symptoms, a statistically significant difference. The prevalence of major depression at any point during lifetime was 22 percent in the Fort Devens group, 10 percent in the New Orleans group, and 4 percent in the control group of troops deployed to Europe. The rates of current major depression were 7 percent in the Fort Devens and 4 percent in the New Orleans group. There were no cases of major depression among the veterans who had served in Germany. The frequency of major depression (lifetime and current) was significantly greater in the Gulf War veterans from Massachusetts than in the Louisiana cohort or among the troops sent to Germany. The only other mood disorder diagnosed in this sample was dysthymia (4 percent in the Fort Devens group and 5 percent among troops from New Orleans). There were no cases of dysthymia diagnosed among the military personnel not deployed to the Persian Gulf.

The highest frequency of current (7 percent) and lifetime (8 percent) post-traumatic stress disorder was recorded in the group of Gulf War veterans from Louisiana. By comparison, the Fort Devens group had a lifetime prevalence of 6.5 percent and a current prevalence of 6.5 percent. There were no cases of post-traumatic stress disorder among the group deployed to Germany, a difference that reached statistical significance with both groups of Gulf War veterans. Other anxiety disorders (generalized anxiety disorder, panic disorder, agoraphobia, social phobia, and obsessive-compulsive disorder) were distinctly uncommon in all three groups of veterans, with the highest frequencies recorded for these disorders being 7 percent for social phobia (Louisiana group), 4 percent for panic disorder (Louisiana group), 1 percent for generalized anxiety disorders (Fort Devens group), 1 percent for agoraphobia (Fort Devens Group), and 1 percent for obsessive-compulsive disorder (Fort Devens group).

The Fort Devens and New Orleans cohorts were then combined and a hierarchical multiple regression was performed in order to establish the correlation between deployment to the Persian Gulf and the presence of somatic complaints. The study found an inverse correlation with the level of education and prior military service. The veterans reporting the largest number of somatic symptoms were less educated and more likely to have no prior military experience. A significant correlation existed between the presence of a psychiatric disorder (major depression and/or post-traumatic stress disorder) and the number of somatic symptoms. Among troops reporting ten or more symptoms, the lifetime prevalence of major depression was 61 percent and that of posttraumatic stress was 19 percent. In contrast, the lifetime prevalence of major depression was only 5 percent, and there were no cases of post-traumatic stress disorder among Gulf-deployed veterans who reported no somatic symptoms at the time of entry into the study. After controlling these findings for cohort and prior military service, the authors found that only current post-traumatic stress disorder, but not major depression, had a significant impact on the number of somatic complaints.

Veterans diagnosed with current post-traumatic stress disorder had an average of five more somatic symptoms than troops without this anxiety disorder. The comorbid association between post-traumatic stress disorder and the other psychiatric disorders did not change the strength of the statistical correlation with the number of somatic complaints. A number of observations pointed out that somatic complaints were clustered by organ or system. For example, of the four symptoms from the neurological clusters (headaches, numbness of the arms or legs, dizziness, and lightheadedness), the Gulf-deployed veterans with current major depression or post-traumatic stress disorder reported an average of 3.8 symptoms, while the Gulf-deployed troops without these mental illnesses reported an average of two symptoms. Substantial differences were also found with regard to the neuropsychological cluster (difficulty learning new material, difficulty concentrating, and confusion) and the gastrointestinal cluster (stomach cramps or excess gas, nausea or upset stomach, and diarrhea or constipation), for which Gulf-deployed veterans with major depression and post-traumatic stress disorder reported at least three times more symptoms than Gulf veterans without these diagnoses and ten times more than the troops serving in Germany.

Investigators from the University of Iowa, Iowa City, and the Centers for Disease Control and Prevention, Atlanta, Georgia, carried out an epidemiological study of 29,010 individuals who had served in the U.S. military during the time of the Persian Gulf conflict and had listed Iowa as their home state at the time of entry into the service (Doebbeling et al., 2000). Deployed and nondeployed subjects were randomly selected using a stratified procedure aimed to match the study groups with regard to age, gender, ethnic group, rank, and service branch. Of the 4,886 eligible veterans, 3,695 (76 percent) participated in the study. The subjects had served in 889 deployed and 893 nondeployed military units.

Data were collected during computer-assisted telephone interviews from September 1995 through May 1996. The core of the structured instrument used during the interviews was 78 symptoms. These items were rated on a scale ranging from "not present" to "extremely bothersome." Data were also obtained regarding the presence of 35 additional symptoms and 24 medical problems. The symptoms were recorded only if they had been present during the year preceding the interview and only if their onset occurred during or after the Gulf conflict.

The analysis of the data was carried out in three main stages. First, the frequency distribution of each symptom was compared between the two groups. Second, the group of veterans deployed to the Persian Gulf was randomly divided into a "derivation" and a "validation" sample, and factor analysis was used to detect reproducible clusters of symptoms specific for the deployed group. Third, factor analysis was employed to compare groups of symptoms in the deployed and nondeployed veterans' groups.

Compared with the nondeployed subjects, the veterans who had served in the Persian Gulf were slightly more likely to be younger than 25 years of age (55 versus 47 percent), of male gender (93 versus 89 percent), of enlisted rank (91 versus 87 percent), and to have only a high school education (92 versus 42 percent).

The most common symptoms reported by the Gulf War veterans and nondeployed military personnel were feeling tired (38 versus 19 percent), lacking in energy (35 versus 17 percent), needing to rest more (32 versus 17 percent), and feeling extreme fatigue almost every day (23 versus 9 percent). A substantial number of veterans also reported joint pains (37 versus 16 percent), muscle soreness or stiffness (31 versus 17 percent), back pain (30 versus 16 percent), and headaches (23 versus 8 percent). Many subjects suffered from sleep disturbances that were described as feeling unusually sleepy or drowsy (27 versus 13 percent) or having trouble falling or staying asleep (26 versus 13 percent). Common cognitive difficulties included forgetfulness (22 versus 8 percent) and impaired concentration (17 versus 7 percent). A substantial proportion of participants reported numbness or tingling sensations (27 versus 14 percent) and feeling weak in parts of the body (23 versus 10 percent). Overall, significantly more of the deployed veteran group (50 versus 14 percent) reported continuing health problems considered by them to be related to service during the Gulf War period. Of the 137 symptoms recorded in this study, 123 were more frequently reported by the deployed veterans.

In the derivation subsample of the Gulf War veterans, the factor analysis isolated three groups of symptoms. The first was called "somatic distress" and had as its key symptoms items such as joint stiffness and pain, muscle pain, headaches, numbness or tingling, and nausea. The second focused on symptoms indicating "psychological distress," i.e., depression, loss of interest in pleasurable activities, worrying, and feeling distant or cut off. The third group of symptoms was aggregated under the label of "panic" and described complaints common during panic attacks or states of sympathetic arousal such as episodic diaphoresis, chest pain, and palpitations. The three groups of symptoms were reliably confirmed in the validation subsample. The total variance attributed to these factors was 37 percent in the derivation group and 35 percent in the validation group. Moreover, the intercorrelation scores of the three factors, a measure of their conceptual strength, were very good at 0.88 for "panic," 0.89 for "psychological distress," and 0.90 for "somatic distress." The same three factors were identified among the nondeployed veterans. In this population, the common variance explained by the three factors was 29 percent. The authors interpreted their findings as a rejection of the existence of a morbid condition specific to Gulf War veterans, because the broad range of symptoms was considered "difficult to explain pathophysiologically as a single illness" (Doebbeling et al., 2000, p. 702). It appears that being a member of the U.S. military at the time of the conflict in the Persian Gulf determined a high prevalence of medically unexplained symptoms in later years. The question as to whether this pattern of reporting was similar to other combat-induced illnesses or was analogous to traditional somatoform disorders was left unanswered by these data.

The similarity between the symptoms reported by deployed and nondeployed veterans of the U.S. military after the Gulf War conflict was confirmed by investigators from the Naval Health Research Center, San Diego, and University of California at San Diego, La Jolla, California (Knoke et al., 2000). The sample studied consisted of the 8,500 U.S. naval mobile construction personnel (Seabees) who had been on active duty from September 1990 through 1994. Research data were obtained from the 1,496 of these individuals who agreed to participate and were in residence in the United States at the time of the study. After excluding the 39 women Seabees, the final study groups comprised 524 personnel who had been deployed to the Persian Gulf during the conflict and 935 nondeployed (control) subjects. The participation rate was 65 percent for deployed Seabees, but only 46 percent for the nondeployed personnel. As in the Iowa cohort (Doebbeling et al., 2000), the deployed participants were younger, had less education, and were less likely to have officer rank. The ethnic origin of the subjects was similar in the two groups.

The primary data collection instrument was a list of 98 symptoms, which included 57 symptoms evaluated by a standard instrument, the Hopkins Symptom Checklist (Derogatis et al., 1974), and 41 symptoms selected by the authors as representative of the common complaints after deployment for the Gulf War. The complaints evaluated by the Hopkins Symptom Checklist were clustered to identify somatization, obsessive-compulsive states, interpersonal sensitivity, depression, and anxiety. Statistical processing used factor analysis to identify clusters of symptoms in both groups.

The most common complaints were headache (55 percent in the deployed group versus 43 percent in the nondeployed group), trouble remembering things (51 versus 29 percent), lower back pain (51 versus 40 percent), slowed down/low in energy (51 versus 33 percent), muscle soreness (36 versus 26 percent), worrying about things (35 versus 24 percent), worried about sloppiness (35 versus 23 percent), difficulty sleeping (34 versus 21 percent), trouble concentrating (32 versus 16 percent), joint pain (14 versus 5 percent), and rash or skin ulcer (14 versus 4 percent). Overall, significantly more deployed men reported significantly more symptoms than the nondeployed control subjects.

Factor analysis identified five groups of symptoms with minimal overlap in the deployed group. The first was named "insecurity or minor depression" and included items such as feeling lonely, feeling blue, feeling inferior to others, asking others what to do, worrying about things, feeling hopeless about the future, feeling trapped, feeling fearful, being shy or uneasy about the opposite sex, and finding it tough to make decisions. The second factor was named "somatization" and relied on symptoms of weakness in parts of the body, heavy arms and legs, trouble getting breath, soreness in muscles, numbness or tingling, faintness or dizziness, and headache. The third factor was named "depression" and was based on reports of unusual irritability, loss of interest in life, marital stress, trouble sleeping, and unusual fatigue. The "obsessive-compulsive" factor took into account symptoms such as feeling confused, forgetfulness, double-checking oneself, and doing things slowly. The fifth and final factor was named "malaise" and included tender lymph nodes, fever, sore throat, night sweats, and sudden hair loss. All together, they accounted for 80 percent of variance in the symptoms retained in the model. A similar analysis of the data provided by the nondeployed Seabees produced five similar factors, which accounted for 89 percent of the variance.

The direct comparison of the two groups indicated that three of the five groups of symptoms, i.e., somatization, depression, and obsessive-compulsive, had significantly greater scores in the deployed group. The factor malaise, based on symptoms considered specific for the Gulf War illness, had a significantly greater score in the nondeployed group ($p < 0.0001$). The factor insecurity was similarly scored in the two groups. A multivariate analysis excluded malaise from the model. The three factors that emerged from this complex evaluation, somatization, depression, and obsessive-compulsive, had higher scores among the deployed Navy men. The study's conclusion showed a striking similarity to that of previous work (Doebbeling et al., 2000): veterans of the Gulf War and nondeployed controls have the same symptoms and the same illnesses, but the former report more of both.

The presence of posttraumatic stress was the focus of a study carried out by investigators affiliated with the Portland (Oregon) Environmental Hazards Research Center and the Oregon Health Sciences University (Ford et al., 2001). The authors used a large database provided by the Department of Defense to conduct a cross-sectional study of these symptoms and their relationship to the somatic and psychological dimensions of this syndrome. A total of 2,002 randomly selected eligible veterans from the states of Oregon and Washington were mailed a screening questionnaire, and the 1,119 who returned it were offered a comprehensive medical evaluation of their chronic symptoms. The process identified 237 individuals with persistent symptoms that had started after their service in the Persian Gulf and could not be attributed to a physical disorder. The subjects had symptoms from at least one of the following categories: cognitive, fatigue, musculoskeletal pain, gastrointestinal distress, and skin or mucous membrane lesions. The symptoms had to have their onset during or after the Gulf War, last at least one month, and be present within three months of entry into the study.

Of the 237 cases, 207 had cognitive symptoms, 100 had fatigue, 92 had muscle and joint pains, 25 had gastrointestinal symptoms, and four had skin lesions. The final study group comprised 119 veterans with cognitive symptoms plus fatigue or musculoskeletal pain. A control group of 112 veterans without persistent symptoms was also recruited. Ill and control groups were similar with respect to gender, ethnic background, marital status, and current income.

The participants were assessed with a 19-test battery administered during a four-hour session. The instruments measured psychiatric symptoms, current severity of anxiety and depression, presence and severity of personality pathology, psychosocial stressors, functional impairment, alcohol and drug use, war zone exposures (e.g., wounding or death of others, threat of injury, physical abuse, and experience as a prisoner of war), and service-related posttraumatic stress symptoms. A preliminary analysis indicated no significant overlap between cognitive symptoms and posttraumatic stress findings and confirmed the validity of full-sample logistic regression evaluation of the data.

The ill veterans were younger (mean 32 versus 34 years) and had a lower educational level (13 versus 14 years) than the control group. Univariate logistic regression tests indicated that the ill veterans had more posttraumatic stress symptoms, reported more war-related traumatic exposures, and had significantly higher levels of somatic preoccupation and distress ($p < 0.0001$) than the veteran control group. They were also more depressed and more anxious ($p < 0.0001$) and had more health problems, pain, and fatigue ($p < 0.0002$). In a multivariate logistic regression model, the two groups were distinguished by four variables: posttraumatic stress symptoms ($p < 0.004$), traumatic war-zone exposures ($p = 0.007$), severity of somatic preoccupation and distress ($p < 0.001$), and severity of current depression ($p = 0.003$). The model had a sensitivity of 90 percent, a specificity of 77 percent, and classified correctly 86 percent of the participants. Cross-validation analyses conducted on a randomly selected half-sample produced evidence that the severity of somatic preoccupation and posttraumatic symptoms were the two replicable indicators of caseness. The authors stressed the fact that in most cases the number of post-traumatic symptoms did not support a full-fledged diagnosis of post-traumatic stress disorder. Nonetheless, they felt that psychological factors specifically related to trauma are "robustly associated with the presence of persistent somatic problems that could be medically documented but not diagnostically explained" (Ford et al., 2001, p. 848).

A further contribution to the discovery of post-traumatic stress disorder in Gulf veterans has been made by investigators associated with Center for the Study of War-Related Illness, Veterans Administration Medical Center in East Orange, New Jersey (Natelson et al., 2001). The authors restricted their investigation to a group of 76 ill Gulf veterans who met criteria for chronic fatigue syndrome ($N = 65$) or idiopathic chronic fatigue ($N = 11$) as defined by an international collective (Fukuda et al., 1994). Data were collected with a structured diagnostic interview for psychiatric disorders (Marcus et al., 1990) and a validated symptom checklist (Keane et al., 1988).

The structured psychiatric interview diagnosed post-traumatic stress disorder in 23 of the 76 participants (30 percent). The condition was currently active in all but one of these patients. The symptom checklist identified the presence of posttraumatic stress in 26 (41 percent) of the ill Gulf veterans. Twelve veterans (21 percent) met criteria for post-traumatic stress disorder on both the interview and the symptom checklist. The authors conclude that the "stress of deployment and combat did play a significant role in producing the alterations in health" (Natelson et al., 2001, p. 795) reported by many Gulf veterans with medically unexplained physical complaints.

In summary, the evidence indicates that Gulf War illness is characterized by multiple bodily complaints, somatic preoccupation, and somatic distress. The magnitude of somatization phenomena correlates with the presence and severity of posttraumatic stress symptoms. Fatigue, sleep disturbance, cognitive deficits, and panic symptoms are also commonly reported by ill veterans, but a direct relationship with depressive or anxiety disorders has not been established.

PART III:
THE PSYCHOBIOLOGY
OF FUNCTIONAL SOMATIC
SYNDROMES

Chapter 8

Neuroanatomy and Brain Perfusion in Functional Somatic Syndromes

Neuroimaging methods have been extensively used to help define structural and functional abnormalities in psychiatric and functional illnesses. Particular attention has been devoted to the neuroanatomy of depression and anxiety, and the prefrontal and parietal cortex, anterior cingulate, and the amygdala have emerged as critical components of dysfunctional circuitry in these conditions (Davidson et al., 1999). The best-replicated finding in mood disorders is an increased frequency of periventricular and white matter hyperintensities on magnetic resonance images (Soares and Mann, 1997). Static imaging in unipolar depression has also demonstrated a decrease in the size of the frontal lobe, cerebellum, caudate, and putamen (Soares and Mann, 1997), while functional neuroimaging has identified a decrease in the prefrontal cortical function and an increase in subcortical anterior paralimbic activity (Ketter and Wang, 2002). In this chapter we review the controlled neuroimaging studies performed in patients with functional somatic syndromes to determine whether these conditions are associated with neuroimaging abnormalities, whether these abnormalities are similar to those of mentally ill controls, and whether the anatomical and functional changes correlate with the clinical manifestations of the functional illness.

MAGNETIC RESONANCE AND SINGLE PHOTON EMISSION IMAGING IN CHRONIC FATIGUE SYNDROME

The first study of magnetic resonance abnormalities in patients with chronic fatigue syndrome evaluated a cluster of cases seen in a general internal medicine practice located in Incline Village, Nevada (Buchwald et al., 1992). Magnetic resonance scans were obtained on 144 of the 259 patients enrolled in the cross-sectional investigation. Their mean age was 39 years, 72 percent were female, and 43 percent had completed at least four years of post-high school education. Compared with the remainder of study cohort, patients sent for magnetic resonance imaging of the brain were more likely to consider themselves unable to hold full-time jobs (67 versus 37 percent), and to have chronic headaches (91 versus 78 percent), paresthesias (75 versus 47 percent) and nausea (63 versus 38 percent). The neurological events recorded for this cohort included transient ataxia (ten patients), transient paresis (eight patients), and seizures (seven patients). The control data were obtained from an evaluation of magnetic resonance images obtained on 47 gender- and age-matchedpatients without chronic fatigue. The control subjects had been neuroimaged in another state with similar equipment, i.e., a 1.5 Tesla magnet programmed to obtain transaxial spin echo scans at 5 mm intervals from the foramen magnum to the vertex. Forty-two of the control subjects were healthy, four had been referred for evaluation after head trauma, and one had neck pain. A neuroradiologist not involved with the original examination evaluated all the scans but was not blinded to the clinical status of the subjects.

Magnetic resonance abnormalities were identified in 78 percent of patients with chronic fatigue syndrome and 21 percent of the healthy control subjects. The abnormalities consisted of punctate hyperintensities in the subcortical white matter. Larger hyperintense areas were also occasionally seen, but the frequency of these abnormalities was not reported. The location of hyperintense signals correlated with the patients' symptoms in only 8 percent of the cases; seven patients with unspecified visual complaints had abnormalities in the occipital cortex, one patient with ataxia had cerebellar high-intensity signals, and one patient with ataxia had a contralateral internal capsule hyperintensity. The authors noted that "the clinical significance of these 'incidental' areas of high signal intensity in the white matter is not known" (Buchwald et al., 1992, p. 109).

One year after the publication of the Incline Village data (Buchwald et al., 1992), investigators from the New Jersey Medical School in Newark reported the results of a study of brain magnetic resonance imaging in 52 patients with chronic fatigue syndrome and 52 age-

and gender-matched control subjects (Natelson et al., 1993). The patients with chronic fatigue (46 women and six men; mean age 38 years) were diagnosed with the syndrome according to standard criteria (Holmes et al., 1988). The illness had been present for at least 12 months and was accompanied by at least a 50 percent reduction in activity in all participants. Self-administered instruments were used to assess the presence of current mood disorders. All patients had a completely normal neurological examination and had tested negatively for Lyme disease on multiple occasions. The control group comprised subjects undergoing diagnostic evaluation of headaches or neuroimaging following head trauma. Other than to indicate that none of these subjects had a space-occupying lesion, the authors did not provide any other clinical or psychometric data.

All of the control subjects and 27 of the 52 patients with chronic fatigue syndrome underwent brain imaging at the same location. The remaining patients with the syndrome had their magnetic resonance scans obtained at four other sites. Each of the five imaging centers used a different data acquisition system. After each center's neuroradiologist read the images, the identifying data were obliterated and scans read by a second neuroradiologist. Observer agreement was recorded for 39 of the chronic fatigue syndrome cases and 44 control subjects.

Magnetic resonance abnormalities were identified in 14 patients (27 percent) with chronic fatigue syndrome and one of the control subjects (2 percent). Among the fatigue patients, the abnormalities consisted of small areas of increased signal intensity in the corona radiata area of the white matter (seven patients); ventricular or sulcal enlargement (five patients); a single pontine calcium or hemosiderin deposit (one patient); and a single, small periventricular hyperintensity (one patient). The control subject had a small abnormality in the pons. Twelve of the 14 chronic fatigue patients with magnetic resonance abnormalities had completed the psychometric evaluation and were compared with 12 fatigue patients without neuroimaging abnormalities. The frequencies of depression in these subsamples were 58 percent and 25 percent, respectively. Due to the small sample size, the difference did not reach statistical significance. In their analysis of the data, the authors pointed out that clinical follow-up of eight patients with magnetic resonance abnormalities reclassified two with multiple sclerosis and one patient with collagen vascular disease. Two other patients from this subgroup were thought to have abnormalities related to a discrete vascular lesion or severe head trauma. Therefore, the revised prevalence of abnormalities in the chronic fatigue syndrome group was 17 percent, significantly lower than the 78 percent prevalence reported by Buchwald et al. (1992). Of note also is the fact that Buchwald et al. (1992) reported ten times more abnormalities in their control group (21 versus 2 percent). The significance of the abnormalities remained unknown, but the authors wisely suggested the need to include control subjects with depression in future neuroimaging studies of chronic fatigue syndrome.

The third study of magnetic resonance abnormalities in chronic fatigue syndrome was performed by an interdisciplinary group from the Brigham and Women's Hospital in Boston (Schwartz et al., 1994). Two of the investigators were among the authors of a previous report (Buchwald et al., 1992). The researchers used the database generated by the clinical evaluation of 251 patients to select 16 cases (mean age 42 years) who had had both magnetic resonance and single photon emission tomographic studies within a period not exceeding ten weeks. Fifteen age- and gender-matched healthy subjects (mean age 39 years) formed the control group for the magnetic resonance study. Fourteen other healthy subjects (mean age 49 years) constituted the control group for the single photon emission tomography portion of the data. The neuroimaging was performed using standard techniques at the authors' institution and the computer-generated films submitted in random order for blinded interpretation by three neuroradiologists. A consensus conference was held to reach closure regarding the number, size, and location of the identified abnormalities.

Magnetic resonance abnormalities were present in 50 percent of patients with chronic fatigue syndrome and 20 percent of healthy control subjects. The difference between these proportions did not reach statistical significance. The findings consisted of small areas of signal hyperintensity involving the subcortical and periventricular white matter, the internal capsule, centrum semiovale, and corona radiata. The largest such area of increased signal intensity was 1 cm in diameter. The average number of hyperintense foci was statistically similar in the two groups (2.06 versus 0.8).

Single-photon emission tomographic images were interpreted to show perfusion abnormalities in 81 percent of patients with chronic fatigue syndrome and 21 percent of the healthy control subjects ($p <$ 0.01). The number of hypoperfused areas was substantially greater in the patient group (7.3 versus 0.4, $p < 0.001$). The regions most affected in chronic fatigue syndrome were the lateral frontal cortex, the lateral temporal cortex, and the basal ganglia. This distribution did not match the location of hyperintense signals found on magnetic resonance imaging. Without giving details, the authors indicated that "the majority of patients with abnormalities on SPECT [single photon emission tomography] had normal findings on MR [magnetic resonance] images" (Schwartz et al., 1994, p. 937).

European researchers added to the growing popularity of magnetic resonance assessments in chronic fatigue syndrome a controlled study performed at the University College, London Medical School, London (Greco et al., 1997). Their patient group comprised 43 patients with chronic fatigue syndrome. Structured psychiatric evaluations identified lifetime psychiatric disorders in 28 patients. Fourteen cases had a current or past history of depression, and 14 had anxiety or somatization disorder. An age and gender-matched control group was recruited from among individuals with a diagnosis of benign positional vertigo. All of the control subjects had normal findings on neurological examination. Images were obtained with a 1.0 Tesla magnet for the patients with chronic fatigue syndrome. A 1.5 Tesla magnet was used to image the control subjects. The difference in equipment was not explained in the report, and probably contributed to the fact that the neuroradiologist who read the images was apparently blinded only to the psychiatric diagnoses of the chronic fatigue syndrome patients.

Magnetic resonance abnormalities were identified in 13 patients (32 percent) with chronic fatigue syndrome and 12 control subjects (28 percent). Eleven of the 13 chronic fatigue cases had punctate foci of hyperintensity in corona radiata, centrum ovale, frontoparietal subcortical white matter, and external capsule. The remaining two fatigue patients had periventricular hyperintensities compatible with demyelination. Chronic fatigue patients older than 50 years of age had a much higher prevalence of abnormalities than younger sufferers (64 versus 21 percent, $p < 0.01$). In the younger group the hyperintensities were nonspecific, while those identified in older patients were interpreted to suggest age-related small vessel disease. A similar pattern was detected in the control group. The prevalence of abnormalities was 40 percent in the chronic fatigue subgroup without psychiatric disorders, 36 percent in those with associated depression, and 14 percent among fatigue patients with other psychiatric diagnoses. The difference between these proportions did not reach statistical significance. Based on these findings, the authors appropriately concluded "no MR [magnetic resonance] pattern of abnormalities is specific to CFS [chronic fatigue syndrome]" (Greco et al., 1997, p. 1269).

A few years later, the investigators from the New Jersey Medical School, Newark, evaluated again the significance of brain magnetic resonance imaging abnormalities and their relationship to the psychiatric morbidity of patients with chronic fatigue syndrome (Lange et al., 1999). Thirty-nine patients with chronic fatigue syndrome were recruited for this project. All patients met established diagnostic criteria (Fukuda et al., 1994). Only patients without psychiatric disorder (American Medical Association, 1987) prior to the onset of the fatigue illness were included in the study group. The 19 control subjects contacted the investigators in response to advertisements and had no history of medical or psychiatric illnesses. A structured psychiatric interview (Markus et al., 1991) was administered to all participants and identified a psychiatric disorder in 18 of the 39 chronic fatigue patients. In this subgroup, 89 percent of patients had major depression, 6 percent had dysthymia, 11 percent had generalized anxiety disorder, and 6 percent had somatoform disorders. All of these disorders had their onset after the start of the functional illness.

Magnetic resonance imaging was performed on all participants at a single location, using a 1.5 Tesla magnet. The images were read independently by two neuroradiologists who were unaware of the subjects' status as patients or controls. The readers had been trained to identify and score the severity of lateral ventricular enlargement, subcortical white matter hyperintensity, gray matter and brainstem hyperintensity, cerebral atrophy, and right-left cerebral asymmetry. Their interpretations of the data were in agreement for 19 of the 39 patients with chronic fatigue syndrome and 11 of the 19 control subjects. The two readers met and reached consensus on 27 of the discrepant results, while a tie-breaking third neuroradiologist adjudicated the remaining cases. The disputed findings were the number of hyperintensities and the decision to diagnose atrophy or asymmetry.

Magnetic resonance abnormalities were identified in the brains of 18 patients (46 percent) with chronic fatigue syndrome and six control subjects (32 percent). The difference between these proportions was not significant. The duration and severity of the fatigue illness did not correlate with the radiological findings. The analysis of clinical subsets revealed abnormalities in 14 of the 21 chronic fatigue patients without a current psychiatric disorder and in four of the 18 patients with this comorbid association (70 versus 22 percent, $p < 0.01$). The difference was explained in large part by a higher incidence of hyperintensities in the subcortical white matter (less than 5 mm in diameter), present in 48 percent of chronic fatigue syndrome patients without psychiatric disorder, as compared with 17 percent in the other patients and 11 percent in the healthy control group ($p = 0.04$). All participants with these abnormalities had at least one such hyperintensity in the frontal lobe, and in two-thirds of these cases the hyperintensities were confined to the frontal lobe. Periventricular white matter hyperintensities, gray matter hyperintensities, lateral ventricular enlargement, and atrophy were uncommon in both groups. None of the intergroup differences reached statistical significance. The pathophysiological significance of the magnetic resonance abnormalities was not elucidated.

Two years later, the same group of investigators from the New Jersey Medical School at Newark focused their attention on the magnetic resonance assessment of cerebral ventricular volumes (Lange et al., 2001). The authors hypothesized that patients with chronic fatigue syndrome have white matter loss and recruited for their study 28 patients with this condition and 15 healthy control subjects. The groups were similar with regard to age, gender distribution, handedness, and level of education. The patients had a mean duration of illness of three years and no history of psychiatric disorder within the five years preceding the onset of their fatigue. Structured psychiatric interviews identified current psychiatric disorders in 11 of the 28 patients. The most common psychiatric disorder was major depression, diagnosed in ten subjects. Three patients had anxiety disorders, which in two cases were comorbid to major depression.

Magnetic resonance examinations were performed at a single center using a 1.0 Tesla magnet. In each case, fifty 3-mm adjoining slices were obtained. The volumes of different tissue types (i.e., brain and cerebrospinal fluid) were calculated using an algorithm that required visual estimation of the size and intensity of each area and automatic morphometric measurements. The data were collected independently by two raters who were unaware of group membership or other characteristics of the cases. Other measurements included self-ratings of the severity of 16 symptoms and of the overall level of discomfort.

Compared with healthy subjects, patients with chronic fatigue syndrome were found to have larger volumes of the lateral ventricles. The significance of the differences was given as $p = 0.06$ for the entire ventricular system and as $p = 0.07$ for the separate comparisons of the left and right ventricles, respectively. The ventricle-to-brain ratios were also statistically similar in the two groups, as was the degree of brain asymmetry. Coexisting psychiatric diagnoses, severity of symptoms, and duration of the fatiguing illness did not correlate with the cerebral ventricular volumes. The authors attributed the lack of significant differences to the small sample size by noting that the study had only a 46 percent chance to detect true differences at the $p < 0.05$ level. Be that as it may, the hypothesized brain mass loss in patients with chronic fatigue syndrome was not confirmed by this work.

A further attempt to elucidate the relationship between magnetic resonance abnormalities and clinical dimensions of chronic fatigue syndrome was made by the same group of investigators from the New Jersey Medical School, Newark (Cook et al., 2001). This time, the authors hypothesized that patients with neuroimaging abnormalities would report impaired physical functioning. Data were obtained from 48 subjects with chronic fatigue syndrome. The majority of the subjects had been included in a previous study (Lange et al., 1999). Images were obtained with 1.0 Tesla magnet that produced 5-mm thick slices. The films were read independently by two neuroradiologists who identified them as abnormal based on the detection of enlargement of the lateral ventricles; hyperintensities in the gray matter or brainstem; cerebral atrophy; and left-right hemispheric asymmetry. Functional impairment was measured with the physical functioning subscale and the physical component summary of the self-administered short form of the Medical Outcome Study questionnaire (Stewart et al., 1988).

Twenty-five of the 48 chronic fatigue syndrome patients included in this study had brain magnetic resonance abnormalities. As a group, they were significantly older than patients with normal neuroimaging studies (43 versus 33 years, $p < 0.001$). Patients with magnetic resonance abnormalities reported more impairment in physical functioning than the remainder of the study cohort ($p < 0.03$). However, analysis of covariance with age indicated that the difference in physical functioning had only marginal significance ($p < 0.05$) for one subscale and lacked significance for the summary score ($p < 0.66$). The data did not support a clinically meaningful correlation between magnetic resonance abnormalities and physical functioning. The findings were similar with those obtained in studies showing that white matter abnormalities discovered during neuroimaging studies are not associated with detectable impairment in healthy adults without neuropsychiatric disorders (Tupler et al., 1992; Schmidt et al., 2000).

Single photon emission tomography was used to evaluate patients with chronic fatigue syndrome and compare them to control groups with major depression and viral encephalitis (i.e., dementia complex associated with acquired immune deficiency syndrome) by a research group from the Brigham and Women's Hospital and Harvard Medical School, Boston (Schwartz et al., 1994). The 45 patients with chronic fatigue syndrome were selected from among 251 subjects with this diagnosis. Although the selection criteria were not detailed in the published report, it appears that all patients had symptoms suggestive of neurological disturbance. Ten patients had had an acute event whose neurological origin was inferred because of seizures, weakness, or transient visual impairment. The remaining 35 patients had been complaining of chronic disequilibrium, paresthesias, or photophobia. Compared with chronic fatigue syndrome patients not selected for this study, the participants had a greater prevalence of ataxia and a shorter duration of illness. The 14 control subjects with major depression had been diagnosed according to the accepted standard (American Psychiatric Association, 1987). They had been recruited from an inpatient unit and had no significant abnormalities on a neurological examination. The 27 patients with human immunodeficiency virus (HIV) encephalopathy were diagnosed according to criteria established by the American Academy of Neurology (Janssen et al., 1989). All had focal neurological signs or cognitive impairments and CD4+ counts less than $500/mm^3$. The third control group comprised 38 healthy individuals who had a negative physical examination. The samples differed substantially with regard to age, which averaged 43 years in the chronic fatigue syndrome group, 40 years in the HIV encephalopathy group, 70 years in the depressed patients, and 62 years in the healthy control group. The proportion of women in the HIV encephalopathy group was 11 percent, while in the other three groups it ranged from 61 to 64 percent.

The neuroimaging procedures were carried out 10 minutes after the administration of 925 to 1,110 MBq of 99m Tc-hexamethyl propyleneamine oxime, and the image acquisition lasted 30 minutes. Standard coronal, axial, and sagittal planes were used to reconstruct and analyze the data contained in 14 summed-up slices that were each 8 mm thick. The presence of abnormalities was established by consensus among three radiologists.

Patients with chronic fatigue syndrome and major depression had a similar average number of perfusion defects (6.5 versus 6.3), and both groups were quite different from subjects with HIV encephalopathy, who averaged 9.1 defects per subject. The healthy volunteers had only 1.7 defects per subject. The regional distribution of hypoperfusion defects was also similar between chronic fatigue syndrome and depressed patients, the average number of defects being 1.7 versus 1.4 in the frontal lobes and 2.8 versus 2.5 in the temporal lobes. The authors suggested that the similar regional distribution of defects was related to common symptoms of depression and irritability and to the cognitive impairment experienced by their patient groups. The possibility of an association between the severity of perfusion abnormalities and that of depressive symptomatology was not explicitly addressed in the published report.

The perfusion of the brain stem in chronic fatigue syndrome was the focus of a controlled study performed at the University College Medical School, London (Costa et al., 1995). The authors recruited 43 patients with chronic fatigue syndrome (29 women), 20 patients with major depression (12 women), and 16 healthy control subjects (five women). Structured psychiatric evaluation were used to confirm the diagnosis in the depressed group and to subdivide the chronic fatigue group into subsamples with no lifetime history of psychiatric disorder ($N = 16$), past or current major depression ($N = 13$), and other psychiatric conditions, including dysthymia, anxiety, and somatization disorders ($N = 14$).

Brain perfusion was assessed on three contiguous slices reconstructed for each region of interest, defined as a volume of 2 cm^3 of the basal ganglia, thalamus, brain stem, and cerebellum. Compared to patients with major depression, brain stem perfusion was significantly decreased in the chronic fatigue syndrome group, particularly among those without psychiatric disorders.

The cerebral perfusion of patients with chronic fatigue syndrome and major depression was also evaluated by investigators from the Free University of Brussels, Belgium (Fischler et al., 1996). The 16 chronic fatigue syndrome patients (14 women; group mean age 35 years) had been diagnosed according to a working case definition proposed by Holmes et al. (1988). Thirteen of the 16 chronic fatigue syndrome patients had a past history of major depression, and three patients had a current depressive disorder. The major depression control group included 19 inpatients (15 women; group mean age 40 years) diagnosed according to standard U.S. criteria (American Psychiatric Association, 1987). For the healthy control group, the authors recruited eight women and 12 men, with a mean age of 36 years with no history of psychiatric or neurological disorders. With only one exception, all patients had been off psychotropic drugs for at least one week prior to the study. A validated instrument (Mowbray, 1972) was used to determine the severity of depressive symptomatology in the major depression and chronic fatigue syndrome groups.

Single photon emission computerized tomography was performed in all subjects 15 and 30 minutes after administration of 900 MBq of 99m Tc-hexamethylpropyleneamine oxime. Data were collected at a rate of 30 seconds per view in 64 angular increments. The perfusion was measured in four consecutive slices each for the lower, middle, and upper cerebral regions. Separate reconstructions allowed the estimation of cerebellar perfusion.

The most important finding was the discovery that the 13 chronic fatigue patients without a current mood disorder showed a positive correlation between frontal lobe perfusion and the severity of current depressive symptomatology. The areas involved in this relationship involved both the left frontal lobe (superior and inferior slices) and the right frontal lobe (superior slice only). Global measures of perfusion were not different in the chronic fatigue syndrome and healthy control subjects. Compared with chronic fatigue syndrome and healthy subjects, inpatients with major depression showed a decrease in the left frontal lobe perfusion and less asymmetry in the regional (right versus left) perfusion.

The evaluation of cerebral perfusion in chronic fatigue syndrome was continued by investigators from Edinburgh University and Royal

Edinburgh Hospital, Scotland, and Warneford Hospital, Oxford, England (MacHale et al., 2000). The authors recruited 24 patients with chronic fatigue from an infectious disease outpatient clinic and 76 individuals from a local self-help group. A total of 30 subjects fulfilled diagnostic criteria for chronic fatigue syndrome (Fukuda et al., 1994). The subjects were found to score below the threshold for caseness on a validated scale measuring the severity of anxiety and depression (Zigmond and Snaith, 1983) and had no evidence of psychiatric disorders on a structured interview. The two control groups included 12 patients diagnosed as suffering from current major depression with melancholia and 15 healthy volunteers recruited from among friends of patients and hospital personnel.

The imaging procedure required the administration of 500 MBq of technetium-99m hexamethylpropylamine oxime in the chronic fatigue syndrome patients, followed by head scanning at the rate of 2.5 minutes per slice. The control subjects received 250 MBq of the radioactive material and were scanned for 5 minutes per slice. Image acquisition started approximately 2 cm above the orbitomeatal plane and proceeded at 1-cm intervals thereafter. Image analysis used the slices obtained at 4 and 6 cm above the orbitomeatal plane. The lower slice allowed the visualization of the caudate, putamen, thalamus, and portions of the frontal, temporal, and occipital cortex. The upper slice imaged the frontal, parietal, and occipital cortex. The perfusion of the brain stem was not assessed.

The 30 patients with chronic fatigue syndrome (19 women) had a mean age of 44 years and had been ill for an average of six years. Ten patients were treated with antidepressant drugs at the time of recruitment in the study, and five of these patients had a past history of a depressive disorder.

The only patient with a currently active psychiatric diagnosis among patients with chronic fatigue syndrome had somatization disorder. The 12 patients from the depressed group (six women) had a mean age of 44 years and had suffered their current episode for an average of one year. Ten depressed patients were on psychoactive medications, including antidepressants in eight patients, neuroleptics in three, hypnotics or anxiolytics in three, and lithium in two patients. Five depressed patients had been treated with electroconvulsive therapy within the six months preceding the study. The 15 healthy volunteers (11 women) had a mean age of 41 years and were medication free, with the exception of three subjects on hormones for replacement or contraception. The severity of fatigue was statistically similar in the chronic fatigue syndrome and depressed groups, but the latter showed a significantly greater burden of depressive symptomatology.

Compared with healthy control subjects, the patients with chronic fatigue syndrome and those with depression had significantly increased uptake in the right thalamus, pallidum, and putamen. The only difference between currently depressed patients and chronic fatigue syndrome subjects was the decreased perfusion of the left prefrontal cortex observed in the depressed group. The authors' interpretation of the findings relied on the crucial contribution made by the thalamic output to the cortical functions such as discrimination of painful stimuli (Davis et al., 1996; Lenz et al., 1998); regulation of sleep and wakefulness (Contreras and Steriade, 1995; Kiss et al., 1995; Steriade and Contreras, 1995); and vigilance and attention (Kinomura et al., 1996; Weese et al., 1999). The findings were interpreted to support the overlap between depression and chronic fatigue syndrome. The fact that the prefrontal perfusion was decreased in patients with major depression but not in those with chronic fatigue syndrome was thought to be a neuroimaging corollary of the more severe cognitive deficits present in the depressed subjects.

CEREBRAL PERFUSION IN FIBROMYALGIA

Investigators from Sahlgren Hospital, Göteborg, Sweden, were the first to assess the presence of cerebral dysfunction in fibromyalgia using measurements of regional cerebral blood (Johansson et al., 1995). The study group comprised 20 fibromyalgia patients (16 women and four men with a mean age of 45 years) admitted to a rehabilitation center for pain management or vocational retraining. In addition to the standard criteria for fibromyalgia (Wolfe et al., 1990), all participants had to have evidence of hallucinosis or cognitive impairment that could not be explained by a comorbid psychiatric disorder. Eighteen of the 20 patients had stopped working at least one year before the study because of their pain syndrome. As ascertained by specialty consultations, none of the participants had a neurological disorder. Seven patients had dysphoria and five had psychomotor retardation. Eight patients were treated with psychotropic drugs and six patients were taking benzodiazepines. Nineteen healthy subjects without a history of psychiatric disorders were recruited for the control group. The regional cerebral blood flow was measured after the inhalation of the radioactive isotope 133Xe (70 MBq/L). The gamma radiation was measured ten minutes later.

The mean cerebral perfusion was identical in fibromyalgia and healthy subjects (53.5 versus 53.4 mL/100 g/min). Regional flow abnormalities were detected in 12 of 19 patients with fibromyalgia. Seven patients had evidence of a decreased flow in the frontal areas. Five patients had mild to moderate decreased perfusion of the temporal, central, or parietal areas. Areas of hypoperfusion were detected in both hemispheres in eight of these 12 cases. In three of the remaining four cases, the perfusion abnormalities were restricted to the left hemisphere. Compared with the healthy control group, fibromyalgia patients had decreased flow to the dorsolateral frontal areas and the left temporal area.

The evaluation of cerebral perfusion in fibromyalgia was continued at the University of Alabama, Birmingham (Mountz et al., 1995), by a group of researchers who studied ten female patients and seven healthy control subjects. The authors sought to determine whether the groups differed with regard to blood flow to the thalamus and caudate nuclei, areas known to be involved in the perception and integration of pain signals. The diagnosis of fibromyalgia (Wolfe et al., 1990) was established after a careful examination that excluded the presence of rheumatic disorders and chronic fatigue syndrome. Fibromyalgia and control subjects were similar with respect to age, ethnic background, and level of education.

Pain threshold levels were measured using a standardized direct pressure technique at a total of ten paired anatomical sites. Five of these sites were traditional tender points (e.g., the second rib at the costochondral junction and the medial fat pad of the knee). The other five were control points above and below the waist (e.g., the midshaft of the ulna and anteromedial surface of the tibia). One hour after the examination, the patients completed a questionnaire assessing their pain perception. Psychological distress was assessed with self-administered instruments measuring depression and anxiety. Single photon emission computerized tomographic brain scans were obtained after intravenous injection with 99m technetium hexamethylpropylene amine oxime. The scans were obtained after all discomfort caused by the intravenous canullation had ceased.

Patients with fibromyalgia had significantly more pain at both the diagnostic and control anatomical sites than the healthy subjects ($p <$ 0.001). They also experienced significantly more psychological distress, as evidenced by much higher scores on the scales assessing depression and anxiety ($p < 0.001$). A substantial majority of the patients (80 percent) had scores indicating moderate or severe depression, and half of the patients had scores suggesting clinically significant anxiety. In contrast, only one control subject was classified as psychiatrically impaired. The measured and self-perceived severity of pain and the pain threshold did not correlate with the severity of psychological distress, age, or educational level.

The regional blood flow was significantly decreased in the four regions of interest studied. The most marked difference involved the right thalamus ($p < 0.003$), followed by the left thalamus ($p < 0.01$), the left caudate ($p < 0.01$), and the right caudate ($p < 0.02$). The blood flow to the thalami of fibromyalgia patients was 16 to 20 percent lower than in the control group. The difference in the perfusion of the caudate nuclei amounted to 12 to 14 percent. Further analyses indicated an 8 percent reduction in the total cortex perfusion of fibromyalgia patients. The reduction was evenly distributed in the anterior, lateral, and posterior regions of the cortex. The decrease in perfusion did not correlate with age or with the levels of anxiety and depression.

The third investigation of the regional cerebral blood flow in fibromyalgia was carried out by researchers from the University of Adelaide, Australia (Kwiatek et al., 2000). The clinical sample comprised 17 women diagnosed with fibromyalgia by community-based rheumatologists. A control group of healthy women was recruited through newspaper advertisements. All participants were examined by one of the authors to confirm the diagnosis and establish the absence of any other physical illness. The 18 anatomical sites recommended by the American College of Rheumatology for the detection of fibromyalgic tender points (Wolfe et al., 1990) and 18 control sites (e.g., middeltoid, thumbnail, and midtibia) were manually assessed by a rheumatologist on two separate occasions. The examiner was blinded to the group status of the subjects. The 14 fibromyalgia patients who were treated with antidepressants, benzodiazepines, or narcotic analgesics were asked to discontinue the use of these medications for at least four days prior to scanning.

Single photon emission computed tomography was performed on all participants after intravenous injection with 500 MBq of 99m Tc-hexamethylpropyleneamine oxime. The images were matched with magnetic resonance scans to within 1.2 mm. Data were examined independently by three investigators and the average of their regional blood flow estimates used for final statistical processing. Other measurements were performed with self-administered instruments assessing the impact of illness and the severity of pain, depression, and anxiety.

Patients with fibromyalgia and healthy control subjects were similar with regard to age and level of education. As expected, the clinical sample had significantly more lethargy, pain, stiffness, sleep disturbance, depression, and anxiety than the healthy control group ($p < 0.001$ for all comparisons). The tender point scores were also significantly higher in the fibromyalgia group and remained statistically constant on the second examination.

Single photon emission scans showed significant reduction in the regional blood flow of patients with fibromyalgia. The area most affected extended from the upper right lentiform nucleus to the left putamen and included the upper thalami. Other sites included the right internal capsule, the pontine tegmentum, and the cerebellar peduncles. The caudate and the lentiform nuclei were not significantly affected. A quantitative analysis of the blood flow indicated significant reductions only for the pontine tegmentum (12 percent) and right thalamus (8 percent). These changes did not correlate with any of the clinical and psychometric variables. Specifically, the regional blood flow reductions were not statistically related to the number of tender points or to treatment with antidepressant drugs. With the available data, the authors "were unable to generate a discriminant equation that reliably separated the conditions of fibromyalgia and health on the basis of regional cerebral blood flow" (Kwiatek et al., 2000, p. 2830).

MAGNETIC RESONANCE IMAGING AND PREMENSTRUAL BRAIN VOLUME

For the only neuroimaging study of premenstrual abnormalities (Grant et al., 1988), researchers from Southern General Hospital,

Glasgow, Scotland, recruited 20 menstruating women and compared their cranial cerebrospinal fluid volume with that of a control group comprising ten postmenopausal women and ten men. All participants were asymptomatic and had normal findings on neurological examination. Magnetic resonance images were obtained midcycle and premenstrually in the study group and two weeks apart in the control group.

The total cranial cerebrospinal volumes averaged 107 mL in the menstruating group, 120 mL in the postmenopausal control group, and 134 in the male control group. The volume increased during the luteal phase by an average of 12 mL or 11 percent. The second examination of the control group indicated a small increase (5 mL/subject) in the postmenopausal group and a nominal decrease (2 mL/subject) in the male group. The data were interpreted to indicate that the brain does not swell during the premenstrual phase, and that premenstrual symptoms are unlikely to be produced by brain edema. The validity of the findings is severely limited by the fact that none of the menstruating women had active symptoms of late luteal phase dysphoric disorder.

FUNCTIONAL MAGNETIC RESONANCE IN IRRITABLE BOWEL SYNDROME

Functional magnetic resonance imaging was used by investigators from Vanderbilt University, Nashville, Tennessee, to study central nervous system changes during painful stimulation in patients with irritable bowel syndrome (Mertz et al., 2000). The technique measured the ratio of oxyhemoglobin to deoxyhemoglobin, which was considered a marker for the local blood flow and metabolic activity. The activated area produced a magnetic resonance signal of higher intensity and allowed the precise definition of the activated anatomical site. The subjects recruited for the study included 16 patients with irritable bowel syndrome (14 women and two men with a mean age of 33 years) and 18 age- and gender-matched healthy individuals. The control subjects were free of abdominal pain and other complaints attributable to the gastrointestinal tract. Organic disease was ruled out in all participants by history and physical examination, comprehensive laboratory testing, and sigmoidoscopy or other endoscopic procedures.

Blood oxygen level-dependent imaging was performed with a 1.5 Tesla magnetic resonance unit as the patients underwent rectal distention with a barostat pump. A plastic bag was advanced into the subjects' rectal vault and inflated to pressures of 15 mm Hg, 30 mm Hg, and 55 mm Hg. The levels were selected to induce sensation of gas, stool, and pain, respectively. At each level of pressure the distention was maintained constant for 40 seconds, and each set contained four repetitions. The participants rated the intensity of pain after each set.

The analysis of the functional magnetic resonance data concentrated on three regions of interest: the anterior cingulate cortex, the prefrontal cortex, the thalamus, and the insular cortex. An experienced neuroradiologist who was kept unaware of the participants' group distribution identified these areas on the high-resolution anatomical images. The intensity of the activated voxels was averaged for these areas for each rectal pressure level.

Compared with data obtained in the healthy control group, the severity of pain and the expanse of the painful abdominal surface produced by a 55-mm Hg rectal distention were significantly higher in the irritable bowel syndrome group. Rectal distention produced significant activation of the four brain regions of interest in both groups. In patients with irritable bowel syndrome, but not in the control subjects, the 55-mm Hg (i.e., painful) rectal distention produced greater regional cerebral activation in the anterior cingulate cortex and thalamus than a 30-mm Hg distention. The phenomenon remained constant throughout the series of four distensions at 55 mm Hg, suggesting lack of sensitization or anticipatory response to pain. In the irritable bowel group, the subjective rating of pain severity did not correlate with the degree of cerebral activation. In contrast, the activation of the anterior cingulate cortex correlated significantly with the pain perceptions of the healthy control subjects.

The authors' interpretation of the data was based on their understanding of the functional differences in the pain-processing centers of the human brain. They believed that the thalamus is a relay station in the connection between the gastrointestinal tract and cortical centers; that the insular cortex is the processing area for all visceral inputs; and that the prefrontal cortex has the executive function with regard to pain perception. The anterior cingulate cortex was thought to integrate or produce the emotional response to visceral stimuli. The findings did not clarify "whether the anterior cingulate cortex itself is abnormally responsive [in irritable bowel syndrome], or merely responding appropriately to heightened visceral afferent signals" (Mertz et al., 2000, p. 846) and "did not rule out psychological causes of increased pain sensitivity" (p. 847). The lack of coupling between subjective assessment of pain and the degree of brain activation was interpreted as the result of cognitive and emotional factors.

MAGNETIC RESONANCE AND SINGLE PHOTON EMISSION TOMOGRAPHY IN GULF WAR SYNDROME

Investigators from the University of Texas Southwestern Medical Center at Dallas, Texas, conducted a carefully controlled evaluation of neurological function in ill Gulf War veterans (Haley, Hom, et al., 1997). The patient group ($N = 23$) was selected from a cohort of 249 veterans who had participated in a study that had identified three strongly clustered groups of symptoms (Haley, Kurt, et al., 1997). The 23 veterans recruited for the current nested case-control study were the highest scorers in the clusters named confusion-ataxia (13 patients), impaired cognition (five patients) and arthro-myo-neuropathy (five patients). A healthy control group included ten deployed and ten nondeployed veterans. Magnetic resonance imaging of the entire brain was performed with a 1.5 Tesla device before and after the administration of gadolinium. Single photon emission images were obtained 90 minutes after the intravenous infusion of the standard technetium 99m-labeled oxime. One control subject did not complete the neuroradiological evaluation. A panel of three experts who were kept unaware of the cases' group status interpreted all radiological data. Other tests included a clinical neurological evaluation, brain stem auditory potentials, visual evoked potentials, and two measures of neuropsychological function.

Seven ill veterans (30 percent) and five healthy control veterans (26 percent) had small foci of increased signal intensity in the subcortical white matter. None of these abnormalities were enhanced after the administration of gadolinium. The single photon emission images revealed no additional pathological findings. A majority of veterans had neuropsychological and brain stem auditory abnormalities, but the study did not identify an association between these findings and the high-intensity white matter foci. The appropriate conclusion was that "neuroimaging studies, such as MRI and SPECT, do not appear useful in differentiating cases and controls" (Haley, Hom, et al., 1997, p. 229).

CONCLUSION

Nonspecific structural abnormalities are relatively common in patients with chronic fatigue syndrome and Gulf War illness, but do not correlate with the severity of neuropsychiatric symptoms. Regional brain hypoperfusion has been identified in patients with chronic fatigue syndrome, fibromyalgia, and irritable bowel syndrome. The functional neuroimaging defects in the frontal lobe and subcortical structures of patients with chronic fatigue and fibromyalgia correlate poorly with the severity of depressive symptoms, but are often associated with reports of pain and cognitive difficulties.

Chapter 9

Neuropsychological Deficits in Functional Somatic Illness

Poor memory and difficulty with attention and concentration are among the most common symptoms of patients with functional somatic syndromes. In this chapter, we review the neuropsychological research to determine the objective severity of these deficits and their relationship with psychiatric symptoms. The intellectual framework for our analysis is provided by the progress made in the cognitive research on patients with mood disorders. Only a few years ago, attentional deficits in patients with depression were seen as a final common pathway of impaired cognition similar to that observed in schizophrenia or dementias (Mialet et al., 1996). Recent findings have challenged the assumption that the cognitive deficits in depression are a simple epiphenomena of the disorder and have identified specific memory and executive impairment that are independent of age, severity of the clinical syndrome, motivation, and response bias (Austin et al., 2001). These abnormalities have been linked to dysfunction in the prefrontal cortex, considered a key structure for the integration of cognition and emotion in negative mood states (Liotti and Mayberg, 2001). The frontal lobe dysfunction has been specifically designated as the cause of changes in executive functions such as episodic memory, dealing with novelty, selecting strategies, inhibiting incorrect responses, problem solving, and planning (Fossati et al., 2002).

CHRONIC FATIGUE SYNDROME

The influence of depression on the cognitive performance of patients with chronic fatigue syndrome was first assessed in a controlled study performed by researchers from the State University of New York at Stony Brook and the Albert Einstein College of Medicine, New York (Krupp et al., 1994). The chronic fatigue syndrome group comprised 20 patients diagnosed according to a modification of the criteria proposed by Holmes et al. (1988). The diagnosis required the presence of cognitive disturbance and at least five other symptoms. A group of 20 patients with multiple sclerosis complaining of fatigue as one of their most bothersome symptoms and 20 healthy volunteers served as controls. None of the subjects had any other detectable physical cause for fatigue and all had normal results on a comprehensive laboratory evaluation. Five patients from the chronic fatigue syndrome group and one patient with multiple sclerosis carried the diagnosis of major depression or dysthymia. They were retained in the study because the psychiatric disorder was considered secondary to the main diagnosis. A standard depression severity scale (Radloff and Locke, 1986) was used to make sure that none of the participants were overwhelmingly depressed.

The main measurements relied on a battery of neuropsychological tests assessing premorbid verbal ability (Wechsler, 1981; Jastak and Wilkinson, 1984); spatial-constructional skills (Wechsler, 1981); attention and concentration (Golden, 1978; Wechsler, 1981); visuomotor search (Smith, 1973; Wechsler, 1981; Reitan and Wolfson, 1985); ability and flexibility in shifting from one assignment to another (Smith, 1973); abstract reasoning (Adams and Trenton, 1981); verbal and visual memory (Buschke and Fuld, 1974; Benton, 1974; Wechsler, 1987); verbal fluency (Benton and Hamsher, 1983); and motor speed (Reitan and Wolfson, 1985; Bornstein, 1986).

The two patient groups (chronic fatigue syndrome and multiple sclerosis) and the healthy control group were statistically similar with regard to age and educational achievement. The subjective assessments of fatigue were similar for patients with chronic fatigue syndrome and multiple sclerosis. Both had significantly greater levels of fatigue than the healthy control subjects. Direct comparisons of the depressive symptomatology revealed a statistical difference only between chronic fatigue syndrome and healthy control subjects. Mood disorders were diagnosed in eight of the 20 patients (40 percent) with chronic fatigue syndrome. Three patients had a history of major depression, three current major depression, and one each current dysthymia and atypical depression. In the multiple sclerosis group, mood disorders were diagnosed in three of the 18 patients (17 percent).

Chronic fatigue syndrome and multiple sclerosis patients had similar scores on neuropsychological testing. Compared with healthy control subjects, multiple sclerosis patients scored lower on five of the nine specific tasks. In contrast, patients with chronic fatigue syndrome demonstrated abilities similar to those of control subjects for all the tests measuring verbal memory, attention, verbal fluency, and abstract reasoning. The finding was remarkable given that all chronic fatigue syndrome patients complained of difficulty with concentration and memory loss. The data did not support a significant influence of depression on cognitive performance in chronic fatigue syndrome.

Investigators from the University of Minnesota Medical School and Hennepin County Medical Center, Minneapolis, tested the hypothesis that the primary neuropsychological disturbance in chronic fatigue syndrome is a decrease in the speed of cognitive processes (Marshall et al., 1997). Their hypothesis was based on the common observation that patients with this condition complain of deterioration in the working memory, a function that is dependent on the ability to remember a large number of specific information units, and on the efficiency of the cognitive operations. The methodology employed in this exemplary work included a direct comparison of nondepressed chronic fatigue syndrome patients with healthy control subjects and patients with major depression, as well as an evaluation of the effect of cognitive exertion on further performance.

The 20 patients with chronic fatigue syndrome were recruited from among individuals 25 to 50 years of age diagnosed with this condition at the Hennepin County Medical Center after a thorough medical, psychiatric, and psychometric evaluation. All patients met standard diagnostic criteria (Holmes et al., 1988). Prior to enrollment in this study, a psychiatrist unaware of the results of previous psychometric testing interviewed the patients and retained for the study group only those without a psychiatric disorder. The only exception was a patient who had dysthymia and major depression at least six months prior to the start of the study. The 13 women and seven men included in the final study group were matched for age, gender, level of education, and level of intelligence with 20 healthy subjects and 14 patients with mood disorders. The diagnoses given to the patients with mood disorders were major depression in remission (eight patients); current major depression and dysthymia (four patients); current major depression (one patient); and dysthymia (one patient).

The assessments of intelligence were based on the Block Design and Vocabulary subtests of the Wechsler Adult Intelligence Scale (Wechsler, 1987). Each patient completed a six-test battery assessing cognitive function. The first measured long-term retrieval, long-term storage, and delayed recall (Buschke, 1973). The second was a test of sustained selective attention (Cornblatt et al., 1988). The third test was a measure of the paced auditory serial addition task assessing working memory, sustained and divided attention, and cognitive processing speed (Roman et al., 1991). The fourth measure was a test of focused attention and motor and cognitive processing speed (Golden, 1978). The fifth test measured reaction time as indicated by decision and motor speed (Jensen, 1987). The sixth procedure assessed working memory by evaluating the storage of items (words) for further retrieval and processing (Salthouse, 1994). Finally, all participants took the portions of the Scholastic Aptitude Test that measure verbal and reading comprehension, vocabulary, and verbal abstraction (College Entrance Examination Board, 1993) and completed a standard depression inventory (Beck et al., 1961).

Patients with chronic fatigue syndrome and affective disorders had statistically similar results on tests of working memory, sustained selective attention, short-term and recent verbal memory, and cognitive processing. Chronic fatigue syndrome patients performed similarly to healthy control subjects on short-term and recent verbal memory and sustained selective attention, but had poorer results on most tests of cognitive processing. As a general rule, the performance of chronic fatigue syndrome patients was about one standard deviation below that of healthy control subjects. Eight of the 20 chronic fatigue patients and their matched control subjects exercised on a treadmill (30 minutes at a speed of 2 miles/hour) immediately after the first afternoon of testing. There was no decline in performance on the second day of testing. The combined cognitive and physical exertion did not significantly change the scores obtained the following day.

Most of the differences between chronic fatigue syndrome patients and healthy control subjects were covariates of the difference in the depressive symptomatology reported by the two groups. The only measure among the intergroup comparisons not subject to change according to the severity of depressive symptomatology was decision and motor speed. However, comparisons of chronic fatigue patients with only mild depressive symptoms and those with moderate or severe symptoms did not reach statistical significance. The investigators underlined the fact that the psychomotor retardation of patients with chronic fatigue syndrome may be explained by reactive depression rather than a specific mood disorder, but no test data were offered to support this distinction. They also raised the issue of low effort, but discarded it as an explanation of the relatively slow cognitive speed. This judgment appears questionable given the fact that the patients with chronic fatigue syndrome performed poorly on tests requiring little effort, but not on more difficult learning trials.

The impact of poor effort on the cognitive performance of patients with chronic fatigue syndrome was the focus of a controlled investigation carried out at the University Hospital Nijmegen, Nijmegen, the Netherlands (Van der Werf et al., 2000). The authors started from the position that "the behavior of a small proportion of CFS patients was indicative of psychological distress or poor motivation" (p. 199) and decided to study the response to a test able to detect fictitious memory impairment (Schagen et al., 1997). The patient cohort comprised 144 individuals diagnosed with chronic fatigue syndrome according to standard criteria (Fukuda et al., 1994). Sixty-seven patients from this cohort were matched for gender, age, and level of education with a control group of 40 patients diagnosed with definite multiple sclerosis (Poser et al., 1983).

The instrument used to assess short-term memory was a forced-choice verbal recognition task. The 30 items presented were from common semantic categories (e.g., countries). After a distracting simple numerical task, the subjects were given listings of words from the same categories and asked to recognize the three out of each five words per item that had already been presented in the initial phase. The normative standard allowed for only four mistakes in the recognition of the 90 words. Cognitive deterioration was measured with the Dutch version of the Symbol Digit Test of the Wechsler Adult Intelligence Scale (Stinissen et al., 1970) and the results appropriately corrected for age, gender, and level of education. Finally, a standard test was used to measure the severity of current depressive symptomatology (Beck et al., 1961). As most results on the short-term memory test were close to the normal range, the analysis of data employed nonparametric methods.

Twenty of the 67 chronic fatigue syndrome patients (30 percent) scored below the norm on the short-term memory test. In contrast, only five of the 40 patients with multiple sclerosis (13 percent) did so; the difference was statistically significant. On the test of cognitive deterioration, the two groups had similar performance (16 percent versus 18 percent with subnormal results). However, it is important to note that 13 percent of patients with chronic fatigue syndrome scored abnormally low on the easy short-term memory test, but had normal results on the substantially more difficult test of cognitive performance. None of the multiple sclerosis patients showed this testing pattern, a difference that was again statistically significant. Severe or moderately severe depressive symptoms were reported by 25 percent of the chronic fatigue syndrome group, but by only 3 percent of the group of patients with multiple sclerosis. The severity of depressive symptomatology did not correlate with the results of the tests of short-term memory or cognitive deterioration in either of the two groups. The authors interpreted their findings to indicate that some patients with chronic fatigue syndrome put less effort into solving an easy task for fear of having their illness ignored. The motivational basis of these findings was inferred from data demonstrating that patients with known cognitive deficits after closed-head injuries scored within the normal range on this test of short-term memory, while postwhiplash patients involved in litigation had poor performance on this test despite normal cognitive function (Schmand et al., 1998).

The cognitive difficulties reported by patients with chronic fatigue syndrome were also studied by investigators from the National Jewish Medical and Research Center, who hypothesized that the discrepancy might be related to an enhanced tendency to respond to suggestions (DiClementi et al., 2001). The authors postulated that a more suggestible individual is likely to engage in selective processing of suggestions that conform with their physical explanation of illness and pay less attention to reality-based stimuli. The study cohort included 21 patients (18 women and three men; mean age 40 years) diagnosed with chronic fatigue syndrome after a careful examination and structured psychiatric interview. The patients selected for the study had no past or current psychiatric disorder. A control group (17 women and four men; mean age 33 years) with no physical or psychiatric illness was recruited from among the medical center's nursing and research staff. The groups were similar with regard to ethnic background and educational level.

The experimental procedure comprised suggestibility tasks, tests of cognitive functioning, and a global assessment of psychological symptoms. The main measure of suggestibility required listening to a neutral story and then answering questions purportedly assessing recall (Loftus et al., 1989). In actuality, the questionnaire provided eight items of false information about the story. A forced choice recall test was administered at a later time to determine the amount of false information incorporated by the subjects in their rendition of the story. Half of the false information items were health related. Misinformation scores were calculated separately for health and non-health-related items. A second measure of suggestibility was the ease of induction and stability of a hypnotic experience leading to perception of floating and arm levitation (Spiegel and Spiegel, 1978). Cognitive functioning was assessed with the Stroop Neuropsychological Screening Test (Trenerry et al., 1989) and the Logical Memory Subtest of the Wechsler Memory Scale (Wechsler, 1987). Finally, the Brief Symptom Inventory (Derogatis and Melisaratos, 1983) was used as a global measure of emotional distress.

The hypnotic induction profile indicated significantly greater suggestibility in the chronic fatigue syndrome group ($p < 0.001$). This group also performed less well on the measure of automatic processing ($p < 0.05$). The suggestibility and automatic processing scores were negatively correlated ($p < 0.05$). The groups were similar with regard to premorbid intellectual functioning, logical memory, and processing of misinformation. Suggestibility correlated positively with the number of errors produced by the misinformation task and with number and severity of psychological symptoms ($p < 0.01$). The data were considered to indicate that patients with chronic fatigue syndrome "have relative difficulty attending to relevant, if peripheral information" and that this anomaly could "be subjectively experienced as memory or cognitive deficits" (DiClementi et al., 2001, p. 684).

Investigators from the University Medical Center Nijmegen, Nijmegen, the Netherlands, made another contribution to the understanding of the cognitive deficits in chronic fatigue syndrome (Van der Werf et al., 2002). The authors hypothesized that cognitive complaints, information processing speed, and motor speed are correlated with body consciousness and somatic symptoms. Data were collected from 57 patients with chronic fatigue syndrome (44 females and 14 males; mean age 35 years; mean duration of illness two years). Body consciousness was assessed with a five-item questionnaire (e.g., "I am sensitive to internal bodily tensions," "I am very aware of changes in my body temperature," and "I can often feel my heart beating"). Somatic symptoms were recorded with a somatization subscale of a known symptom checklist (Derogatis, 1992). Neuropsychological testing of motor and mental speed relied on the completion of reaction time tasks. Additional data were obtained with instruments assessing self-reported problems with memory and concentration.

Thirteen of the 57 patients had evidence of malingering. The data generated by the remaining 44 subjects were analyzed with structural equation modeling techniques, which assumed the information processing speed to be inversely correlated with body consciousness and somatic symptoms.

Body consciousness ($p < 0.01$) and the somatic burden of illness ($p < 0.04$) influenced the information processing speed in this sample of patients with chronic fatigue syndrome. The motor speed did not correlate with body consciousness, but showed a direct relation to somatic symptoms. Overall, the model explained 46 percent of the variance in information processing speed and 27 percent of the variance in motor speed. Self-reported memory and concentration problems correlated strongly with the somatic burden of illness, but not with body consciousness. The findings led the authors to suggest that "instead of labeling slowing of information processing [as] a direct result of cerebral impairment or deficit, it could also be interpreted as a consequence of affective processing of symptoms or a too strong attention for bodily sensations" (Van der Werf et al., 2002, p. 7).

GULF WAR ILLNESS

The first attempt to correlate neuropsychological performance with somatic complaints, environmental exposure, and clinical findings in veterans with Gulf War illness was carried out by investigators affiliated with the Veterans Administration Medical Centers in Detroit, Michigan, and San Diego, California, and with the Behavioral

Healthcare Group in Southfield, Michigan (Sillanpaa et al., 1997). The 48 participants were recruited from among an 82-member Army Reserve Military Police unit. The group's age, gender, level of education, and premorbid level of intelligence were similar to those of the 33 veterans who chose not to participate in this research.

The study was carried out two years after the end of the conflict. The subjective complaints were collected with the somatization component of the Hopkins Symptom Checklist (Derogatis, 1992). A comprehensive questionnaire assessed exposure to a large variety of potential hazards, including shell explosions, oil fire smoke, sandfly bites, inadequately refrigerated foods, unpurified water, prisoners, and corpses. A composite index of objective abnormalities was constructed based on the presence of rash, lymphadenopathy, and evidence of viral or fungal infection as well as the monocyte count and the blood levels of aspartate amine transferase and alanine amino transferase. All participants were tested with a comprehensive battery of neuropsychological tests measuring sustained attention, motor coordination, executive function, memory, and general cognitive functioning. Additional information regarding levels of depression and anxiety were also collected. Data were analyzed by logistic regression to determine whether cognitive ability correlated with emotional functioning or with the demographic, exposure, and clinical characteristics of the sample.

The model, which included age, education, level of potentially noxious exposure, and the clinical signs index failed to predict neurocognitive functioning. Subjective complaints correlated strongly with anxiety and depression. The psychological distress predicted poorer performance in the domains of general cognitive functioning, executive functioning, sustained attention, and motor coordination. A backward elimination procedure indicated the unique specificity of depression as a predictor of impaired executive functioning and motor coordination. The anxiety trait had unique specificity as a predictor of decreased ability to sustain attention.

The cognitive functioning of patients with Gulf War syndrome was also studied by investigators from the Center for Environmental Hazards Research, Department of Veterans Affairs, New Jersey Health Care System, East Orange, and New Jersey Medical School, Newark (Lange et al., 2001). The authors focused their research on 48 individuals whose postwar illness also fulfilled the definition of chronic fatigue syndrome (Fukuda et al., 1994) or multiple chemical sensitivity (Fiedler et al., 1996). These syndromes are characterized by self-reported decreases in physical endurance and cognitive ability. Inclusion criteria required that the participants be younger than 57 years of age; have no history of mania, schizophrenia, or eating disorder; deny alcohol abuse or dependence during the two years prior to the study; and have no history of prolonged loss of consciousness. Twenty-seven of the 49 subjects met diagnostic criteria for chronic fatigue syndrome, four were diagnosed with multiple chemical sensitivity, and 17 had both conditions. The control group comprised 39 healthy Gulf War veterans. The groups were similar with regard to age, gender, and proportion of nonwhites.

Main measurements relied on a battery of neuropsychological tests administered by trained master-level psychologists who were unaware of the subjects' clinical status. The battery included 15 tests assessing attention, information processing, and concentration; abstraction and conceptualization; visual and verbal memory; visual-perceptual and perceptual motor function; and fine motor function. All participants were also administered a computerized structured psychiatric interview (Marcus et al., 1990) and a detailed questionnaire assessing drug and alcohol use (Bates and Tracy, 1990).

The lifetime psychiatric morbidity of veterans with symptoms of Gulf War syndrome was significantly more severe than that of their healthy comrades, as reflected by the fact that 32 of the 48 members (75 percent) of the study group, but only 5 of the 39 control subjects (13 percent) met criteria for a postwar psychiatric diagnosis. The most common psychiatric diagnoses in the two groups were major depressive disorder (42 versus 3 percent, $p < 0.001$), anxiety disorders (29 versus 5 percent, $p < 0.005$), and post-traumatic stress disorder (21 versus 3 percent, $p < 0.02$). The prevalence of past alcohol abuse or dependence was similar for the two groups of Gulf War veterans (12 versus 8 percent).

The estimated premorbid intellectual quotient was essentially identical in the two groups. Veterans with Gulf War syndrome and those from the control group also had similar cognitive abilities with respect to visual and verbal memory, visual-perceptual and perceptual-motor function, and fine motor function. However, the ill veterans demonstrated significantly lower ability in three of five tests of attention, concentration, and information processing and in one of two tests of abstraction and conceptualization. The cognitive functions most affected were the simple and complex reaction time and the complex working memory tasks. The presence of postwar major depressive disorder was a significant predictor of slower simple and complex reaction time. Postwar anxiety disorders were significant predictors of impaired ability to perform complex working memory tasks. The diagnosis of post-traumatic stress disorder was not a predictor for impairment in these two domains. The authors concluded that while a role of environmental exposure in the etiology of Gulf War illness cannot be excluded, "evidence is strong that Gulf War illness symptoms, including fatigue and cognitive difficulties may be due to emotional distress experienced as consequence of war" (Lange et al., 2001, p. 247).

A comprehensive study of the neuropsychological function of Gulf War veterans and its relationship to psychiatric morbidity was conducted by investigators from the Boston Environmental Hazards Center, Veterans Administration Boston Healthcare System, in collaboration with faculty members from Boston University, Tulane University in New Orleans, Louisiana, and University of Southern Denmark, Odense, Denmark (White et al., 2001). The Gulf War veterans who participated in the study were U.S. Army and National Guard personnel based at Fort Devens, Massachusetts ($N = 142$) and U.S. Army, Navy, Marine, and Air Force personnel deployed from New Orleans, Louisiana ($N = 51$). At both locations, the participants were recruited according to a stratified randomized procedure from among the veterans who completed a survey of physical and psychological well-being carried out two years after their return from the Persian Gulf area. The control group ($N = 47$) was chosen from among a National Guard air ambulance company deployed from Maine to Germany during the conflict. These troops' main activities consisted of providing assistance to transport and evacuation missions undertaken by German civilian authorities. The Gulf-deployed and Germany-deployed groups were similar with respect to gender distribution, educational level, prior history of occupational exposure to neurotoxicants, and history of alcohol problems. The Gulf-deployed veterans were older and less likely to have served in Vietnam than the cohort deployed to Germany.

The main measurements relied on the administration of a comprehensive battery of neuropsychological tests and a structured psychiatric interview. The battery employed 15 standard procedures similar to those used by Lange et al. (2001), including one test of general intelligence; six tests of attention and executive function; one test of visuospatial processing; three tests of verbal and visual memory; two tests of motor function; one test of motivation; and one test assessing the mood state. The psychiatric evaluation focused on the diagnosis of major depression and post-traumatic stress syndrome. In addition, the subjects completed questionnaires assessing the self-perceived exposure to environmental toxins and combat experiences, including specific items such as being placed on alert for chemical or biological weapon attack, being exposed to pesticides and smoke from burning oil wells, and taking anti-nerve gas drugs.

The diagnosis of current depression was made in 5 percent of the Gulf-deployed veterans. In the same cohort, 2.6 percent of subjects were diagnosed with post-traumatic stress disorder. None of the Germany-deployed veterans met criteria for these diagnoses, but the differences did not reach statistical significance. However, the groups differed substantially with regard to mood states, as evidenced by the fact that the Gulf-deployed veterans had significantly higher scores ($p < 0.003$) for depression, fatigue, tension, anger, and confusion. The results of neuropsychological testing of cognition were statistically similar in the two groups of veterans. The veterans who reported perceived exposure to neurotoxicants displayed more tension and confusion, as well as subtle memory and attention deficits. The same subgroup of veterans had higher scores on tests of malingering, a finding interpreted by authors to raise "the question of whether malingering or motivation to perform well contributed to findings on the tests" (White et al., 2001, p. 48). Although a primary gain might have been inferred from the fact that the proportion of veterans seeking disability rating or an upgrade in a previously established level of disability was significantly higher in the Gulf-deployed group (17 versus 4 percent, $p < 0.006$), the analyses of the data set did not support the presence of a conscious effort to fake the test results.

Another in the series of studies addressing the neurobehavioral deficits of Persian Gulf veterans was carried out by investigators from the Portland Veterans Administration Medical Center and the Oregon Health Sciences University at the Portland Environmental Hazards Research Center in Portland, Oregon (Storzbach et al., 2001). The authors obtained the list of all veterans from the states of

Oregon and Washington who had been deployed to the Persian Gulf during the year starting August 1, 1991, and mailed a questionnaire to a randomly selected sample of 1,934 individuals listed. The questionnaire assessed the presence of symptoms consistent with Gulf War illness and exclusionary diagnoses (e.g., epilepsy, malignancy, schizophrenia, malaria, diabetes, and hepatitis). The authors identified 517 potential cases and 213 potential controls and invited them to report for a clinical and laboratory evaluation. After the evaluation, a multidisciplinary clinical committee identified 239 cases and 112 controls who agreed to participate in the study. The groups were similar with regard to gender distribution and mental ability at the time of induction into the military service. Almost all participants (94 percent in each group) were currently employed. The ill veterans were slightly younger (mean age 32 versus 34 years) and had less education (13 versus 14 years in school) than control subjects.

Data were collected with a battery of six neurobehavioral tests and 12 psychological tests developed and validated by some of the authors of the current report (Anger, 1990; Kovera et al., 1996). The neurobehavioral tests provided objective information regarding response speed, memory, concentration, and complex cognitive processing. The results on one of the tests of motivation, attention, and memory, the Oregon Dual Task Procedure (Binder et al., 2001), was used to select a subgroup of outliers with very poor performance. The psychological questionnaires assessed the presence and severity of symptoms of anxiety, depression, post-traumatic stress syndrome, substance abuse, and abnormal personality traits.

As a group, veterans diagnosed as cases of Gulf War illness performed poorly on all neurobehavioral tests and appeared more distressed on psychological testing than the control subjects. A total of 30 participants (27 cases and three control subjects) were identified as statistical outliers on the Oregon Dual Task Procedure. These individuals had significantly lower mental aptitude scores prior to the Gulf War. About three-quarters of them (73 percent) had sought medical care during their service in the Gulf, as compared with 54 percent of the other cases and 28 percent of the control subjects.

The data were analyzed separately for the outlying subgroup, the other cases, and the control group. This procedure enabled the investigators to demonstrate that the neurobehavioral performance of ill Gulf War veterans was similar to that of control subjects when the subgroup of outliers was excluded. A principal component analysis strengthened the conclusion that the neurobehavioral performance of cases of Gulf War illness had a bimodal distribution. In contrast, the level of psychological distress remained higher among cases even after the exclusion of the outlying group. Objective evidence to suspect poor motivation was found in only two participants. The findings indicated that a substantial majority (895) of veterans with Gulf War illness suffer from significantly more psychological distress than other Gulf-deployed veterans, but have no evidence of objective functional cognitive impairment.

In summary, the neuropsychological evaluation of patients with chronic fatigue syndrome and Gulf War illness provides contradictory evidence regarding the role of psychopathology in the genesis and maintenance of cognitive deficits. An emerging common denominator for difficulties with memory, attention, and concentration appears to be somatic burden of illness, which in turn correlates with depression and anxiety.

Chapter 10

The Hypothalamic-Pituitary-Adrenal Axis in Functional Somatic Illness

Activation of the hypothalamic-pituitary-adrenal axis has been linked with depressive illnesses and chronic pain as part of a stress response that produces loss of affective and cognitive flexibility, anxiety, activation of the autonomic nervous system, sleep disturbance, and diminished sexual interest (Blackburn-Munro and Blackburn-Munro, 2001; Gold and Chrousos, 2002). However, the pattern of response is variable. The classical manifestations of melancholic depression such as restlessness, insomnia, loss of appetite, and morning worsening of dysphoria are associated with an activation of the corticotropin-releasing hormone system. In contrast, patients with atypical depression present with fatigue, hypersomnia, hyperphagia, and increased responsiveness to environment and have a deficiency of corticotropin-releasing hormone and a downregulated hypothalamic-pituitary-adrenal axis (Gold and Chrousos, 2002). Other factors influencing the axis's response in mental illness include age, gender, and psychiatric family history (Birmaher and Heydl, 2001). The axis has been extensively explored in functional somatic syndromes, and the output of this work has been summarized here in an attempt to detect whether these illnesses show consistent hormonal abnormalities and whether these abnormalities suggest similarities with typical or atypical presentations of psychiatric disorders.

HYPOTHALAMIC-PITUITARY-ADRENAL AXIS DYSFUNCTION IN CHRONIC FATIGUE SYNDROME

The first study of the functional integrity of the hypothalamic-pituitary-adrenal axis in patients with chronic fatigue syndrome was carried out by a group of experienced investigators from the National Institute of Mental Health and the National Institute of Allergy and Infectious Diseases, Bethesda, Maryland (Demitrack et al., 1991). The authors used a research protocol that successively measured the basal function of the axis, the adrenal response to direct and indirect stimulation, and the activity of the pituitary corticotrophic cells.

The patient group comprised 30 subjects (18 women and 12 men) with a mean age of 37 years and an average duration of illness of seven years. Eighteen of the 30 patients were unemployed and considered themselves disabled by their condition. The participants were recruited from among a cohort of 127 patients diagnosed with chronic fatigue syndrome (Holmes et al., 1988) at the National Institutes of Health. The selection of subjects was based on willingness and ability to participate. All patients had a comprehensive medical evaluation, an extensive battery of laboratory tests, a structured psychiatric interview, and psychometric testing. Twelve patients had suffered at least one episode of major depression, seven patients had a lifetime history of anxiety disorder, and three patients were given the diagnosis of somatization disorder. Overall, 16 of the 30 patients had a lifetime history of at least one psychiatric disorder. In ten of these 16 subjects, the mental illness preceded the onset of chronic fatigue syndrome. The healthy control group comprised 72 subjects (43 women and 29 men) matched for age with the patient group. All participants abstained from tobacco and alcohol and were medication free for the two weeks prior to the hormonal assays. The number of subjects participating in the three components of the study ranged from 45 (19 patients and 26 control subjects) who agreed to lumbar puncture to 122 (12 patients and 110 healthy volunteers) who had infusion studies with adrenocorticotropin hormone. The assays included plasma cortisol, cortisol-binding globulin, and adrenocorticotropin hormone levels; 24-hour urinary free cortisol; response to synthetic adrenocorticotropin hormone infusion with randomly selected doses ranging from 0.003 to 1 µg/kg; response to ovine corticotropin-releasing hormone infusion (1 µg/kg); and cerebrospinal fluid levels of corticotropin-releasing hormone and adrenocorticotropin hormone. The samples were tested in blinded fashion.

Patients with chronic fatigue syndrome had significantly lower levels of plasma cortisol at baseline than healthy control subjects (89 versus 148 nmol/L, $p < 0.01$). This observation was supported by the finding of a higher concentration of cortisol-binding globulin (490 versus 418 nmol/L, $p < 0.03$) and decreased urinary free cortisol (123 versus 203 nmol/24 hours, $p < 0.001$) in chronic fatigue patients as compared with healthy control subjects. The basal levels of adreno-corticotropin hormone were higher in the patient sample (2.7 versus 1.6 pmol/L, $p < 0.02$). The chronic fatigue syndrome group showed a significant response to low-dose infusions of synthetic adrenocorticotropin hormone, while similar doses failed to elicit a response in the control group. Higher doses of adrenocorticotropin hormone did not stimulate the cortisol production of patients, but did so for the control group.

The administration of ovine corticotropin-releasing hormone produced significantly less adrenocorticotropin hormone in the patient group (net integrated values 128 versus 225 pmol/L, $p < 0.04$). On the other hand, the increase in cortisol levels following the ovine hormone infusion was similar in the two groups. The concentration of corticotropin-releasing hormone in the cerebrospinal fluid was virtually identical in the two groups. The self-assessed severity of fatigue correlated strongly with the severity of depressive symptomatology and the basal plasma level of adrenocorticotropin hormone. The attenuated production of adrenocorticotropin hormone in response to corticotropin-releasing hormone was explained as a hypothalamic deficiency of the latter hormone.

Although the work performed by Demitrack and his colleagues (1991) did not allow a direct comparison between chronic fatigue syndrome and major depression, substantial inferences can be made from data published by investigators from the same laboratory at the National Institute for Mental Health, in Bethesda, Maryland (Gold, Loriaux, et al., 1986). The patient sample comprised 44 patients with major affective disorder. Thirty subjects were depressed at the time of the study; the remaining 16 had recovered from depression. For the control group, the authors recruited 34 healthy subjects. The main measurements were assays for cortisol and adrenocorticotropin hormone after an infusion of ovine corticotropin-releasing hormone ($1\mu g$/kg of body weight).

Depressed patients had significantly higher plasma cortisol levels (i.e., nearly twice those of control subjects), but similar levels of adrenocorticotropin hormone at baseline. Compared with healthy control subjects, currently depressed patients showed marked blunting of the adrenocorticotropin hormone response to the infusion of ovine corticotropin-releasing hormone. Despite the modest adrenocorticotropin response, cortisol levels increased significantly in response to the releasing hormone infusion. Patients who had recovered from depression had normal basal and postinfusion levels of cortisol and adrenocorticotropin hormone. The authors suggested that the findings were best explained by an undefined brain abnormality, at or above the level of the hypothalamus, that leads to increased secretion of corticotropin-releasing hormone. However, evidence for the increased secretion of corticotropin-releasing hormone was not provided. We infer from these data that the only difference between patients currently depressed and those with chronic fatigue syndrome studied by Demitrack et al. (1991) appears to involve the basal cortisol levels, which were elevated in the former group and decreased in the latter.

In this context, it is also important to examine the work conducted at the Clinical Psychobiology Branch, National Institute of Mental Health, on ten patients (five women) with seasonal affective disorder (Joseph-Vanderpool et al., 1991). The authors noted that the condition shares clinical features such as lethargy and hypersomnia with chronic fatigue syndrome. The sample studied was in good physical health and medication free for the month preceding the study. The study was conducted in the winter and the patients had psychometric evidence of moderate depression. A well-matched control group included 13 gender- and age-matched healthy volunteers. The main measurements consisted of the assessment of 24-hour pattern of basal plasma cortisol levels and assays of cortisol and adrenocorticotropin hormone levels after a stimulation test with ovine corticotropin-releasing hormone (100 μg).

Plasma cortisol levels were significantly lower in patients with seasonal affective disorder than in the group of healthy control subjects (47 versus 134 nmol/L, $p < 0.02$). The response to the ovine corticotropin-releasing hormone was significantly blunted in the seasonal affective disorder group. The postinfusion cortisol levels averaged 508 nmol/L in the patient group and 584 nmol/L in the control group ($p < 0.01$), while the mean adrenocorticotropin hormone levels were 4.4 pmol/L and 8.1 pmol/L, respectively ($p < 0.02$). At least with regard to the adrenocorticotropin hormone response, the results indicate again a similarity between patients with seasonal affective disorder and chronic fatigue syndrome. Taken together, the data suggest a common central defect in chronic fatigue syndrome, major depression, and seasonal affective disorder. The difference between these conditions seems to be related to the peripheral level of corticosteroids, which has been the focus of other research reviewed in this section.

The urinary free cortisol excretion of patients with chronic fatigue syndrome was assessed in a carefully controlled study by investigators from St. Bartholomew's Hospital and the Royal London School of Medicine (Scott and Dinan, 1998). The research aimed to evaluate the difference between chronic fatigue syndrome and nonpsychotic depression, a condition known to be associated with increased excretion of cortisol in a substantial majority of patients (Rosenbaum et al., 1983; Kathol et al., 1989; Thase et al., 1996; Maes et al., 1998). The study group comprised 21 patients (14 women) with chronic fatigue syndrome diagnosed according to the accepted standard (Fukuda et al., 1994). Clinical interviews identified major depressive disorders in five subjects. In the depressed control group, the authors enrolled ten patients (six women) with major depressive disorder, melancholic subtype (American Psychiatric Association, 1994). These patients were physically healthy, had normal weight, and had no history of disabling or prolonged tiredness, substance abuse, or personality disorders. A second control group included 15 healthy subjects (nine women) without a significant past medical or psychiatric history. Care was taken to make sure that none of the participants took any drugs known to affect the function of the hypothalamic-pituitary-adrenal axis during the month preceding the study. The only biochemical measurement was free cortisol in the urine, collected over one 24-hour period.

The mean age of patients with chronic fatigue syndrome was 36 years. Patients with depression were older (mean age 43 years) and healthy control subjects younger (mean age 33 years) than the participants with fatigue. The free cortisol excretion averaged 181 nmol/24 hours in the healthy subjects and 116 nmol/24 hours in the depressed group. Patients with major depression and chronic fatigue syndrome excreted an average of 95 nmol/24 hours. The free cortisol excretion of nondepressed chronic fatigue syndrome patients averaged 123 nmol/24 hours, but the difference between subgroups did not reach statistical significance. The severity of depressive symptomatology did not correlate with the cortisol excretion. The authors were appropriately cautious in interpreting their findings and acknowledged the limitations imposed by a single measurement. They were particularly puzzled by the fact that depressed chronic fatigue syndrome patients had the lowest average cortisol excretion and emphasized that symptoms traditionally associated with hypothalamic-pituitary-adrenal hypofunction, such as hyperphagia and hypersomnia, were conspicuously absent in this subgroup.

The confirmation of decreased cortisol production in patients with chronic fatigue syndrome as compared with patients suffering from major depression was attempted in a study assessing salivary cortisol levels (Strickland et al., 1998). Salivary cortisol titers correlate well with serum cortisol levels (Burke et al., 1985). Other research using salivary cortisol measurements had demonstrated increased adrenal secretion in patients with current mood disorders (Goodyer et al., 1996) and past history of major depression (Young et al., 2000).

The chronic fatigue syndrome group comprised 14 female patients diagnosed according to British criteria (Sharpe et al., 1991). Ten of the 14 chronic fatigue syndrome patients were diagnosed to be in the midst of a depressive episode. Twenty-six female subjects with a diagnosis of current depressive disorder and 131 healthy women were enrolled as controls. The subjects were free of any significant physical disorder and were not taking any medications. Saliva samples were collected at home at 11 a.m. and 9 p.m. for two consecutive days. In premenopausal women, the samples were collected during the follicular phase of their menstrual cycle.

The evening salivary cortisol levels averaged 1.5 nmol/L in the healthy control and depressed group and 1.0 nmol/L in the chronic fatigue syndrome group ($p < 0.02$). The morning cortisol values were 7.0 nmol/L among healthy control subjects, 6.0 nmol/L in the depressed group, and 5.8 nmol/L in the chronic fatigue syndrome group. The differences were not significant. However, the authors pointed out that the chronic fatigue syndrome patients with and without depression had substantially different median morning salivary cortisol levels (3.3 versus 6.3, $p < 0.001$). Sleep disturbance, physical fitness, and social and occupational impairment did not correlate with the morning cortisol levels in this sample of patients with chronic fatigue syndrome. Although the authors believed that the findings indicate a meaningful difference between patients with chronic fatigue syndrome and healthy or severely depressed individuals, the report is problematic given the large disparity in the size of the samples, and the subsequent statistical amplification of observed differences.

In contrast to data obtained in studies of urinary and salivary cortisol measurements stand findings that have relied on plasma levels (Scott, Salahuddin, et al., 1999). The principal investigators were based at the Royal College of Surgeons and Trinity College Medical School, Dublin, Ireland. The study group comprised 15 chronic fatigue syndrome patients (eight women and seven men, average age 41 years) who met standard diagnostic criteria (Fukuda et al., 1994) and had no current psychiatric disorders. They were compared with 15 gender-matched patients with major depression (American Psychiatric Association, 1987) who were otherwise healthy. A second control group included 11 age-matched nonobese subjects (five women and six men, average age 36 years) without a history of prolonged fatigue or mental illness. None of the participants had a personality disorder. All subjects were free of any medications known to influence the function of the hypothalamic-pituitary-adrenal axis for at least four weeks prior to the study.

Blinded radioimmunoassays for cortisol, adrenal androgens (dehydroepiandrosterone and dehydroepiandrosterone sulfate), and hydroprogesterone were performed on plasma specimens obtained between noon and 2 p.m. A direct correlation was established between age and cortisol level only in the depressed group. The mean plasma cortisol levels were 10.4 µg/dL in the chronic fatigue syndrome group, 14.5 µg/dL in the depressed group, and 13.6 µg/dL in the healthy control subjects. The difference did not reach statistical significance. The mean dehydroepiandrosterone level in the chronic fatigue syndrome group (6 ng/mL) was significantly lower than that observed among depressed patients (10 ng/mL) and healthy control subjects (11 ng/mL). For the sulfated metabolite of this hormone, the values were similar for the chronic fatigue and depressed groups (137 versus 150 µg/dL). These values were significantly lower than the average (258 µg/dL) recorded for the healthy control group. The severity of depressive symptomatology reported by the participants did not correlate with the levels of any of the hormones measured.

These results were supported by the findings of a study conducted by investigators from Warneford Hospital, Oxford, and Royal Victoria Infirmary, Newcastle upon Tyne, United Kingdom (Young et al., 1998). For their study of salivary and urinary cortisol measurements, the authors selected 22 patients (12 men and ten women) who were diagnosed to have "pure" chronic fatigue syndrome, i.e., fulfilled standard requirements (Fukuda et al., 1994) and had no current psychiatric disorders. Twelve subjects (55 percent) had a history of depressive or anxiety disorders. The patients had suffered the fatigue illness for an average of 2.5 years and were functionally impaired. A control group included 22 healthy subjects who matched the gender, age, and weight of the chronic fatigue syndrome patients. As is customary in this type of study, the participants did not take any medications for one month prior to the study.

Saliva samples were collected at four-hour intervals from 8 a.m. to 8 p.m., and urine was collected during the same 24-hour period. The data were reported as the area under the curve after subtraction of the baseline area. The salivary cortisol values were 138 nmol/L in the chronic fatigue syndrome group and 141 nmol/L in healthy control subjects. The corresponding urinary cortisol levels were 161 pmol/L versus 160 pmol/L. These findings indicate that the basal activity of the hypothalamic-pituitary-adrenal axis was normal in this sample of patients with chronic fatigue syndrome.

Two studies have explored the function of the hypothalamic-pituitary-adrenal axis in chronic fatigue syndrome by assessing its response to vasopressin (Altemus et al., 2001) or desmopressin, its synthetic analogue (Scott, Medbak, et al., 1999). For the first of these studies, investigators from the St. James' Hospital, Trinity College Medical School and Royal College of Surgeons in Dublin, Ireland (Scott, Medbak, et al., 1999) recruited 13 patients (seven females and six males) with chronic fatigue syndrome and no comorbid psychiatric disorder. An age-matched healthy control group comprised nine males and four females. None of the participants were taking medications known to alter the hypothalamic or adrenal function and none had a history of drug or alcohol abuse.

The patients were randomly assigned to receive an intravenous infusion of either desmopressin (10 µg) or ovine corticotropin-releasing hormone (100 µg) or the combination of the two hormones. The subjects who received the combination were first given desmopressin as an intravenous bolus followed two minutes later by the infusion of corticotropin-releasing hormone. Blood samples were drawn at baseline and six times during the two-hour interval following the hormone administration and assayed for cortisol and adrenocorticotropin hormone levels. Statistical analyses processed the baseline levels and the maximum increase from baseline in the concentration of these hormones.

The mean basal cortisol and adrenocorticotropin levels were similar in the patient and control groups. The administration of ovine corticotropin-releasing hormone produced a significant increase in cortisol and adrenocorticotropin hormone in all of the healthy participants. In contrast, the infusion failed to change the cortisol level in five and the adrenocorticotropin hormone level in four of the chronic fatigue syndrome patients ($p < 0.01$). Compared with healthy subjects, the magnitude of the change compared with baseline was significantly lower for both cortisol (158 versus 303 nmol/L, $p < 0.01$) and adrenocorticotropin hormone (29 versus 58 ng/L, $p < 0.005$) in the chronic fatigue syndrome group. The response to the infusion of desmopressin was statistically similar in the two groups. The change in the levels of hormones after the simultaneous administration of desmopressin and corticotropin-releasing hormone was also similar in the chronic fatigue syndrome patient and healthy volunteer groups. The authors noted that the chronic fatigue patients who did not respond to the ovine corticotropin infusion showed significant changes when desmopressin was added to the hormone-releasing stimulus. The basal cortisol level did not correlate with the type and magnitude of response. The data were interpreted as a confirmation of the blunted adrenocorticotropin hormone response to ovine corticotropin-releasing hormone in chronic fatigue syndrome (Demitrack et al., 1991).

A further effort to clarify the mechanism of a postulated hypoactivation of the hypothalamic-pituitary-adrenal axis in chronic fatigue syndrome was made by researchers from Weill Medical College, Cornell University, New York, and National Institutes of Health, Bethesda, Maryland (Altemus et al., 2001). The study investigated the response to vasopressin infusion, an effect known to correlate with the hypothalamic output of corticotropin-releasing hormone. The initial cohort comprised 25 patients (19 women and six men) recruited by the staff of the National Institute of Allergy and Infectious Diseases. Six female patients developed abdominal pain during the vasopressin infusion and were excluded. The 19 patients who completed the experiment had a mean age of 40 years and an average duration of illness of four years. Ten of the 19 patients were disabled by their condition. Structured psychiatric interviews identified current psychiatric disorders in 14 patients. Eleven patients had somatoform pain disorder, two had social phobia, and one patient met criteria for generalized anxiety disorder. The lifetime psychiatric disorders diagnosed among the 19 participants consisted of somatoform pain disorder (13 patients), anxiety disorders other than simple phobia (six patients), and depressive disorders (five patients). Past substance use disorders included nicotine dependence (six patients), alcohol abuse (four patients), and cocaine abuse (one patient). Five patients had to discontinue antidepressant medications two weeks prior to the study. The control group comprised 19 age- and gender-matched healthy volunteers.

The experiment was carried out after an all-night fast. Four blood samples were drawn at 15-minute intervals to establish the baseline concentration of vasopressin, cortisol, and adrenocorticotropin hormone. The procedure continued with an arginine vasopressin (aqueous pitressin) intravenous infusion at a dose of 1 mIU/kg/minute over one hour. Blood was sampled at 15-minute intervals during the infusion and for one hour afterward. Additional data were collected with questionnaires assessing mood states, arousal levels, and functional well-being.

The mean basal cortisol levels were essentially identical in chronic fatigue syndrome patients and healthy control subjects (9 versus 8 μg/dL). There was also no difference between the means of basal adrenocorticotropin hormone levels of the two groups (15 versus 14 pg/mL). The cortisol levels declined steadily during the baseline hour in both groups. Basal and peak vasopressin levels were identical in patients and healthy control subjects at 0.6 pg/mL and 92 pg/mL, respectively.

The change in the levels of adrenocorticotropin after vasopressin suggested a blunted response in patients with chronic fatigue syndrome. However, there were no significant differences in the mean adrenocorticotropin concentrations of the two groups at any single time point. Similar observations were made with regard to changes in cortisol levels after vasopressin infusion. The cortisol response was described as faster in the chronic fatigue syndrome group, but the raw data and the level of significance of the difference were not provided.

The maximal change in the cortisol level was similar in the chronically fatigued and healthy subjects (13 versus 12 µg/dL). None of the hormonal measures correlated with duration of illness, level of activity, severity of fatigue, and depression score. The authors interpreted their data to signify a subtle impairment of the hypothalamic secretion of corticotropin-releasing hormone leading to mild adrenal insufficiency in patients with chronic fatigue syndrome. The authors stressed the fact that their patient sample did not show decreased basal cortisol levels. They felt that the findings suggested that a "failure of adaptive restoration of homeostasis in the hypothalamic-pituitary-adrenal axis may mediate symptom development in chronic fatigue syndrome as well as in patients with chronic mood and anxiety disorders" (Altemus et al., 2001, p. 183) and other conditions characterized by fatigue or anergic depression. However, the authors pointed out that the results could also be attributed to physical deconditioning, as demonstrated by Luger et al. (1987) in work performed at the National Institutes of Health in Bethesda, Maryland. Nonetheless, the connection to psychopathology remains, because Purba et al. (1996) have shown a clear activation of the vasopressin neurons in depression, illustrated by the fact that postmortem examination of the brains of patients with major depression showed 56 percent more vasopressin-expressing neurons than in nondepressed control individuals. The same group has also identified a fourfold increase in the number of corticotropin-releasing hormone-expressing neurons in the hypothalamic paraventricular nucleus of six depressed patients as compared with ten control subjects (Raadsheer et al., 1994).

THE REACTIVITY OF THE HYPOTHALAMIC-PITUITARY-ADRENAL AXIS IN FIBROMYALGIA

The function of the hypothalamic-pituitary-adrenal axis in fibromyalgia has attracted considerable research interest over the last decade. The first study to focus on this issue was the result of a collaboration between clinicians from Rijnstate Hospital, Arnhem, and pharmacologists from the University of Leiden, Leiden, the Netherlands (Griep et al., 1993). The participants were ten outpatients with fibromyalgia and ten healthy and sedentary control subjects who were drug free and without evidence of adrenal insufficiency. The groups were similar with respect to age, body mass, and arterial blood pressure. All subjects underwent three procedures: dexamethasone (1 mg) suppression, a human corticotropin-releasing hormone (100 μg) infusion, and insulin-induced hypoglycemia (0.1 unit of insulin/kg of body weight).

The administration of dexamethasone suppressed the cortisol production to less than 60 nmol/L in all participants. Basal cortisol and adrenocorticotropin hormones were similar in the two groups. The infusion of corticotropin-releasing hormone produced significantly more adrenocorticotropin hormone in the fibromyalgia group. In contrast, the cortisol levels after the infusion were essentially identical in the two groups. The same pattern was observed after insulin-induced hypoglycemia. The authors interpreted the data to indicate "hyperreactivity of hypothalamic CRH [corticotropin-releasing hormone] upon stressful challenges" (Griep et al., 1993, p. 472).

Investigators from the National Institutes of Health studied the hypothalamic-pituitary-adrenal function in 12 female patients with fibromyalgia and age-matched healthy volunteers (Crofford et al., 1994). The duration of illness averaged six years in the fibromyalgia group. Three of the fibromyalgia patients met criteria for major depression. Measurements included assays for free cortisol in 24-hour urine samples and hormonal assays for adrenocorticotropin hormone and cortisol after an infusion of 1 μg/kg of ovine corticotropin-releasing hormone. A total of 14 blood samples were tested; six were obtained during the two hours prior to the infusion and eight during the three hours after the infusion. The researchers also measured the plasma level of arginine vasopressin and neuropeptide Y after postural change from the supine position. These two measurements were chosen because arginine vasopressin stimulates the pituitary release of adrenocorticotropin hormone and because neuropeptide Y is a marker of sympathetic response to stress.

Morning plasma cortisol levels were similar in patients with fibromyalgia and healthy control subjects (276 versus 283 nmol/L). Evening plasma cortisol levels were significantly higher in the patient group (301 versus 138 nmol/L, $p < 0.04$). The 24-hour urinary free cortisol mean was significantly lower in fibromyalgia patients (116 versus 196 nmol, $p < 0.002$). Before the stimulation test with infused ovine corticotropin-releasing hormone, the basal cortisol levels were significantly higher in the fibromyalgia group (222 versus 92 nmol/L,

$p < 0.02$). The postinfusion peak cortisol (694 versus 702 nmol/L) and adrenocorticotropin hormone levels (14 versus 8 pmol/L) were similar in the two groups, but the net change in cortisol was decreased ($p < 0.02$) in subjects with fibromyalgia. The levels of arginine vasopressin were similar at baseline and after postural change in the two groups. The levels of neuropeptide Y were lower in the fibromyalgia group, both at baseline and after postural change. The authors interpreted their data to reflect adrenal hyporesponsivity to adrenocorticotropin hormone and proposed that this state might be explained by a chronic understimulation resulting from deficient or inappropriate brain production of corticotropin-releasing hormone, an effect similar to that described by Demitrack et al. (1991) in chronic fatigue syndrome. The low neuropeptide Y levels were attributed to physical deconditioning or to decreased function of the adrenergic stress response. The findings were also considered similar to those observed in atypical depression, seasonal affective disorder, post-traumatic stress disorder, and nicotine withdrawal.

The baseline activity of the hypothalamic-pituitary axis of patients with fibromyalgia, as reflected by 24-hour urinary cortisol excretion, was examined in a well-controlled study by investigators from the University of Antwerp, Belgium, in collaboration with researchers from Vanderbilt University, Nashville, Tennessee, and University La Sapienza, Rome (Maes et al., 1998). The authors recruited 14 patients (11 women and three men, mean age 51 years) diagnosed with fibromyalgia according to the accepted standard (Wolfe et al., 1990). The subjects had no significant past psychiatric history (i.e., affective disorders, psychosis, alcoholism, or drug abuse); had not taken anti-inflammatory drugs for at least four weeks; and had been off any psychotropic medications for at least one week prior to being studied. For the three control groups, the authors obtained the cooperation of 10 hospitalized patients with major depression, ten subjects with post-traumatic stress disorder, and 17 healthy volunteers. Patients with major depression (seven women and three men, mean age 45 years) met U.S. diagnostic criteria (American Psychiatric Association, 1987), had no significant other lifetime psychiatric disorder, and were taken off all psychotropic drugs one week before they were tested. The ten post-traumatic stress disorder patients (seven women and three men, mean age 51 years) had been the victims of two witnessed events, a flash fire at a hotel and a multiple automobile collision. An unspecified number of these patients had developed a depressive disorder after the traumatic event. The group of healthy subjects included 11 women and six men and had a mean age of 42 years. All participants had normal laboratory tests. Urine samples were tested on the same day, using a single batch of reagents. Other data collected by the authors included the severity of depressive symptomatology, pain, and posttraumatic symptoms.

The 24-hour urine cortisol excretion averaged 8 µg/dL and 118 µg/24 hours in the healthy control group, 9 µg/dL and 158 µg/24 hours in the fibromyalgia group, 41 µg/dL and 591 µg/24 hours in the group of patients with major depression, and 49 µg/dL and 840 µg/24 hours in the post-traumatic stress disorder group. The difference between the fibromyalgia group and the patients with major depression or post-traumatic stress disorder was highly significant ($p = 0.0002$). Age, gender, urine volume, and renal function (i.e., creatinine excretion) did not correlate with the cortisol excretion and diagnostic group. Cortisol excretions greater than 240 µg/24 hours were observed in 80 percent of patients with major depression and post-traumatic stress disorder, but in only one patient (7 percent) with fibromyalgia. The severity of depressive symptomatology did not correlate significantly with the cortisol excretion measured in the fibromyalgia and major depression groups. Among patients with fibromyalgia, the 24-hour urinary cortisol excretion was statistically independent of the duration of illness, number of tender points, and subjective assessments of pain and stiffness.

The function of the hypothalamic-pituitary-adrenal axis was also investigated by a group of Dutch researchers in a controlled study that evaluated the response to corticotropin-releasing hormone in 40 patients with fibromyalgia, 28 patients with chronic noninflammatory back pain, and 14 healthy subjects (Griep et al., 1998). The patients with fibromyalgia (36 women and four men; mean age 43 years) were randomly recruited from a list maintained by a nationwide patients' network. Their diagnosis was confirmed by one of the investigators in accordance with standard criteria (Wolfe et al., 1990). The control subjects with low back discomfort had chronic pain affecting only the area between the lower rib cage and the gluteal folds. Those selected for the study (25 women and three men; mean age 41 years) matched the age and gender distribution of the fibromyalgia group. The duration of the pain syndrome averaged 11 years in the fibromyalgia group and ten years in the low back pain group. The authors also specified that the intensity of pain was similar in these two patient groups. The healthy control group (12 women and two men; mean age 38 years) was selected from among acquaintances of patients with low back pain. They had no complaints of pain or fatigue and did not engage in sustained physical activities. None of the participants had overt evidence of adrenal disease, obesity, hypertension, or abnormal laboratory test results.

The research protocol started with a standard dexamethasone suppression test, which consisted of the administration of 1 mg of dexamethasone at 11 p.m. and the determination of the serum cortisol level ten hours later. This test was followed by adrenal stimulation with intravenous synthetic adrenocorticotropin hormone at a dose of either 0.025 µg or 0.1 µg/kg of body weight. Blood samples were drawn 60 minutes and 90 minutes later for cortisol assays. The third procedure required the intravenous administration of 100 µg of human corticotropin-releasing hormone followed by the determination of blood levels of adrenocorticotropin hormone and cortisol six times during the three hours after infusion. All participants had cortisol excretion assayed in urine collected over a 24-hour period.

The 24-hour urinary cortisol levels were similar in the fibromyalgia and low back pain groups (192 versus 185 nmol/24 hr). These values were significantly lower than the mean cortisol excretion of 254 nmol/24 hr recorded for healthy sedentary subjects. The basal plasma cortisol levels were also similar in the two patient groups (399 versus 410 nmol/L) and only marginally lower than the mean level of 441 nmol/L observed in the healthy control group. The basal free cortisol and adrenocorticotropin hormone levels were similar in the three groups. The dexamethasone suppressed cortisol secretion in 95 percent of patients with fibromyalgia, 86 percent of those with low back pain, and 100 percent of healthy subjects. The response to the administration of synthetic adrenocorticotropin hormone revealed no differences between groups. Patients with fibromyalgia had a significantly greater secretion of adrenocorticotropin hormone in response to the infusion of corticotropin-releasing hormone than did low back patients ($p < 0.02$) and healthy control subjects ($p < 0.0002$). Despite the increased adrenocorticotropin response in fibromyalgia patients, the postinfusion cortisol levels were essentially identical in the three groups. The authors interpreted their findings to indicate that fibromyalgia and low back patients had evidence of mild hypothalamic-pituitary-adrenal axis dysregulation. A characteristic of the fibromyalgia group appeared to be the attenuated adrenal response to the increased adrenocorticotropin levels that followed an infusion of corticotropin-releasing hormone. However, the results of the direct stimulation of adrenal with synthetic adrenocorticotropin hormone were within the expected range, thereby excluding adrenal insufficiency.

An important contribution to the clarification of the role played by the hypothalamic-pituitary-adrenal axis in fibromyalgia has been made in a study carried out by investigators from the State University of New York at Stony Brook (Catley et al., 2000). The unique feature of this work was a longitudinal design that studied the impact of acute stressors and correlated them with salivary cortisol secretion and psychosocial and lifestyle variables. A community rheumatology practice was the source for recruiting 21 patients with fibromyalgia and 18 control subjects with rheumatoid arthritis. The participants met standard criteria for the diagnosis of their condition. The exclusion criteria were pregnancy, endocrine disorders, treatment with glucocorticoids, and night shift work. Data collected from 22 healthy individuals involved in a previous research with similar design (Ockenfels et al., 1995) were used as normal control. The technique of ecological momentary assessment was used to collect samples of saliva for cortisol assays six times each day. The collection was prompted by a signal transmitted via a programmable watch. At the same time, the participants completed short questionnaires that recorded situational and psychological variables, identified stressors, and rated their severity. Data were collected over a two-day period for each participant. The response rate was adequate, with 81 percent of the saliva samples and 85 percent of the timed questionnaires available for processing. Statistical analyses were performed on the results provided by the 74 percent of the saliva and questionnaire pairs collected within 18 to 32 minutes of each other.

Patients with fibromyalgia were somewhat younger than control subjects with rheumatoid arthritis (48 versus 53 years), had a shorter duration of illness (3 versus 8 years), and were less likely to have retired (10 versus 44 percent). The groups were similar with respect to gender distribution, educational level, and ethnicity. Sleep quality was significantly poorer in the fibromyalgia group. Patients with fibromyalgia and rheumatoid arthritis had similar mean cortisol levels at 7.1 and 6.5 nmol/L, respectively. Both groups had higher cortisol levels than the value of 4.7 nmol/L observed among the healthy control subjects. The differences retained statistical significance after adjustment for demographic variables. The same observation was made after adjusting for sleep quality. The effect of psychosocial stress was statistically insignificant. The results suggested that important dimensions of the illness experienced by patients with fibromyalgia, i.e., poor quality sleep and increased sensitivity to daily hassles, do not result in measurable changes in the activity of the hypothalamic-pituitary-adrenal axis.

CORTISOL LEVELS IN IRRITABLE BOWEL SYNDROME

The relationship between hypothalamic-pituitary-adrenal axis function and psychopathology in irritable bowel syndrome was assessed by investigators from the University La Sapienza, Rome (Patacchioli et al., 2001). The study sample comprised 54 outpatients (33 women and 21 men; mean age 33 years). They had been diagnosed with irritable bowel syndrome after a clinical evaluation that included in all cases fecal testing for blood and bacteria, a lactose tolerance test, and a barium enema. The 28 healthy control subjects were hospital employees or medical students. The groups were similar with regard to age, gender distribution, educational level, and marital status. None of the subjects had clinical evidence of hypercortisolism and none reported significant menstrual abnormalities. All participants were kept medication-free for four weeks prior to the study. Adrenal activity was assessed by measuring salivary cortisol levels at 8 a.m. and p.m. The burden of psychopathology was measured with self-administered questionnaires recording the severity of depression and anxiety. Additional questionnaires investigated the severity of mental/emotional and physical exhaustion and the levels of stress in the personal and social domains.

Compared with healthy control subjects, the salivary cortisol levels of patients with irritable bowel syndrome were significantly higher in the morning (30 versus 22 ng/mL; $p < 0.001$) and lower in the evening (3.6 versus 6.4 ng/mL; $p < 0.001$). The psychometric tests indicated that the irritable bowel syndrome group suffered significantly more depression and physical fatigue. The self-reported levels of mental fatigue, anxiety, and stress were similar in the two groups.

Researchers from the Lynn Institute for Healthcare Research and the Veterans Administration Medical Center, Oklahoma City, Oklahoma, made an important contribution to this field by assessing the effect of experimentally induced stress on the symptoms and cortisol levels of patients with irritable bowel syndrome (Elsenbruch et al., 2001). The 24 patients and 20 control subjects recruited for the study were all women without evidence of organic gastrointestinal disorders, other physical illnesses, or current psychiatric disorders. None of the participants were taking psychotropic drugs. The diagnosis of irritable bowel syndrome was established in accordance with standard criteria (Thompson et al., 1989). The mean age of patients with irritable bowel syndrome was 33 years, and the duration of illness averaged 13 years. The groups were statistically similar with respect to age, ethnicity, educational level, and marital status. The body mass index and blood pressure readings were virtually identical in the two groups. The group of women with irritable bowel syndrome had more depressive and gastrointestinal symptoms ($p < 0.001$) and consumed more alcohol ($p < 0.05$) than the healthy control subjects.

The study was designed as a two-day examination. On the "stress day," the patients ingested a standardized meal and were then administered a test requiring a quick answer to a visual signal. Failure to answer correctly within 0.6 seconds led to a loud burst of noise delivered into headphones and to score deduction. The aversive auditory and visual signals were also sent in a random manner regardless of the reaction time. Salivary samples for cortisol and data regarding cardiac rhythm changes and gastrointestinal and affective symptoms were collected at baseline, after the meal, after stress induction, and at the end of the recovery period. The same data were collected during the second day of the study, during which the stress induction was replaced by a passive relaxation period.

Patients with irritable bowel syndrome and healthy control subjects had similar cortisol levels at baseline and in response to the stressful experience. Likewise, no change in gastrointestinal symptoms occurred after stress induction. There was no difference in the degree of sympathetic and cardiovascular activation after stress. Patients with irritable bowel syndrome had a negative affective response to stress ($p < 0.05$), which persisted throughout the recovery period. The findings indicated that "these affective responses do not appear to be closely related to autonomic or cortisol abnormalities," but were "consistent with the increased incidence of psychopathology and may determine other aspects of IBS [irritable bowel syndrome] such as illness experience, healthcare seeking and coping strategies" (Elsenbruch et al., 2001, p. 811).

ASSESSMENT OF THE HYPOTHALAMIC-PITUITARY-ADRENAL AXIS IN PREMENSTRUAL SYNDROME

The function of the hypothalamic-pituitary-adrenal axis in premenstrual syndrome was thoroughly assessed by investigators from the National Institutes of Health, Bethesda, Maryland (Rabin et al., 1990), in seven patients. None of the patients had psychiatric disorders identifiable with a comprehensive structured interview. A group of age-, height-, and weight-matched healthy subjects formed the control group.

The participants had two stimulation tests with ovine corticotropin-releasing hormone. The tests were performed during the first week after the onset of menstruation and three weeks later. The hormone (1 µg/kg body weight) was administered as an intravenous bolus. Blood samples obtained at baseline and six times during the two hours after infusion were assayed for cortisol, cortisol-binding globulin, adrenocorticotropin hormone, and progesterone. Daily urinary free cortisol measurements were conducted for the duration of an entire menstrual cycle in five of the seven patients and in the seven control subjects.

Patients with premenstrual syndrome had significantly lower basal plasma cortisol levels than healthy control subjects during the follicular phase (64 versus 132 nmol/L, $p < 0.05$) and luteal phase (80 versus 143 nmol/L, $p < 0.05$) of the menstrual cycle. The means of urinary free cortisol excretion of the two groups were not different (149 versus 140 nmol/day during the follicular phase and 156 versus 156 nmol/day during the luteal phase). Plasma concentrations of cortisol-binding protein, adrenocorticotropin hormone, and progesterone were similar in the two groups. In response to the infusion of corticotropin-releasing hormone, patients with premenstrual syndrome and healthy subjects had slight and statistically similar increases in the level of adreno-corticotropin hormone. The patients also had higher postinfusion cortisol levels than healthy subjects ($p < 0.05$) The data were interpreted to indicate subtle and transient alterations of the hypothalamic-pituitary-adrenal axis in premenstrual syndrome. The authors contrasted the heightened cortisol secretion induced by corticotropin-releasing hormone infusion in these patients with the blunted response obtained when similar experiments were carried out by them in patients with melancholic depression (Gold, Loriaux, et al., 1986) and anorexia nervosa (Gold, Gwirtsman, et al., 1986). The existence of two types of response to corticotropin-releasing hormone in depression, strongly implied by the discordant data presented here, was confirmed unequivocally by Thalen et al. (1993). Working at St. Goran's Hospital in Stockholm, Sweden, these investigators were able to show that depressed patients with normal dexamethasone suppression tests had a significantly higher average adrenocorticotropin response to human corticotropin-releasing hormone than nonsuppressors, a difference that did not correlate with the severity of the affective illness.

Cortisol production during the premenstrual phase was more recently studied by researchers from the Royal Edinburgh Hospital, University of Edinburgh, and Medical Research Council Reproductive Biology Unit, Edinburgh, Scotland (Odber et al., 1998). The authors chose to measure salivary cortisol levels, a stress-free, convenient and specific way to assess the physiologically active hormone. The participants were selected from among women enrolled with a local premenstrual syndrome clinic. Daily ratings obtained at the clinic enabled the categorization of the subjects as having premenstrual depression and bloating, premenstrual bloating only, and menstrual symptoms only. Control subjects were recruited from among the patients' co-workers, employees of local businesses, and regional women's groups. All participants had regular menstrual cycles and did not use oral contraceptives or psychotropic agents.

To assess the diurnal variation in salivary cortisol pre- and postmenstrually, 2 mL samples were collected hourly from 10 a.m. to 11 p.m. during the two days prior to the expected onset of the menstrual cycle and for seven days afterward. A standard inventory of depressive symptomatology was filled out in the evening of these two premenstrual days. In a second phase of the study, the sample of women with premenstrual symptoms and healthy control subjects collected saliva each evening for an entire cycle. Statistical analyses compared the groups of women with premenstrual depression ($N = 19$), other premenstrual symptoms, primarily bloating ($N = 24$), symptoms restricted to menstrual period ($N = 12$), and no symptoms ($N = 26$). Only a minority of the subjects (19 patients and 13 control subjects) participated in both phases of the study.

The cortisol levels of healthy control subjects were higher during the premenstrual period. In contrast, in patients with premenstrual complaints, the premenstrual cortisol secretion levels were lower than the postmenstrual values. The diurnal variation was absent among premenstrually depressed women. The findings suggested that the pattern of cortisol secretion of women with premenstrual depression is similar to that observed in seasonal affective disorder (Joseph-Vanderpool et al., 1991).

In conclusion, the majority of research reports indicate that patients with functional somatic syndromes have evidence of mild and variable dysfunction of the hypothalamic-pituitary-adrenal axis. The changes are clearly different from those seen in major depression with melancholic features. Some of the studies have identified dysfunctional patterns similar to those discovered in other mental illnesses, such as seasonal affective disorder and eating disorders. However, the common denominator of this body of work is the absence of a biological gradient correlating hormonal abnormalities with depressive symptomatology and environmental stressors. Overall, the findings do not support a robust analogy between functional somatic syndromes and affective disorders.

Chapter 11

Serotonin Metabolism in Functional Somatic Illness

The monoamine hypothesis of depression, which was proposed more than 30 years ago, states that the biological basis of affective disorders is a deficiency in serotonergic and noradrenergic neurotransmission (Hirschfeld, 2000). Most research activities have focused on the serotonergic system, a complex neurofunctional apparatus with dozens of receptor subtypes in cortical and subcortical structures (Mann, 1999). Impairments in the serotonergic system occur at many levels and may involve decreased concentrations of serotonin, altered affinity and numbers of serotonin receptors and uptake sites, and postreceptor abnormalities (Leonard, 2000). In this chapter, we review the work testing the components and function of the serotonergic system in functional illnesses to determine whether patients with functional somatic syndromes show evidence of serotonergic deficiency and whether such deficiency correlates with the somatic and psychological manifestations of these conditions.

SEROTONERGIC NEUROTRANSMISSION IN CHRONIC FATIGUE SYNDROME

The first investigation of serotonin metabolism in chronic fatigue syndrome was carried out at the National Institutes of Health, Bethesda, Maryland (Demitrack et al., 1992). The work assessed the central monoaminergic activity involved in serotonergic, noradrenergic, and dopaminergic neurotransmission. Nineteen patients (13 women and six men) with this syndrome and 17 healthy control subjects (eight women and nine men) underwent lumbar puncture and had their blood and cerebrospinal fluid tested for 5-hydroxyindoleacetic acid (the main metabolite of serotonin), 3-methoxy-4-hydroxyphenylgly-col (the main metabolite of norepinephrine), and homovanillic acid (the main metabolite of dopamine). All patients were also adminis-tered a structured psychiatric interview.

Compared with healthy control subjects, patients with chronic fa-tigue syndrome had higher levels of the serotonin metabolite in pe-ripheral blood (67 versus 37 pmol/mL; $p < 0.002$). The metabolite's concentration in the cerebrospinal fluid was statistically similar in the two groups (112 versus 95 pmol/L). The norepinephrine metabolite concentrations were significantly lower in the plasma samples ob-tained from patients with chronic fatigue syndrome (8 versus 11 pmol/mL) and essentially identical with those of healthy subjects in the cerebrospinal fluid. The dopamine metabolite was found in simi-lar concentrations in both types of specimens obtained from the two groups. Thirteen of the 19 chronic fatigue patients had one or more psychiatric disorders, but the levels of monoamine metabolites did not discriminate them from patients without detectable psychiatric morbidity. The biochemical pattern identified in this sample of pa-tients with chronic fatigue syndrome was different than that consid-ered typical for melancholic depression, in which the levels of seroto-nin metabolites are reduced. The evidence led the authors to state that "a disturbance in central serotonin metabolism in patients with chronic fatigue syndrome seems unlikely" (Demitrack et al., 1992, p. 1072).

Three years later, British investigators from Maudsley Hospital and King's College Hospital, London, conducted a well-designed study evaluating central serotonergic neurotransmission in chronic fatigue syndrome (Cleare et al., 1995). The innovative dimension of this study was to stimulate the serotonergic pathways in the hypothal-amus with challenge with fenfluramine, a serotonin-agonist sub-stance. The fenfluramine challenge is known to elevate the level of both cortisol and prolactin in healthy individuals (O'Keane et al., 1991; Feeney et al., 1993; Gorard et al., 1993). In contrast, the change in prolactin and cortisol levels in response to this neuroendocrine challenge is almost undetectable in patients with major depression (O'Keane and Dinan, 1991).

The investigators assembled a ten-patient chronic fatigue syn-drome group (40 percent women) and a 15-patient depressed group (60 percent women) from among referrals to the specialty outpatient psychiatry clinics of the participating hospitals. The chronic fatigue syndrome patients were diagnosed according to standard criteria extant at the onset of the study (Holmes et al., 1988) and care was taken to make sure that they did not have a comorbid depressive disorder (American Psychiatric Association, 1987). Each patient was matched for age (within ten years), gender, and weight (within 10 kg) with a healthy control subject selected from among staff and students. All of the participants had stopped taking medications for at least three months prior to the study.

The experimental procedure was carried out after an overnight fast. First, blood was drawn to determine the baseline levels of cortisol and prolactin and the subject given 30 mg of *d*-fenfluramine by mouth. Venous blood samples were then obtained at hourly intervals for the next five hours. Technicians unaware of the subjects' status performed the hormonal measurements. For the analyses of the data, particular attention was paid to the phase of the menstrual cycle and only the measurements performed during the follicular phase were considered valid.

Baseline prolactin levels were similar in the three groups. The prolactin response, measured as mean change from baseline, reached 90 mU/L in the control group, 21 mU/L in the depressed group, and 141 mU/L in the chronic fatigue syndrome group. The differences between patients with chronic fatigue syndrome and depression were statistically significant ($p < 0.01$). The mean baseline cortisol level recorded for all of the control subjects was 305 nmol/L. The value recorded for the depressed group (428 nmol/L) was significantly higher, while that observed in the chronic fatigue syndrome group (226 nmol/L) was significantly lower. The magnitude of change in cortisol level after *d*-fenfluramine challenge was similar in the three groups. The findings did not support the presence of serotonergic deficiency in chronic fatigue syndrome and highlighted the psychobiological difference between this illness and major depression.

A similar assessment of the serotonin function in chronic fatigue syndrome was published the same year by Canadian investigators from Dalhousie University, Halifax, Nova Scotia (Yatham et al., 1995). The sample comprised 11 patients and 11 age- and gender-matched healthy control subjects. Nine of the 11 chronic fatigue patients had a current or past psychiatric diagnosis. The experimental procedure required the oral administration of 60 mg of *dl*-fenfluramine. Blood samples for prolactin and cortisol were obtained at baseline and hourly for five hours after the ingestion of fenfluramine.

Baseline prolactin and cortisol levels were essentially similar in the patient and control groups. The analysis of the published graphs indicates an average prolactin level of 8 µg/L at baseline and 12 to 14 µg/L four hours after fenfluramine. The difference between groups was insignificant. Similarly, the postchallenge cortisol levels were statistically similar at most data points. The baseline and postchallenge levels of prolactin and cortisol did not correlate with the severity of depressive symptomatology. The data were prudently interpreted to indicate that the "depressive symptoms in patients with CFS are perhaps not due to an alteration in 5-HT [serotonin] function" (Yatham et al., 1995, p. 95).

Investigators from St. Bartholomew's Hospital, London, and Southern General Hospital, Glasgow, Great Britain, also studied the serotonin-mediated activation of the hypothalamic-pituitary-adrenal axis in chronic fatigue syndrome (Dinan et al., 1997). The authors employed a neuroendocrine challenge with ipsapirone, a moderately selective serotonin agonist, in 14 patients with chronic fatigue syndrome and 14 age-, gender-, and weight-matched healthy control subjects. All patients were medication free at the time of the study and had no evidence of past or current psychiatric or endocrinological disorder. Blood samples were collected at baseline and after the oral administration of ipsapirone (20 mg) and assayed for cortisol and adrenocorticotropin hormone levels.

Baseline levels of cortisol (433 versus 453 nmol/L) and adrenocorticotropin hormone (19 versus 21 ng/L) were statistically similar in the chronic fatigue and control groups. A postchallenge increase in the adrenocorticotropin hormone levels was observed in six of the 14 chronic fatigue patients and in 13 control subjects. The difference in postchallenge cortisol levels was insignificant. The response to the ipsapirone challenge did not correlate with the duration of illness, age, or weight. The blunted response was tentatively attributed to a decreased responsivity of hypothalamic serotonin receptors in chronic fatigue syndrome.

In a more recent attempt to evaluate serotonergic neurotransmission in chronic fatigue syndrome, investigators from Warneford Hospital, Oxford, England (Vassallo et al., 2001), used the m-chlorophenylpiperazine challenge in 20 patients (16 women) with chronic fatigue syndrome and 21 healthy control subjects (16 women). The molecule is a directly acting serotonin receptor agonist, and its oral administration at a dose of 0.25 mg/kg should increase prolactin levels at a rate corresponding to the sensitivity of postsynaptic serotonin receptors. The participants underwent two challenges (active and placebo) separated by a two-week interval. Biochemical assays for plasma prolactin, cortisol, tryptophan, and neutral amino acids (leucine, isoleucine, valine, phenylalanine, and tyrosine) measured the postchallenge response.

The prolactin and cortisol responses were significantly greater after the active challenge in both groups. The groups were also similar with regard to baseline plasma total tryptophan and neutral amino acids, but free tryptophan levels were significantly lower in the chronic fatigue syndrome group. The data were interpreted to indicate that the prolactin response was not related to an increase in the sensitivity of the postsynaptic serotonin receptors. The authors deduced that "the neuroendocrine responses revealed by fenfluramine challenge are probably due to enhanced presynaptic release of 5-HT [serotonin]" (Vassallo et al., 2001, p. 589) and "unlikely to be due to increased peripheral availability of tryptophan" (p. 585). Taken together, the findings did not support serotonergic deficiency as an etiologic mechanism for chronic fatigue syndrome.

SEROTONIN METABOLISM IN FIBROMYALGIA

Research carried out at the University of Texas Health Sciences Center, San Antonio, Texas, focused on establishing the presence of a serotonin-deficient state by assessing serum serotonin levels and platelet 3H-imipramine uptake receptor density (Russell, Michalek, et al., 1992). These receptors are specific for serotonin, and the number of binding sites had been found to be significantly smaller in patients with untreated depression than in healthy control subjects (Paul et al., 1981; Zarifian et al., 1982). Additional support for the specificity of these receptors has been provided by work finding that the number of sites increases after treatment with antidepressants (Suranyi-Cadotte et al., 1984; Marazziti et al., 1988). These data suggested that an acquired deficiency of serotonin transport mechanisms might be involved in the pathogenesis of depression (Paul et al., 1981) and chronic pain (Magni et al., 1987; Mellerup et al., 1988).

The Texas investigators recruited 22 patients with primary fibromyalgia and 22 pain-free healthy control subjects. The groups were well matched for age, gender, and ethnic background. Four of the fibromyalgia patients had been treated with tricyclic drugs (i.e., amitriptyline or cyclobenzaprine) during the month prior to the study. The blood specimens from patients and control subjects were processed in randomly interspersed order for high-affinity binding of the 3H-imipramine. Serum serotonin levels were measured in nine participants from each group. The patients rated the severity of their pain and were examined by an experienced rheumatologist for tenderness at 16 specified anatomical sites. Additional data documented physical disability and the presence and severity of depression and anxiety.

The baseline pain measures indicated significantly more muscle tenderness and stiffness in the fibromyalgia group. The psychometric data indicated that four patients (18 percent) were depressed and that 13 (59 percent) had significant anxiety. The means for imipramine binding in the fibromyalgia and control groups were 836 and 694 fmol imipramine/mg platelet membrane protein, respectively ($p = 0.012$). The serum serotonin levels were significantly lower in the fibromyalgia group (84 versus 126 ng/mL, $p = 0.011$). The data did not provide support for a functional serotonin deficiency in fibromyalgia.

Similar assays were used in a well-designed study performed at the Rush-Presbyterian-St. Luke's Medical Center, Chicago, and Rush North Shore Medical Center, Skokie, Illinois (Kravitz et al., 1992). The study groups included ten nondepressed women with fibromyalgia, 14 patients (eight men and six women) with major nonpsychotic depression, and ten healthy individuals (three men and seven women). Two of the fibromyalgia patients had a history of major affective illness. All participants had their platelets tested at least twice with a standard imipramine-binding assay.

The fibromyalgia and healthy control groups showed no difference with regard to imipramine binding. Compared with depressed women, the imipramine binding was significantly lower in patients with fibromyalgia and in men with depression. The imipramine binding did not correlate with the severity of pain reported by fibromyalgia patients. The data were interpreted to indicate that serotonergic function in fibromyalgia is essentially normal. The results also challenged the assumption that biologically mediated negative mood states are connected with the pain symptoms of fibromyalgia.

Another test of the serotonin deficiency hypothesis was designed and executed by investigators from the University of Texas Health Sciences Center, San Antonio, in collaboration with European investigators based at the University of Bergen, Norway, and University of Uppsala, Sweden (Russell, Vaeroy, et al., 1992). The study design was similar to that employed by Demitrack et al. (1992) in chronic fatigue syndrome. The investigators set out to compare the levels of the biogenic amines serotonin, norepinephrine, and dopamine by measuring their metabolites in the cerebrospinal fluid of 17 female patients with fibromyalgia, five female patients with rheumatoid arthritis, and seven healthy control subjects. All of the subjects were of Scandinavian descent and none were receiving treatment with psychotropic agents or opioid analgesics at the time of the study.

Approximately 16 mL of spinal fluid were obtained by lumbar puncture from each participant and submitted for high-performance liquid chromatography assays of the serotonin metabolite 5-hydroxyindoleacetic acid; the norepinephrine metabolite 3-methoxy-4-hydroxyphenethylene glycol; and the dopamine metabolite homovanillic acid.

The mean concentration of the serotonin metabolite identified in the cerebrospinal fluid was 18 ng/mL in patients with fibromyalgia, 40 ng/mL in patients with rheumatoid arthritis, and 21 ng/mL in healthy control subjects. The corresponding group levels for the metabolite of norepinephrine were 5.8 ng/mL, 7.5 ng/mL, and 7.9 ng/mL. For the metabolite of dopamine, the levels were 26 ng/mL in the fibromyalgia group, 42 ng/mL in the rheumatoid arthritis group, and 42 ng/mL in the healthy control group. The statistical significance of the differences was calculated for fibromyalgia versus non-fibromyalgia participants; the p values were 0.005 for the dopamine metabolite, 0.03 for the norepinephrine metabolite, and 0.06 for the serotonin metabolite. A lower serotonin metabolite concentration in the cerebrospinal fluid was usually associated with a lower concentration of the dopamine metabolite. There was no correlation between age and the serotonin metabolite's concentration in the fibromyalgia group. The results indicated that the turnover of biogenic amines is lower in patients with fibromyalgia, but the data did not support the hypothesized serotonin-deficient state.

The strength of these observations was also supported by data reported by investigators associated with the Wichita Arthritis Research and Clinical Center, University of Kansas at Wichita, and the University of Texas Health Sciences Center in San Antonio (Wolfe et al., 1997). The unique feature of this well-designed research effort was the community-based sample, for which the authors hypothesized a direct correlation between decreased serum serotonin levels and severity of pain. The initial cohort comprised 3,150 residents of Wichita, Kansas, who were interviewed about the presence of pain. After further clinical and psychometric evaluations, 292 subjects were recruited for the current study. Of these, 63 had no pain, 87 had regional (nonwidespread) pain, and 142 had widespread pain. Thirty-one of the 142 patients with widespread pain fulfilled the standard criteria for the diagnosis of fibromyalgia. The data collected included an assessment of tender points, dolorimetric tenderness at six specified musculoskeletal locations, and subjective severity of pain, sleep disturbance, depression, and anxiety. Sera were collected at the time of the interview, frozen at −80°C and submitted in a single batch for serotonin assays by high-performance liquid chromatography.

The mean serum serotonin concentration of the 31 patients with fibromyalgia was 87 ng/mL. The value was significantly lower ($p < 0.03$) than the mean of serotonin levels observed among the other 111 subjects with widespread pain (106 ng/mL) and subjects with regional pain (105 ng/mL). The value recorded for the group of pain-free individuals (100 ng/mL) was statistically similar to that measured in the fibromyalgia group. The serum serotonin concentrations were positively correlated with the tender point count ($p < 0.001$) and with the measures of anxiety and depression ($p < 0.004$). The correlation between the number of tender points and severity of depression, on one hand, and the serum concentration of serotonin, on the other, retained statistical significance after adjustment for age and gender. The authors commented that "serotonin is not correlated with any clinical variables in the general population, and separate pain groups cannot be distinguished" (Wolfe et al., 1997, p. 555). The correlation between pain and serotonin concentration in the fibromyalgia group did not support serotonin deficiency as a valid mechanism for myalgia.

SEROTONERGIC FUNCTION
IN PREMENSTRUAL SYNDROME

The neuroendocrine response to *d*-fenfluramine was used to measure the serotonergic function in premenstrual syndrome in studies conducted in Scotland (Bancroft and Cook, 1995), the United States (FitzGerald et al., 1997), and Canada (Steiner et al., 1999).

In pioneering work, investigators from the Reproductive Biology Unit, Medical Research Council, Edinburgh, Scotland, recruited 27 patients with premenstrual depression and 19 healthy control subjects (Bancroft and Cook, 1995). The oral administration of 15 or 30 mg of *d*-fenfluramine produced the neuroendocrine challenge, with the higher dose given to the participants weighing more than 65 kg. Blood samples were collected at baseline and eight times after the oral intake of fenfluramine. All samples were assayed for cortisol and prolactin levels. Standard scales were used to measure the severity of depressive symptomatology in the clinical sample. Complete data were obtained from 17 patients and 14 control subjects.

The groups were similar with regard to age, but patients with premenstrual syndrome were significantly heavier than control subjects and therefore received more fenfluramine. The postchallenge prolactin levels were similar in patients and controls in all phases of the menstrual cycle. For instance, the premenstrual postchallenge increase in the prolactin means averaged 223 mU/L in the clinical group and 246 mU/L in the control subjects. The baseline cortisol levels were marginally lower in the premenstrual depression group, but the response to neuroendocrine challenge was similar in the two samples. Estradiol levels did not correlate with the neuroendocrine responses. Overall, the data refuted the hypothesized serotonergic deficiency as a specific mechanism for premenstrual dysphoria.

Investigators from the College of Physicians and Surgeons, Columbia University, and the New York State Psychiatric Institute also attempted to test the presence of serotonergic deficiency in premenstrual syndrome by measuring prolactin levels before and after a fenfluramine challenge (FitzGerald et al., 1997). The authors enrolled in the study nine women with premenstrual dysphoric disorder (mean age 33 years) and 11 healthy control females (mean age 27 years). All subjects were physically healthy and none had current psychiatric disorder detectable by structured interviews. However, all of the patients had a past history of major depression or dysthymia. The average body weight was similar in the two groups.

The testing was conducted during two consecutive days in the luteal phase. The participants reported to the laboratory at 8 a.m. after an eight-hour fast. Blood was drawn before the oral administration of 60 mg of fenfluramine or placebo and then hourly for five hours. The blood samples were processed for prolactin levels with a radio-immunometric assay and for fenfluramine and norfenfluramine with gas-liquid chromatography. The outcome of the challenge was the difference between the prolactin levels measured after the administration of fenfluramine and those produced by placebo ingestion.

The baseline prolactin levels were similar in the two groups and did not change significantly from the first to the second day of testing. The maximum net prolactin response measured after fenfluramine challenge was significantly lower in the premenstrual dysphoric disorder group ($p < 0.02$). For instance, three hours after the challenge, the net response averaged 20 ng/mL in the healthy control group, but only 7.5 ng/mL in the group with premenstrual dysphoric disorder. The magnitude of the difference persisted when the data were controlled for age, weight, and fenfluramine and norfenfluramine levels. The authors contended that the central serotonergic deficiency identified in premenstrual dysphoric disorder is specific for this condition and not a consequence of previous episodes of mood disorders. This view is supported by data demonstrating enhanced prolactin response to the fenfluramine challenge in patients with treated (O'Keane et al., 1992) and remitted depression (Shapira et al., 1993). However, data published after the completion of this study indicated that the prolactin response to fenfluramine remained abnormal at least one year after the last major depressive episode (Flory et al., 1998).

An attempt to arbitrate the contradictory results obtained by Bancroft and Cook (1995) and by FitzGerald and her colleagues (1997) was carried out at St. Joseph's Hospital, McMaster University, Hamilton, Canada (Steiner et al., 1999). The investigators were mindful of the main confounding variable of the previous work, i.e., the fact that all of the patients with premenstrual syndrome studied by FitzGerald and her co-workers had a past history of mood disorders. For their study group, the Canadian researchers recruited nine patients with premenstrual dysphoric disorder (mean age 36 years) who had no past or current evidence of mood disorders detected with a structured psychiatric interview. The patients had no physical or laboratory abnormalities suggestive of any physical illness. The control group comprised nine physically healthy women (mean age 39 years) without premenstrual dysphoria or psychiatric disorders. All participants had regular periods, were within 25 percent of the calculated normal weight, and were not taking prescription drugs.

The fenfluramine challenges were carried out during the follicular and late luteal phases of the menstrual cycle. The challenge used the same oral dose of fenfluramine (60 mg) as in the previous study (Fitz-Gerald et al., 1997). Blood samples were obtained at baseline for platelet 3H-imipramine binding levels, and cortisol and prolactin levels. Cortisol and prolactin were also measured in samples drawn hourly for six hours after the administration of fenfluramine. The primary outcome of the challenge was the difference between the mean postchallenge and baseline levels of prolactin.

Baseline cortisol and prolactin levels were similar for patients and control subjects during both phases of the menstrual cycle. Platelet 3H-imipramine binding levels measured during the luteal phase were significantly lower in the patient group (6,889 versus 1,151 fmol/mg protein; $p < 0.008$). The binding levels were similar in the two groups during the follicular phase (1,036 versus 1,023 fmol/mg protein). The finding confirms previous work conducted in patients with premenstrual syndrome (Ashby et al., 1988; Rojansky et al., 1991; Steege et al., 1992) and is similar to data reported in studies of depressed patients (Paul et al., 1981; Raisman et al., 1982). The prolactin response to the fenfluramine challenge was statistically similar in the two groups. The baseline cortisol levels showed an inverse correlation with the postchallenge prolactin levels only in the patient group. This correlation has been identified frequently in patients with mood disorders, most emphatically in work performed in Australia (Mitchell and Smythe, 1990) and Israel (Lichtenberg et al., 1992). However, enthusiasm for such an interpretation of the data must be tempered by evidence showing a similar relationship in a group of healthy subjects challenged with a smaller dose of fenfluramine (Cleare and Bond, 1997). Taken together, the data did not replicate the blunted prolactin response found by FitzGerald et al. (1997). Nonetheless, the authors felt that the "significant negative correlation between prolactin and basal cortisol in patients but not in controls during both phases of the menstrual cycle, suggests an underlying 5-HT [serotonin] dysfunction" (Steiner et al., 1999, p. 114).

The neuroendocrine response to an intravenous L-tryptophan challenge in women with premenstrual syndrome was studied at the School of Medicine, University of California, Los Angeles (Rasgon et al., 2000). The investigators postulated that the administration of L-tryptophan, a serotonin precursor, would affect cortisol and prolactin production. Five patients (mean age 24 years) and five healthy women (mean age 27 years) participated in the study. History and physical examination verified the absence of medical illnesses and obesity in all subjects. None of the patients were taking psychoactive or hormonal preparations. All subjects took nonsteroidal oral contraceptive drugs, abstained from alcohol, and followed a tyramine-free diet during the month of the study.

The L-tryptophan challenges were conducted twice weekly for four consecutive weeks. Ovulation was documented with a urinary kit and the testing period divided into follicular, ovulatory, and luteal phases. The L-tryptophan was administered after an overnight fast at a dose of 7 g diluted in 500 mL of 0.47 percent normal saline infused at a constant rate over a 20-minute period. Blood samples were obtained at baseline and six times during the 90-minute period that followed the start of the challenge. The neuroendocrine outcomes were calculated as the difference between the peak response to the challenge and the baseline value for whole blood serotonin, cortisol, and prolactin.

Compared with healthy control subjects, patients with premenstrual syndrome had blunted whole-blood serotonin responses during the luteal phase. The cortisol and prolactin levels were not affected by the challenge. Baseline cortisol levels were greater during the luteal phase in the premenstrual syndrome group. The data were interpreted to "firmly establish that there is difference in handling the tryptophan in subjects with PMS in the luteal phase compared with the follicular phase and with controls" (Rosgon et al., 2000, p. 448). In contrast with studies of depressed individuals, which have shown a blunted prolactin response to the L-tryptophan infusion (Heninger et al., 1984; Cowen and Charig, 1987), the prolactin levels did not change significantly in this small sample of patients with premenstrual disorder.

Attempts to explain the psychobiology of premenstrual syndrome have focused on the role of allopregnanolone, a neuroactive progesterone metabolite produced in the ovaries and the adrenals (Girdler et al., 2001; Rasgon et al., 2001). The molecule easily crosses the blood-brain barrier and modulates the hypothalamic-pituitary-adrenal axis, the gamma-aminobutyric acid receptors (Girdler et al., 2001), and the central serotonergic tone (Rasgon et al., 2001). Women with premenstrual syndrome have been shown to have lower levels of allopregnanolone than control subjects (Rapkin et al., 1997), and the levels of allopregnanolone were inversely correlated with the severity of premenstrual symptoms (Wang et al., 1996).

In the first of these studies, investigators from the University of North Carolina at Chapel Hill measured the relationship between allopregnanolone levels and premenstrual symptoms and plasma cortisol levels (Girdler et al., 2001). The participants were recruited from a cohort comprising 28 premenstrual syndrome patients and 28 healthy control subjects who were participating in a research project studying neuroendocrine reactivity to stress. Twenty-five patients and 13 control subjects were available for plasma allopregnanolone measurements. The premenstrual syndrome was diagnosed according to established criteria (American Psychiatric Association, 1994) on the basis of daily recording of symptoms over at least two menstrual cycles and a structured psychiatric interview. The subjects included in the control group had only mild emotional changes and moderate physical symptoms on fewer than three days prior to their menstruation. The groups were comparable with respect to age (33 versus 32 years); height and weight; current use of alcohol, coffee, and tobacco; prior major depression (29 versus 25 percent); prior anxiety disorders (4 versus 0 percent); and prior substance abuse or dependence (20 versus 8 percent). None of the participants had a current Axis I psychiatric disorder and all had stopped medication use at least three months prior to the study.

The experimental procedure comprised follicular and luteal phase assays, i.e., testing during four to eight days after the onset of menstruation and again eight to 12 days after a urine test indicated the increase in luteinizing hormone levels that precede ovulation. Baseline levels of allopregnanolone, progesterone, and cortisol were obtained just before the patients were exposed to verbal and cognitive stressors. The stressors consisted of preparation and delivery of a response to an unpleasant interpersonal situation and the paced auditory serial addition test. The stressors were followed by blood sampling for allopregnanolone and cortisol levels. Data analyses were restricted to values obtained during the luteal phase, as allopregnanolone was undetectable in most of the samples obtained from control subjects tested during the follicular phase.

Patients with premenstrual syndrome had significantly higher levels of allopregnanolone than those recorded for the control group. The intergroup difference was statistically significant ($p < 0.001$) both at baseline (2.6 versus 1 ng/mL) and after stressful tasks (2.3 versus 1.2 ng/mL). Compared with the baseline value, the poststress allopregnanolone level increased in 83 percent of the control subjects and 42 percent of the premenstrual syndrome patients. Patients with greater premenstrual anxiety had significantly lower levels of allopregnanolone than the remainder of the group ($p < 0.01$), and a similar trend was noted for premenstrual irritability ($p = 0.08$) and depression ($p = 0.09$). The cortisol levels were lower in the premenstrual group ($p < 0.05$). A negative correlation between cortisol and allopregnanolone levels was demonstrated for both baseline and poststress conditions in the premenstrual syndrome group ($p < 0.05$). The findings were interpreted to indicate that premenstrual syndrome is associated with higher levels of allopregnanolone, which inhibit the function of the hypothalamic-pituitary-adrenal axis. They also postulated that the hormone alters the receptor sensitivity of neurotransmitters that modulate the anxiety, irritability, and depression of patients with this condition, but direct evidence for this type of effect was not obtained in the study.

A closer evaluation of the interaction between neurotransmitters and allopregnanolone was attempted by researchers from the University of California at Los Angeles and the University of Cagliari, Italy (Rasgon et al., 2001). The study was carried out in Los Angeles and involved five women with premenstrual syndrome and five age-matched (mean age 24 versus 27 years) control subjects. The participants were not married and had no children. Clinical evaluation established the absence of current physical and psychiatric conditions. All subjects had normal weight and regular menstrual cycles and had not been taking psychotropic or hormonal preparations for at least six months prior to the study.

The experimental procedure was an L-tryptophan challenge, which involved the intravenous administration of 7 g of L-tryptophan, diluted in 500 mL of a 0.45 percent saline solution. The infusion was given at a constant rate over a 20-minute period. Blood samples for allopregnanolone, progesterone, pregnenolone, and the 11-deoxy-corticosterone metabolite 3alpha-5alpha-tetrahydrocorticosterone were obtained 15 and 0 minutes prior to the L-tryptophan infusion and 30, 60, and 90 minutes after the infusion. The challenge was administered twice weekly for four consecutive weeks. Data analyses compared hormonal levels obtained during the follicular and luteal phases of the menstrual cycle encompassed by the four-week study period.

The pre-tryptophan challenge data indicated that in the premenstrual syndrome group, the allopregnanolone levels increased from 5 ng/mL in the follicular phase to 11 ng/mL at the time of ovulation and 12 ng/mL during the luteal phase. In contrast, the corresponding levels (5, 5, and 7 ng/mL) measured in the control group were significantly lower in the second half of the cycle ($p < 0.05$). The behavior of pregnenolone and tetrahydrocorticosterone followed a similar pattern. After the tryptophan challenge, only the concentrations of allopregnanolone showed a significant increase. This change was most striking during the luteal phase in the premenstrual syndrome group. The authors felt that this increase "strongly suggests that there is a relationship between central serotonergic activity and circulating allopregnanolone concentrations" and reflects "lower baseline serotonergic activity in this group of women" (Rasgon et al., 2001, p. 145).

In conclusion, a serotonergic deficiency has not been demonstrated in chronic fatigue syndrome and fibromyalgia. This conclusion is supported by the ineffectiveness of serotonin reuptake inhibitors in alleviating chronic fatigue syndrome (Vercoulen et al., 1996; Wearden et al., 1998) and fibromyalgia (Goldenberg et al., 1996). The biological support for serotonergic deficiency in premenstrual syndrome is relatively weak, but certainly not negligible, given the confirmed effectiveness of selective serotonin reuptake inhibition in a majority of patients with premenstrual dysphoria (Steiner et al., 1995; Yonkers et al., 1997; Freeman et al., 1999).

PART IV:
ABNORMAL PERSONALITY
AND ILLNESS BEHAVIOR
IN FUNCTIONAL SOMATIC
SYNDROMES

Chapter 12

Abnormal Personality in Functional Somatic Syndromes

In patients with medically unexplained symptoms, the number of bodily complaints over an individual's lifetime correlates linearly with neuroticism, functional impairment, and coexisting anxiety and depressive disorders (Katon and Walker, 1998). The relationship between personality and somatization is multidimensional: negative affectivity is associated with somatic distress; absorption makes the patient more likely to focus attention on symptoms and enhances illness anxiety; and conscientiousness may lead to failure of medical reassurance (Kirmayer et al., 1994). However, the interpretation of these associations in patients with unexplainable physical complaints is difficult, given the fact that many personality dimensions, including neuroticism, extraversion, dependency, and perfectionism are also powerful predictors of major depressive illnesses (Enns and Cox, 1997). In this chapter, we explore the large body of work that has assessed the personality traits and personality disorders of patients with functional somatic syndromes and attempt to determine their specificity and relationship with psychiatric morbidity.

CHRONIC FATIGUE SYNDROME

The controlled investigation of personality in chronic fatigue syndrome was started by a group of investigators from the Otago Medical School, Dunedin, New Zealand (Blakely et al., 1991). The study group ($N = 58$) was assembled from among the patients evaluated for chronic fatigue at the Mornington Health Centre, Dunedin. Inclusion in the study was restricted to individuals ages 10 to 60 and required an illness duration of no less than six months, relapsing chronic fatigue, myalgias, and exercise-induced muscle weakness. A control group of patients with chronic pain ($N = 81$) was recruited from the pain clinic of the area's hospital. A second control group comprised healthy subjects selected from the registry of a general practitioner to match the gender and age of the chronic fatigue patients.

The main data collection instrument was the Minnesota Multiphase Personality Inventory (Dahlstrom et al., 1972), an extensively validated instrument for assessing personality traits. Psychiatric morbidity was assessed with the General Health Questionnaire (Goldberg and Williams, 1988), an instrument that identified psychiatric caseness, but did not establish precise diagnoses. In addition, the authors measured the severity of depressive symptomatology and the ways in which the subjects were coping with the internal and external demands of stressful situations.

The groups were similar with respect to age, marital status, and socioeconomic class. The proportion of females was 72 percent in the chronic fatigue group, 69 percent among healthy control subjects, and 48 percent in the chronic pain group. The patients with chronic fatigue syndrome had been ill for an average of five years. In the control group of patients with chronic pain, 32 percent had a chief complaint of lower back pain, 17 percent had upper extremity pain, and 10 percent had head and neck pain.

Psychiatric morbidity was similar in the chronic fatigue and chronic pain groups, with 57 versus 46 percent of females and 63 versus 62 percent of males being classified as psychiatric cases. In the healthy control sample, the proportion of psychiatric cases was 11 percent for females and 13 percent for males. A majority of chronic fatigue patients (48 percent of females and 63 percent of males) were found to have moderate or severe depression. These proportions were significantly higher than those recorded in the chronic pain group, in which 33 percent of females and 43 percent of males had this level of depression. In the healthy control group, the frequencies of depression were 10 percent for females and 13 percent for males. The analysis of ways of coping indicated that women with chronic fatigue scored higher on escape/avoidance than healthy control subjects. Men with chronic fatigue scored higher on distancing than chronic pain patients and healthy control subjects. Other coping strategies, including confrontation, self-control, seeking social support, planned problem solving, and positive reappraisal, were essentially similarly represented in the three groups.

The evaluation of personality indicated substantially more abnormalities in the chronic fatigue group. Compared with chronic pain patients and healthy control subjects, the differences reached statistical significance ($p < 0.01$) for seven of the ten basic dimensions measured with the Minnesota Multiphasic Personality Inventory: hypochondriasis, hysteria, depression, paranoia, psychasthenia, schizophrenia, and social introversion. The chronic fatigue patients had a significantly higher level of neuroticism than chronic pain patients and healthy control subjects. They also had elevated scores on guilt and self-criticism, and an obvious inward direction of hostility. In contrast, a tendency for an outward direction of hostility characterized the healthy control subjects.

Two-point classifications of patients in the three groups showed a strong clustering among the chronic fatigue patients. A substantial majority of these patients (70 percent) belonged to one of three categories of codes: hypochondriasis/hysteria (40 percent), hypochondriasis/depression (16 percent), and hypochondriasis/schizophrenia (14 percent). A weaker clustering tendency (50 percent of cases) was noted in the chronic pain group. The distribution of the two-point codes recorded for the healthy controls showed no discrete clusters. Chronic fatigue patients assigned the hypochondriasis/hysteria code had significant elevations on the denial scale compared with the other fatigue patients. The authors interpreted the findings to indicate that the patients from this subgroup did not acknowledge the experience of anxiety or depression, but tenaciously endorsed the somatic symptoms of chronic fatigue syndrome. In contrast, a highly neurotic/emotional subgroup of patients with chronic fatigue ($N = 5$) had the most psychological symptoms and the shortest duration of illness. Their personality abnormalities were essentially restricted to the scales measuring depression and psychasthenia. The data did not support a relationship between emotionality and the somatic burden, meaning that the abnormal dimensions of personality uncovered by the study were permanent traits rather a neurotic reaction to illness.

The first U.S. study to address the issue of abnormal personality in a controlled investigation of patients with chronic fatigue syndrome was conducted by researchers from the State University of New York at Stony Brook (Pepper et al., 1993). The 69 chronic fatigue syndrome subjects were selected from among the referrals to one of the authors of the study, a neurologist known for her interest and expertise in chronic fatigue. The diagnosis was based on a set of criteria similar to the standard in use at the time (Holmes et al., 1988). The complaint of fatigue had to be of new onset, present for at least six months, severe enough to limit daily activities to less than half the premorbid function, and not explained by any past or current medical condition. At least five of 11 specified symptoms or clinical features (fever, myalgia, arthralgia, generalized headache, sore throat, painful lymphadenopathy, muscle weakness, sleep disturbance, neuropsychological symptoms, and abrupt onset of illness) were also required. A control group of 65 patients with multiple sclerosis was selected from among patients referred to the same neurologist. These subjects were included if they met the standard diagnostic criteria for multiple sclerosis (Poser et al., 1983); if they indicated fatigue as one of their three most bothersome manifestations of illness; and if they considered their fatigue severe and requested specific treatment for it. A complete neurological evaluation and a battery of laboratory investigations were used to determine that there were no other significant abnormalities and that the fatigue illness was due solely to chronic fatigue syndrome or multiple sclerosis, respectively. A second control group included 20 patients with major depression recruited by contacting clinical psychologists in private practice and the personnel of the psychiatry outpatient clinic at State University Hospital at Stony Brook, New York. The diagnosis was confirmed by one of the co-authors, a psychologist who interviewed each patient to establish compliance with standard criteria (American Psychiatric Association, 1987). The exclusion criterion for this group was the presence of any other psychiatric or physical disorder.

Data were collected with the Millon Clinical Multiaxial Inventory, a 175-item self-report instrument designed to assess psychiatric symptoms and to establish psychiatric diagnoses (Millon, 1987). Additional questionnaires were used to measure the severity of fatigue and depression. A subsample of patients with chronic fatigue syndrome ($N = 35$) and multiple sclerosis ($N = 53$) were also administered a structured psychiatric interview. Statistical processing relied on logistic regression to determine the variables discriminating chronic fatigue patients from control patients.

The three groups had similar demographic characteristics. The expected predominance of middle-aged women was confirmed by a mean age of 40 years for each clinical sample and a proportion of women that ranged from 65 percent in the multiple sclerosis group to 73 percent among patients with major depression. The level of education averaged 13 years in the major depression group and 15 years in the other two groups. The duration of illness had a mean of seven years in the chronic fatigue syndrome group and eight years in the control groups. A lifetime history of any psychiatric disorder was identified with the Structured Clinical Interview among 51 percent of subsamples of patients with chronic fatigue syndrome and 32 percent of those with multiple sclerosis. Current psychiatric disorders were diagnosed in 23 percent of patients with chronic fatigue syndrome, but only 7 percent of those with multiple sclerosis. A significant difference was also noted with regard to the frequency of psychiatric disorders preceding the diagnosis of fatigue illness. The severity of depressive symptomatology was much greater in the chronic fatigue syndrome group.

The prevalence of personality disorders among the chronic fatigue syndrome patients was established in the subgroup ($N = 45$) who scored above the threshold for severe psychopathology on the Millon Clinical Multiaxial Inventory (Millon, 1987). Obsessive-compulsive personality disorder was identified in 16 percent of patients, histrionic in 13 percent, dependent in 11 percent, passive-aggressive in 9 percent, narcissistic in 7 percent, antisocial in 7 percent, and borderline personality disorder in 4 percent of patients. Overall, the instrument detected 36 personality disorders in this group of 45 patients with chronic fatigue syndrome. The logistic regression analysis showed that the chronic fatigue syndrome and major depression groups were essentially identical for schizoid, narcissistic, antisocial, passive-aggressive, self-defeating, and borderline personality disorders, and for somatization and thought disorder. A direct comparison by stepwise regression between chronic fatigue syndrome and multiple sclerosis was not performed. Overall, the results indicate a slight specific excess of obsessive-compulsive, narcissistic, and dependent personality disorders in the chronic fatigue syndrome patients with severe psychiatric symptoms.

An attempt to confirm the findings of the two previous studies was carried out by investigators from the Chronic Fatigue Syndrome Research Center, the Kessler Institute for Rehabilitation, and the University of Medicine and Dentistry of New Jersey (Johnson et al., 1996). The patients with chronic fatigue syndrome ($N = 35$) had to meet the diagnostic criteria proposed by Holmes et al. (1988) and have an illness duration of less than four years. The first of three control groups included patients ($N = 20$) diagnosed with multiple sclerosis according to standard criteria (Poser et al., 1983). These patients had minimal functional disability and no known medical or psychiatric comorbidity. The second control group included 24 patients with depressive disorders (major depression or dysthymia). A third control group comprised 35 healthy subjects. Exclusion criteria for all participants were a history of loss of consciousness, substance abuse, bipolar disorder, schizophrenia, and eating disorder. The control subjects were paid for their participation.

Psychiatric diagnoses were established with the Quick Diagnostic Interview Schedule (Marcus et al., 1990). A written version of the same instrument (Robins et al., 1991) was used to identify somatization disorder and dysthymia. Personality pathology was assessed with the Personality Disorders Questionnaire (Hyler and Reider, 1987), an instrument yielding 14 different diagnoses and a global score of personality disturbance. Personality traits were measured with the neuroticism scale of a widely used personality inventory (Costa and McCrae, 1985). Statistical analyses determined the significance of differences between the chronic fatigue syndrome patients and the three control groups and compared depressed versus nondepressed chronic fatigue subjects.

The four groups studied were similar with regard to female predominance (range of proportions of females 85 to 94 percent), age (range of means 35 to 40 years) and years of education (range of means 14 to 15 years). Current major depressive mood disorders were identified in 34 percent of patients with chronic fatigue syndrome, but in only 11 percent of those with multiple sclerosis. Other diagnoses were dysthymia (6 versus 0 percent), generalized anxiety disorder (9 versus 5 percent), panic disorder (9 versus 0 percent), phobia (11 versus 6 percent), and somatization disorder (6 versus 0 percent). Overall, 45 percent of chronic fatigue syndrome subjects, but only 16 percent of multiple sclerosis cases, had a current psychiatric disorder.

Compared with matched healthy control subjects, patients with chronic fatigue syndrome had an excess of diagnosable personality disorders. Specifically, the five most common personality disorders identified among patients with chronic fatigue syndrome were histrionic (23 versus 6 percent in the healthy control group), borderline (17 versus 0 percent), paranoid (9 versus 3 percent), avoidant (9 versus 3 percent), and obsessive-compulsive disorders (9 versus 3 percent). Other personality disorders diagnosed in the chronic fatigue group but not in the healthy control subjects were self-defeating (6 percent) and schizoid or schizotypal disorders (6 percent). The total scores on the Personality Disorders Questionnaire were similar in the chronic fatigue syndrome and multiple sclerosis groups. The depressed control group had a significantly higher rate of personality disorders. The healthy control group had a negligible rate of personality abnormalities. The authors pointed out that the personality pathologies most closely associated with chronic fatigue syndrome in this study were borderline, histrionic, narcissistic, and antisocial disorders or the so-called dramatic or emotional cluster (Widiger and Rogers, 1989).

The global measurements based on the neuroticism scale indicated the same distribution of personality abnormalities, with the depressed control group having the highest proportion of abnormal results, followed by chronic fatigue syndrome and multiple sclerosis. Subscale comparisons identified vulnerability, depression, and anxiety as traits significantly more abnormal in chronic fatigue syndrome versus healthy control subjects.

An important set of analyses focused on the differences between the chronic fatigue syndrome patients with ($N = 12$) and without ($N = 23$) a concurrent diagnosis of mood disorder. Nondepressed chronic fatigue syndrome patients were similar to the healthy control subjects for all measures of personality pathology. In contrast, the subgroup with a current mood disorder had significantly more personality disorders and prominent abnormalities on the measure of neuroticism.

Two years later, investigators from the University of Edinburgh and Royal Edinburgh Hospital published data on the personality dimensions of 30 patients with chronic fatigue syndrome recruited with the help of a patient support group and from a local infectious disease clinic (Buckley et al., 1998). Care was taken to ensure compliance with standard diagnostic criteria (Fukuda et al., 1994), modified to exclude subjects with current depressive or anxiety disorders. A control group consisting of 20 subjects with a primary diagnosis of major depression was assembled from subjects seeking or receiving inpatient or outpatient care from the authors' academic teaching hospital. These patients suffered from melancholic depression and had no history of manic episodes. A second control group included 15 healthy volunteers from among patients' friends and hospital staff.

Complete data for all three groups of subjects were obtained with the Eysenck Personality Questionnaire, a 90-item self-report measuring neuroticism, psychoticism, extroversion, and lying (Eysenck and Eysenck, 1975). The data collection on patients with chronic fatigue syndrome was modified to allow an assessment of premorbid personality.

The three groups were similar with regard to age and female preponderance. The average duration of the current episode of chronic fatigue syndrome was 5.2 years, while the duration of current episode of illness in the major depression group was 0.8 years. The mean age at the onset of clinical condition was 38 years for the chronic fatigue syndrome patients and 30 years for patients with major depression. Fourteen chronic fatigue patients (47 percent) were taking medications at the time of enrollment; ten patients were taking antidepressants and four were treated with anxiolytics. Fifteen patients (75 percent) with major depression were taking psychotropics: eight were on antidepressants, six were taking neuroleptics and antidepressants, and one patient was treated with lithium.

Patients with chronic fatigue syndrome had significantly higher levels of neuroticism than healthy control subjects, but significantly lower levels than patients with major depression. Compared with the premorbid state, the chronic fatigue illness was associated with increased neuroticism and decreased extroversion. The authors were unable to establish whether these data reflected changes in personality brought about by the illness experience, were perpetuating factors of chronic fatigue syndrome, or were simply the result of biased recall.

The personality characteristics of patients with chronic fatigue syndrome were also evaluated in a carefully controlled cross-sectional study performed by investigators from the New Jersey Medical School, Newark, University of North Carolina, Charlotte, and the Kessler Institute for Rehabilitation, West Orange, New Jersey (Christodoulou et al., 1999). The work represented an expansion of previous research completed by this group and was the first to use a relatively new biosocial construct of personality (Cloninger, 1987a). The study group consisted of 38 chronic fatigue syndrome patients who had presented for evaluation to the CFS Cooperative Research Center at the University of Medicine and Dentistry of New Jersey. Inclusion criteria were a diagnosis of chronic fatigue syndrome (Fukuda et al., 1994); a duration of illness of less than ten years; and no evidence of psychiatric disorder in the five years prior to the onset of the fatigue illness. A control group of 40 patients with a primary diagnosis of multiple sclerosis was assembled from referrals to a specialized clinic at the same institution. For inclusion in this group, the patients had to have been diagnosed with definite multiple sclerosis (Poser et al., 1983); be at least one month after the last exacerbation episode of their illness; and have a moderate degree of neurological disability. A second control group consisted of 40 healthy individuals recruited from the surrounding institutions of higher learning and communities. None of the participants had a history of neurological disorders such as stroke, seizure, significant head injury, prolonged loss of consciousness, or dementia. Care was also taken to exclude subjects with a history of bipolar affective disorder, schizophrenia, and alcohol or drug abuse. Subjects were not included in the study if they were currently treated with corticosteroids or benzodiazepines.

The main data collection instrument was the Tridimensional Personality Questionnaire (Cloninger, 1987b), which measures 12 personality features grouped into the categories of harm avoidance, novelty seeking, and reward dependence. Harm avoidance explores anticipatory worry and pessimism, fear of uncertainty, shyness with strangers, and fatigability and asthenia. Novelty seeking evaluates exploratory excitability, impulsiveness, extravagance, and disorderliness. Reward dependence measures sentimentality, attachment, persistence, and dependence.

The three groups studied comprised a clear majority of females, who represented 87 percent of the chronic fatigue syndrome patients, 82 percent of the multiple sclerosis patients, and 80 percent of the healthy control subjects. The chronic fatigue syndrome patients were significantly younger than the patients in the multiple sclerosis group (mean age 38 versus 45 years). The mean age of the healthy control subjects was 40 years. The groups were well matched with respect to level of education.

Compared with the healthy control group, this sample of chronic fatigue syndrome patients was shown to be significantly more harm avoidant. The difference was due in part to the expected increase in the fatigability and asthenia characteristic of the harm avoidance dimension. However, a significant difference was also noted for the feature measuring shyness with strangers, which indicates the degree to which a person is unassertive in social situations. Chronic fatigue syndrome patients were more shy than controls. Compared with multiple sclerosis patients, the chronic fatigue syndrome patients perceived themselves as having significantly more fatigue and asthenia. They were also more persistent, meaning that they felt stable, hardworking, and industrious despite fatigue and frustration. The authors interpreted the elevation of the harm avoidance scores among chronic fatigue syndrome patients to indicate either a negative mood state or a feature of neuroticism.

The Tridimensional Personality Questionnaire (Cloninger, 1987a) was also used in a study of personality and social attitudes of patients with chronic fatigue syndrome performed by investigators from Maudsley Hospital and the Institute of Psychiatry, London (Wood and Wesseley, 1999). The sample studied consisted of 120 patients recruited from consecutive referrals to an academic outpatient unit dedicated to the diagnosis and treatment of chronic fatigue. To be eligible for inclusion in the study, the subjects had to meet the diagnostic criteria for chronic fatigue syndrome suggested for use in the United Kingdom (Sharpe et al., 1991) and the United States (Fukuda et al., 1994). A control group included 60 patients with the diagnosis of rheumatoid arthritis who were under the care of the rheumatologists from the same medical center.

In addition to the dimensions assessed by the Tridimensional Personality Questionnaire (Cloninger, 1987b), the study also measured the severity of depressive symptomatology, social adjustment, social desirability, defensiveness, perfectionism, and alexithymia, a construct whose salient features indicate deficits in regulation of emotions and cognitive processing (e.g., difficulty in distinguishing between bodily sensations and emotions, and difficulty in describing feelings) and a predominantly concrete and reality-based cognitive style (Taylor, 2000). All patients were also given a structured psychiatric assessment.

Usable data were obtained from 101 patients with chronic fatigue syndrome and 45 control subjects with rheumatoid arthritis. Although composed predominantly of middle-aged white women with long-term illnesses, the groups differed with respect to the proportion of women (60 percent in the chronic fatigue syndrome group versus 80 percent in the rheumatoid arthritis group), mean age (37 versus 42 years), and median duration of illness (6 versus 12 years). Patients with chronic fatigue syndrome were better educated and belonged to more affluent socioeconomic classes.

The severity of depressive symptomatology was significantly greater in the chronic fatigue syndrome group. Patients with chronic fatigue syndrome scored higher than those with rheumatoid arthritis on the fatigability and asthenia subscale of the harm avoidance personality dimension. The individual scores were highly correlated with the severity of depressive symptomatology. Novelty seeking and alexithymia were significantly less prominent among patients with chronic fatigue syndrome and were independent of the mood state. The scores for reward dependence were higher (more abnormal) among females with chronic fatigue syndrome, again independent of mood state. The mood state correlated only with the poorer scores obtained by patients with chronic fatigue syndrome on the social adjustment scale.

The evaluation of self-esteem, emotional control, and perfectionism was the focus of a controlled study conducted at the Queensland University of Technology, Brisbane, Australia (White and Schweitzer, 2000). The patients with chronic fatigue syndrome ($N = 44$) were recruited from the practice of a physician specializing in infectious diseases. Forty-two of these patients met the Australian criteria for the diagnosis of this syndrome (Lloyd et al., 1990). The group included 32 women and 12 men who had a mean age of 43 years and had been ill for an average of ten years. A healthy control group matched for gender and level of education was recruited from the Brisbane area.

The instrument used to measure perfectionism was a 35-item questionnaire addressing issues such as concern over mistakes, personal standards, parental expectations and criticisms, doubts about one's ability to accomplish goals, and importance placed on organization (Frost et al., 1990). A second instrument measured control over reactions produced by anxiety, anger, and depressed mood (Watson and Greer, 1983). A validated scale measuring self-esteem allowed quantifiable insights into characteristics such as loneliness, locus of control, tendency to dissimulate, misanthropy, psychoticism, and neuroticism (Rosenberg, 1965; Shapurian et al., 1987). Finally, a well-established instrument measured social desirability, i.e., the tendency to give socially acceptable answers (Crowne and Marlowe, 1960).

Patients with chronic fatigue syndrome had higher scores on scales measuring concern over mistakes and doubts about actions ($p < 0.01$) than control subjects. They also reported lower self-esteem ($p < 0.01$). On the other hand, chronic fatigue syndrome patients and healthy control subjects were similar with regard to emotional control over feelings of anger, sadness, and anxiety. The authors interpreted the findings to indicate maladaptive perfectionism, a trait thought to be associated with self-critical depression, suicidal preoccupation, procrastination, and compulsivity. Furthermore, they felt that patients with chronic fatigue syndrome "are likely to set high standards for performance and measure their worth entirely in terms of productivity and accomplishments" (White and Schweitzer, 2000, p. 520).

Investigators from the Division of Child and Adolescent Psychiatry at the University of Utah, Salt Lake City, Utah, completed important work comparing the psychosocial dysfunction of chronic fatigue syndrome with that of juvenile rheumatoid arthritis and mood disorders (Gray et al., 2001). The 15 patients with chronic fatigue syndrome (seven males and eight females; mean age 15 years) were recruited from the pediatric infectious disease clinic and from pediatricians practicing in the community. The subjects met standard diagnostic criteria (Holmes et al., 1988), which required the exclusion of previously diagnosed mental illness. Fifteen patients with juvenile rheumatoid arthritis (one male and 14 females; mean age 13 years) were referred from the rheumatology outpatient clinic of a children's hospital. They had no other significant medical problems and had never been diagnosed with a psychiatric disorder. The group of subjects with mood disorders (four males and 11 females; mean age 14 years) was recruited from the outpatient psychiatry clinic of the same institution. These patients had been diagnosed with major depression or dysthymia (American Psychiatric Association, 1987) after a procedure that included a computerized diagnostic interview (Shaffer et al., 1996) and an independent clinical review of the data. The structured diagnostic interview was conducted with the subject and his or her parents, and disagreements were resolved after a discussion with a child psychiatrist. None of these subjects had ever been admitted to a psychiatric ward and none had a history of mania or psychosis.

The main measurements were performed with the computerized psychiatric interview (Shaffer et al., 1996), a standardized parent report of children's behavioral and emotional problems (Achenbach et al., 1987), and a global assessment of psychological, social, and school functioning (Rey et al., 1995). Additional data were obtained with an inventory of depressive symptomatology, a multiphasic personality inventory, an abuse questionnaire, and a school attendance form. The primary parent (i.e., the parent spending most time with the subject) provided family history data and completed scales measuring the parents' anxiety, insomnia, depression, somatic symptoms, and social dysfunction.

Patients with chronic fatigue syndrome missed an average of 72 days each per school year. In contrast, patients with juvenile rheumatoid arthritis missed an average of seven days, and those with major depressive disorder missed 11 days each school year after the onset of their illness. Family data showed that the parents of patients with chronic fatigue syndrome and depression were significantly more symptomatic than the parents of subjects with rheumatoid arthritis. This finding is probably related to the fact that 53 percent of the patients with chronic fatigue syndrome included in the study had relatives diagnosed with either this condition or fibromyalgia.

Four of the 15 chronic fatigue syndrome patients (27 percent) had one or more current psychiatric disorders. These diagnoses were major depression; generalized anxiety disorder and social phobia; generalized anxiety disorder and eating disorder; and attention-deficit hyperactivity disorder and oppositional defiant disorder. The incidence of past physical abuse was significantly greater among the 15 patients with major depression. The severity of depressive symptomatology was statistically similar in the chronic fatigue, juvenile rheumatoid arthritis, and depressed groups. Patients with chronic fatigue syndrome had significantly more somatic complaints than did the subjects with depression and arthritis. The personality inventories were generally similar in the three groups. The only significant difference indicated more conversion hysteria in the chronic fatigue syndrome group. The authors concluded that that the main finding was the high rate of somatization in the chronic fatigue syndrome group. Given the low frequency of psychiatric disorders identified in this group of patients, the results suggested "that personality features play a greater role than psychiatric disorders" (Gray et al., 2001, p. 240).

FIBROMYALGIA

The first controlled investigation of the personality profiles and degree of psychological disturbance of patients with fibromyalgia was carried out at the Presbyterian–St. Luke's Hospital in Chicago, an affiliate of the Rush Medical College (Payne et al., 1982). The participants included 30 inpatients diagnosed with fibrositis on the basis of diffuse and persistent musculoskeletal pain, as well as tenderness at four or more specified anatomical sites (Moldofsky et al., 1975). All patients had a full range of motion of all joints and no other rheumatological or neurological explanation for their illness. The two control groups included 30 patients with rheumatoid arthritis and 30 patients with chronic joint disease, such as ankylosing spondylitis, psoriatic arthritis, systemic lupus erythematosus, and osteoarthritis. Data were collected with the Minnesota Multiphasic Personality Inventory (Dahlstrom et al., 1972).

The groups were similar with regard to age, ethnicity, gender distribution, and education. A clear majority of patients in each group had had pain symptoms for at least two years. The patients with fibromyalgia had substantial abnormalities on the hysteria and hypochondriasis scales. Moreover, high scores were recorded in 33 percent of the patients for schizophrenia, 27 percent for paranoia, and 20 percent for psychasthenia. Compared with the rheumatoid arthritis and the mixed arthritis groups, the fibromyalgia patients had higher scores ($p < 0.01$) on scales assessing hypochondriasis, hysteria, psychopathic deviancy, paranoia, and schizophrenia. The homogeneity of the fibromyalgia sample was established with regard to hysteria, hypochondriasis, and psychopathic deviancy. The scores obtained on the depression scale were not in the pathological range and were similar in the three groups. The data were interpreted to suggest that fibromyalgia patients lack insight; are neurotic, irritable, and difficult to get along with; are unconventional in thought and communication; and are more likely to have a serious psychiatric illness than patients with chronic pain or disability secondary to organic conditions.

The same dimensions of personality were evaluated by investigators from the University of Illinois College of Medicine at Peoria (Ahles et al., 1984) in a study that compared a group of patients with fibromyalgia ($N = 45$) with subjects diagnosed with rheumatoid arthritis ($N = 30$) and healthy individuals ($N = 32$). The work was a direct continuation of Payne et al.'s (1982) research, extended to outpatient samples, to normal control subjects, and to the investigation of social skills and stressful life events. The fibromyalgia patients had been diagnosed according to the standard of the time (Yunus et al., 1981) after clinical and laboratory evaluations that showed no evidence of other rheumatological or posttraumatic musculoskeletal conditions. The rheumatoid arthritis patients met the standard criteria for this diagnosis (Ropes et al., 1958). The healthy subjects were selected from among the neighbors, relatives, and friends of patients with fibromyalgia. The assessment of personality relied on data collected with the Minnesota Multiphasic Personality Inventory (Dahlstrom et al., 1972). The results were used to classify the patients as normal, or as showing a typical chronic pain profile, or as being psychologically disturbed (Bradley et al., 1978). Abnormal scores in the domains of depression, hysteria, hypochondriasis, psychopathic deviancy, and schizophrenia identified the third category. Validated instruments were used to measure aggressiveness and assertiveness (Bakker et al., 1978) and to review life events (Holmes and Rahe, 1967).

Forty-three of the 45 fibromyalgia patients, 28 of the 30 patients with rheumatoid arthritis, and all 32 healthy control subjects were females. The patients from the fibromyalgia group had a mean age of 34 years and had been symptomatic for an average of seven years. The subjects from the rheumatoid arthritis group had a mean age of 37 years. The duration of their illness averaged 6.5 years. The mean age of the healthy control subjects was 35 years.

Patients with fibromyalgia had significantly more abnormalities on the personality inventory than patients suffering from rheumatoid arthritis and healthy control subjects. The difference between the fibromyalgia group and the other participants reached statistical significance for the domains of hysteria, hypochondriasis, psychopathic deviancy, and schizophrenia. The personality inventory classified 31 percent of the fibromyalgia patients as being psychologically disturbed. In contrast, the proportions of psychologically disturbed subjects were 7 percent in the rheumatoid arthritis group and 3 percent among healthy control subjects ($p < 0.001$ for both intergroup comparisons). One-third of the fibromyalgia patients and close to half (48 percent) of the rheumatoid arthritis group, but only 9 percent of the healthy control subjects had a typical chronic pain personality profile.

Patients with fibromyalgia reported more stressful life events than did patients with rheumatoid arthritis and normal control subjects. The difference was due to the high prevalence of these events among fibromyalgia patients classified as psychologically disturbed. Based on the assessment of assertiveness and aggressiveness, the social skills of the three groups were considered to be quite comparable. The authors pointed out the heterogeneity of the abnormal personality features of patients with fibromyalgia, and emphasized the distinctiveness of the subgroups of patients with clear-cut psychopathology as compared to those with a chronic pain personality profile.

IRRITABLE BOWEL SYNDROME

The cross-sectional approach to the evaluation of psychopathology and personality in patients with irritable bowel syndrome was used in a large study carried out by investigators from the Center for Stress and Anxiety Disorders at the University of Albany, Albany, New York (Blanchard et al., 2001). The goal of the study was to establish whether women with this condition experienced greater psychological distress and whether they were more likely to have diagnosable psychiatric disorders than males with this condition. The sample available for this research ($N = 341$) included 238 women (average age 43 years) and 83 men (average age 41 years). A retrospective review of the clinical data established that each participant met the standard diagnostic criteria for irritable bowel syndrome (Thompson et al., 1989).

Psychiatric diagnoses were established with a structured interview, and psychological distress was measured with widely used instruments assessing depression, anxiety, and personality profiles.

Gastrointestinal symptoms were recorded on standardized diaries over a period of at least two weeks.

There were no gender differences with regard to the severity of gastrointestinal symptomatology. The most common mental illnesses of this group of patients with irritable bowel syndrome were generalized anxiety disorder (26 percent), social phobia (10 percent), major depression or dysthymia (10 percent), and panic disorder (7 percent). Somatization disorder was diagnosed in only 1 percent of the sample. Hypochondriasis, mania, bulimia, and alcohol abuse were identified in only one patient (0.4 percent) each. Overall, 66 percent of the sample had at least one psychiatric diagnosis. The frequency of each diagnosis was similar among females and males. In contrast, examination of the psychometric data revealed that the female samples had significantly more trait anxiety ($p < 0.02$) and depression ($p < 0.02$) than the male participants. The multiphasic personality profile provided evidence for increased depression ($p < 0.03$) and hysteria ($p < 0.05$) among women with irritable bowel syndrome.

An important contribution to the understanding of personality profiles in irritable bowel syndrome was made in a controlled study performed at the Changi General Hospital, Singapore (Fock et al., 2001). The authors recruited 43 patients (24 females) with irritable bowel and 20 control subjects (12 females) with organic bowel disorders. The control group comprised 13 patients with ulcerative colitis and seven with Crohn's disease. The groups were well matched with regard to gender distribution, age, marital status, and educational level. The participants were evaluated for the presence of psychiatric morbidity. Personality profiles were established with a widely used instrument (Eysenck and Eysenck, 1968).

Nineteen of the 43 irritable bowel patients and four of the 20 control subjects had a psychiatric diagnosis. Compared with female control subjects, the frequency of psychiatric caseness was significantly greater among women with irritable bowel syndrome (63 versus 17 percent). Psychiatric diagnoses were equally common for males (21 versus 25 percent). Female patients with irritable bowel syndrome scored significantly higher on the neuroticism scale and much lower on the lie scale, a measure of social desirability. The personality profiles of men with irritable bowel were similar to those of their counterparts with organic bowel disorders.

PREMENSTRUAL SYNDROME

The personality traits of patients with late luteal phase dysphoric disorder were carefully assessed in a controlled study conducted by investigators from the University of California at San Diego and the Research Institute of the Scripps Clinic, La Jolla, California (Parry et al., 1996). The authors selected their patients from among 320 individuals who returned a research questionnaire. After a two- to three-month evaluation that included daily mood ratings and weekly structured interviews, the study group included 15 patients who fulfilled standard diagnostic criteria for this condition (American Psychiatric Association, 1987). The control group comprised 15 women matched for age, education, and number of children. This group was selected from among 50 women without personal or family history of psychiatric illness. None of the participants were treated with hormonal contraceptives or psychoactive drugs at entry or during the study. The patients with premenstrual syndrome and the asymptomatic control subjects were similar with regard to age, intelligence quotient, level of education, and number of children. The main data collection instrument was the Millon Clinical Multiaxial Inventory (Millon, 1987). The inventory was administered in randomized order during the follicular and luteal phases. The interval between assessments was at least two months.

Patients with premenstrual syndrome had higher scores on the passive-aggressive-negativistic trait, a category that includes erratic moodiness, frequent irritability, discontented self-image, pessimistic outlook, interpersonal ambivalence, and deficient affective regulatory control. The difference between groups persisted in the follicular phase. They also had significantly higher scores on the borderline-cycloid personality type. The borderline-cycloid category highlights recurring mood shifts (from depression to excitement) alternating with periods dominated by anger, euphoria, or anxiety, as well as disturbances in the sleep-wake cycle and energy levels. The category also includes suicidal and self-derogatory thoughts. Hypomania and psychotic depression were clearly more prominent among patients with premenstrual syndrome than among asymptomatic control subjects. The hypomanic symptoms (unstable mood, impulsiveness, overactivity, and destructiveness) and the features of psychotic depression (disturbance in psychomotor activity, hopeless resignation, and dread of the future) were constant throughout the menstrual cycle. In the authors' judgment, these findings provided additional support for a relationship between premenstrual syndrome and major affective disorders.

The prevalence of personality disorders among patients with late luteal phase dysphoric disorder was evaluated in a carefully controlled study completed at the Institute of Psychiatry, University of Bologna, Italy (De Ronchi et al., 2000). The patient population consisted of 62 women who had sought care for premenstrual symptoms from an outpatient clinic; of these subjects, 49 agreed to participate in the study. The control group comprised 89 women out of 104 self-referrals to the same clinic for gynecological care. Prospective evaluations were carried out over two menstrual cycles to establish that all participants had regular periods and that none of the control subjects had mood changes related to the luteal phase of their cycles.

The diagnosis of late luteal phase dysphoric disorder was based on the data collected daily for two cycles. The structured instrument used for this purpose recorded the presence of symptoms required for the diagnosis, as well as the necessary difference in symptom severity between the follicular and luteal phase of the cycles, and thus allowed diagnoses conforming to the U.S. standard (American Psychiatric Association, 1987). Psychiatric disorders were identified with the Structured Clinical Interview (SCID), a well-validated instrument with high reliability (Williams et al., 1992; Spitzer et al., 1992). A separate interview evaluated the presence of personality disorders with a related diagnostic tool (Spitzer et al., 1987). Depressive symptomatology was assessed with an instrument known to be sensitive to changes produced by physical illness (Montgomery and Asberg, 1979). The Buss-Darkee Hostility Inventory (Buss and Darkee, 1957) was used to assess motor aggression (assault against people, assault against objects, verbal assault, and irritability), hostility (resentment and suspicion), negativism, and guilt.

The initial psychiatric interviews identified major depressive disorders in six of the 49 women with late luteal phase dysphoric disorder. The sociodemographic characteristics of the remaining 43 patients were similar to those of the 85 control subjects. The average age of the participants was 33 years, and they had been in school for an average of 12 years. The majority (more than 80 percent) of subjects in both groups were employed or were continuing their education. The groups were also similar with regard to marital status, as well as the number of children, deliveries, and abortions.

Overall, the 43 patients with late luteal phase dysphoric disorder were given 43 diagnoses of personality disorders. In contrast, there were only 28 diagnoses of personality disorder identified in the control group, or an average of 0.3 diagnoses per patient. Cluster A personality disorders (paranoid, schizoid, and schizotypal) were identified in 16 percent of patients with late luteal phase dysphoric disorders and 5 percent of control subjects. Cluster B personality disorders (antisocial, borderline, histrionic, and narcissistic) were present in 28 percent of patients with premenstrual syndrome, but in only 12 percent of control subjects. Cluster C personality disorders (avoidant, dependent, obsessive-compulsive, and passive-aggressive) were diagnosed in 51 percent of the patient group and 14 percent of the control group. Finally, self-defeating personality disorder was present in two patients in each group. The most common diagnosis was avoidant personality disorder, which was diagnosed in 23 percent of the premenstrual syndrome group, but only in 5 percent of the control group. The personality disorders with the greatest odds ratios in favor of premenstrual syndrome as compared with control subjects were passive-aggressive (odds ratio 8.7), avoidant (odds ratio 6.3), and schizotypal (odds ratio 5.9).

Seventy percent of patients with late luteal phase dysphoric disorder and 20 percent of asymptomatic control subjects reported mild or moderate depressive symptoms. The crude odds ratio of the difference between the groups was 9.2, with a 95 percent confidence interval ranging from 4 to 21. Logistic regression analyses of the interrelations of these variables indicated that the presence of depressive symptomatology was strongly associated with premenstrual syndrome in the subjects 18 to 30 years old ($p < 0.001$). Among women older than 30, the presence of premenstrual syndrome was significantly associated with both depressive symptomatology ($p < 0.01$) and avoidant personality disorder ($p < 0.05$). There were no differences between patients and control subjects on any of the eight scales of the hostility inventory. Neurotic hostility was associated with avoidant, dependent, and schizotypal personality disorders. Overt hostility was associated with passive-aggressive personality.

Investigators from the Behavioral Endocrinology Branch at the National Institute of Mental Health in Bethesda, Maryland, have completed work focused on the relationship between the menstrual cycle phase and personality characteristics of patients with premenstrual syndrome (Berlin et al., 2001). The aim of the study was to determine whether abnormal personality features are state dependent and thus restricted to the luteal phase of the cycle, or represent a trait-linked condition persisting throughout the cycle. The study included 40 patients with premenstrual syndrome, 20 asymptomatic women, and 20 women with brief depressive illnesses occurring during both follicular and luteal phases of their menstrual cycle. The groups were similar in age. The subjects with premenstrual syndrome had their diagnosis confirmed prospectively. A structured psychiatric interview established the absence of other psychiatric disorders during the previous two years. The control group of women with depressive illnesses had mood symptoms associated with functional impairment every month without significant late luteal exacerbation. None of the participants had any physical illnesses, and all were medication free at the time of the study.

The main data collection instrument was the 52-item Personality Diagnostic Questionnaire (Hyler and Rieder, 1986). The instrument produces a global score as well as separate scoring for 11 personality disorders and employs validated cutoff points to indicate probable or possible personality pathology. The questionnaire was completed by all subjects during the luteal phase (days 23 through 28) and follicular phase (days 5 through 10) of their menstrual cycles. Patients with premenstrual syndrome also rated the severity of depression, irritability, and anxiety experienced at the time of personality assessments. The order in which the procedure was carried out was balanced, as shown by the fact that 39 of the 80 subjects completed the first assessment during the luteal phase.

Subjects with premenstrual syndrome had more abnormalities than asymptomatic control subjects at both points during the menstrual cycle. In contrast, there were no significant differences between the premenstrual syndrome and brief depression groups. The burden of personality pathology increased from the follicular phase to the luteal phase only in subjects with premenstrual syndrome. Based on the data obtained during the luteal phase, 33 percent of subjects with premenstrual syndrome, 15 percent of those with brief depressive illnesses, and 5 percent of asymptomatic control subjects had evidence of probable personality pathology. Compared with asymptomatic subjects, women with premenstrual syndrome scored significantly higher on the subscales identifying symptoms of schizoid, schizotypal, narcissistic, passive-aggressive, avoidant, and borderline personality disorders during the luteal phase. Here again, there were no differences between women with premenstrual syndrome and those with brief depressive illnesses in either phase of the menstrual cycle. High scores were noted for both groups on the scales measuring dependent, histrionic, obsessive-compulsive, and self-defeating features. The severity of mood alteration was correlated with the global personality pathology score recorded during the luteal phase in the premenstrual syndrome group. The authors interpreted the data to indicate luteal phase state-related personality changes that "may accompany the nonspecific condition of chronic or recurrent mood disorder" and "may result in symptomatic residua during the otherwise asymptomatic phase of the menstrual cycle" (Berlin et al., 2001, p. 341). The presence of enduring personality disorders in patients with premenstrual syndrome could not be demonstrated in this study, and the authors felt that mood lability, irritability, and social isolation experienced during the luteal phase may exaggerate the perceived personality abnormalities of patients with this condition.

Further work to explore the mood disorder history and personality morbidity of patients with premenstrual syndrome was carried out at the Institute of Psychiatry, Kings College, London (Critchlow et al., 2001). Newspaper advertisements were used to recruit 34 patients with well-characterized premenstrual dysphoric disorder and 22 healthy control subjects. All patients had severe symptoms in the absence of other known medical illnesses or psychiatric disorders. Patients and control subjects had regular cycles and were not using alcohol or prescribed or illegal drugs. The assessment of psychiatric morbidity relied on a validated structured interview (First et al., 1997). Data regarding personality disorders were collected with the International Personality Disorder Examination, a widely tested tool with proven interrater reliability and temporal stability (Loranger et al., 1997).

The two groups were similar with respect to age (35 versus 32 years). The patients included in the study had been suffering the symptoms of premenstrual syndrome for an average of 11 years. Fifteen patients and six control subjects had at least one child. As compared with women without premenstrual symptoms, the patient group had a strikingly higher frequency of psychiatric disorders (77 versus

18 percent). The most common diagnoses were postpartum depression (66 versus 0 percent among the participants who had given birth), major depression, single episode (53 versus 14 percent), personality disorders (24 versus 3 percent), and recurrent major depression (18 versus 5 percent).

The personality traits prominent in the patient group were perfectionism, rigidity, conventionality, and caution. These obsessional symptoms were more prevalent in the patient group ($p < 0.01$) and not restricted to the premenstrual phase. The authors noted that "obsessional symptoms are known to cluster with depressive disorders and may reflect underlying temperamental and biologic vulnerability" (Critchlow et al., 2001, p. 688) to serotonin-deficient affective illness (Hollander et al., 1992; Benjamin et al., 2000).

GULF WAR ILLNESS

The analysis of personality abnormalities of symptomatic Gulf War veterans was performed in a well-controlled study conducted by investigators from the Oregon Health Sciences University and Portland Environmental Research Center, Oregon, in collaboration with the Malcolm Grow Medical Center, Andrews Air Force Base, Maryland (Binder et al., 2000). An important feature of this work was the selection of control subjects, which included patients with a well-defined neurological condition (epileptic seizure) and somatoform disorder (nonepileptic seizure), as well as asymptomatic Gulf War veterans.

The authors obtained from the Department of Defense the list of veterans from the states of Oregon and Washington deployed to the Persian Gulf from September 1990 through August 1991. Questionnaires regarding exposure to hazards and the presence of symptoms were mailed to a random sample of 2,022 veterans, and usable answers were received from 1,119. To qualify as a case of Gulf War syndrome, the veterans had to have at least one of the following symptoms: fatigue, muscle pain, joint pain, skin lesions, and psychological or cognitive complaints. These symptoms had to have no medical explanation; start during or after deployment to the Persian Gulf theater of military operations; persist for at least one month; and be present

206 THE PSYCHOPATHOLOGY OF FUNCTIONAL SOMATIC SYNDROMES

during the three months immediately preceding recruitment into the study.

Seventy veterans were identified as definite cases, and 70 participants formed the noncase control group. The second control group included patients with unequivocal seizure disorder and the third control group patients with nonepileptic seizure. The latter had been diagnosed by electroencephalographic videotelemetry monitoring that captured at least two spells considered typical for the individual's condition. The participants included in the three control groups were matched for age and educational level with the cases of Gulf War syndrome. The proportion of females was 40 percent among the Gulf War cases, 40 percent among noncases, 47 percent among epileptic seizure patients, and 64 percent in the nonepileptic seizure group. Personality assessments relied on the first 370 questions of the Minnesota Multiphasic Personality Inventory administered as part of a standardized battery of psychological measures (Kovera et al., 1996).

Veterans identified as cases of Gulf War syndrome had significantly more personality abnormalities than Gulf veterans classified as noncases, as reflected by substantially higher scores on eight of the ten clinical scales of the personality inventory, including hypochondriasis, depression, hysteria, paranoia, schizophrenia, and social introversion. The comparison of Gulf War cases with the other control groups indicated that the measures of personality were more abnormal among patients with nonepileptic seizures. In contrast, patients with epileptic seizures scored significantly lower on the hysteria scale than Gulf War cases. The data indicated that ill Gulf War veterans exhibit somatic preoccupation, distress about physical symptoms, and a tendency to express emotional disturbance as bodily complaints. The severity of these states was less than that recorded for patients with an unequivocal somatoform disorder (psychogenic seizures) and substantially greater than that of patients with neurological pathology.

Interesting research performed by an interdisciplinary faculty team from the Robert Wood Johnson Medical School, Piscataway, and the New Jersey Medical School, West Orange, sought to evaluate the coping styles and the role of defensive personality adjustments, anxiety, neuroticism, and alexithymia in the expression of somatic distress by Gulf War veterans with a chief complaint of chronic fatigue (Fiedler et al., 2000). The cohort recruited for the study included 206 military personnel deployed to the Persian Gulf during the conflict. Of these, 164 agreed to participate and were able to complete the requirements of the study. After physical examination, laboratory investigations, structured psychiatric assessment, and neuropsychological assessment, 58 veterans with chronic fatigue and 45 healthy veterans formed the final study and control groups. The ill veterans met the diagnostic criteria for chronic fatigue syndrome or idiopathic chronic fatigue (Fukuda et al., 1994). The authors allowed the participation of individuals with concomitant fibromyalgia (Wolfe et al., 1990) and multiple chemical sensitivity. The diagnosis of multiple chemical sensitivity was given to subjects who claimed a time-specific exposure to more than one chemical leading to symptoms in more than one organ system and at least two of four lifestyle changes to avoid exposure (i.e., special diet, clothing, and home furnishings and avoidance of shops and restaurants to prevent exposure).

The 58 ill veterans were diagnosed with chronic fatigue syndrome ($N = 32$), idiopathic chronic fatigue ($N = 7$), and chronic fatigue syndrome and multiple chemical sensitivity ($N = 19$). Four subjects met criteria for fibromyalgia. Thirty-five of the 58 ill veterans had at least one of the psychiatric disorders allowed in conjunction with chronic fatigue syndrome (Fukuda et al., 1994), but no details were made available regarding the type and frequency distribution of these disorders. The subjects received monetary compensation for their participation.

The three main types of measurements assessed personality, stressors, and coping. Personality traits were evaluated with the Neuroticism, Extroversion and Openness Personality Inventory (Costa and McCrae, 1985), the Toronto Alexithymia Scale (Taylor et al., 1988), and the Social Desirability Scale (Reynolds, 1982). The stressors surveyed included combat experiences during Operation Desert Storm/Shield; exposure to contaminated water, air, military debris, and drugs used to combat the effects of chemical weapons; traumatic events during the first 17 years of life; and events perceived as stressful during the war and six month before and after the war. The evaluation of coping focused on the identification of the avoidant style as opposed to the optimal approach based on logical analysis, positive reappraisal, support seeking, and problem solving. The data were collected separately for the ill Gulf War veterans with and without comorbid psychiatric disorders and for the healthy control group.

The three groups were similar in age and gender, but both groups of the ill Gulf War veterans had on average a lower level of education than the healthy control group (13 versus 15 years). The proportion of nonwhites was significantly greater in the group of ill veterans with concomitant psychiatric disorders (37 percent, as compared to 4 percent in the group of chronically fatigued Gulf War veterans without psychiatric disorders, and 18 percent in the healthy veteran group).

Compared with healthy veterans, Gulf War veterans complaining of chronic fatigue had significant abnormalities ($p < 0.0001$) on the three global measures of personality disturbance, i.e., neuroticism, alexithymia, and defensiveness. The differences in the severity of anxiety, depression, and hostility were independent of the presence of psychiatric diagnoses. On the other hand, the neuroticism subscales for self-consciousness, impulsivity, and vulnerability were clearly abnormal only in the ill Gulf War veterans with a comorbid psychiatric illness. The Gulf War veterans with chronic fatigue showed significantly more difficulty identifying and communicating feelings as compared with healthy deployed veterans. Defensiveness was most marked among chronically fatigued Gulf War veterans without psychiatric disorders. For instance, the prevalence of the repressor pattern low anxiety/high defensive was 57 percent in this group, as compared with 9 percent among psychiatrically ill Gulf War veterans and 27 percent in the healthy control group. In contrast, the normal low anxiety/low defensive pattern was observed in only 4 percent of the chronically fatigued Gulf War veterans who had no diagnosable psychiatric disorder, but in 47 percent of healthy veterans. The evaluation of coping styles indicated greater levels of cognitive avoidance and emotional discharge in the chronically fatigued and psychiatrically ill Gulf War veterans ($p < 0.001$). Veterans with current multiple chemical sensitivity did not report more combat or environmental exposure, but had significantly higher levels of alexithymia and neuroticism than healthy control veterans. The severity of neuroticism, defensiveness, self-reported environmental exposure during the Gulf War conflict, and negative coping styles were shown by logistic regression to be significant predictors of decreased functional ability in this cohort.

In their analysis of the data, the authors emphasized that abnormalities in personality and coping styles were prevalent among ill Gulf War veterans and that they seemed to be independent of recognizable psychiatric illness or multiple chemical sensitivity. As a group, these veterans had "a higher stress burden from exogenous war and non-war-related stressors, internal dispositional attributes, and negative coping styles" (Fiedler et al., 2000, p. 533).

CONCLUSION

Abnormal personality features have been amply demonstrated in patients with functional somatic syndromes. The common abnormalities include high levels of hysteria, hypochondriasis, neuroticism, and harm avoidance. In-depth analyses of neuroticism in chronic fatigue syndrome suggest that negative affectivity is a trait, rather than a neurotic reaction to illness. When present, abnormal personality traits correlate better with the somatic manifestations of illness than with the psychiatric symptoms. In contrast, the presence of personality disorders (obsessive-compulsive, narcissistic, dependent, and passive-aggressive) appear to be related to the clinical burden of psychopathology and are considered likely to increase vulnerability to the development of affective illness.

Chapter 13

The Sexual Victimization of Patients with Functional Somatic Syndromes

Victims of sexual assault report significantly more physical symptoms and conditions (Frayne et al., 1999), but usually have normal findings on objective examinations (Holmes et al., 1998). In general population studies, poor subjective health following sexual assault was not related to gender, ethnicity, and depression (Golding et al., 1997). In this chapter, we evaluate the prevalence of sexual victimization in patients with functional syndromes and attempt to establish its relationship with psychopathology, somatic symptoms, and functional impairment.

FIBROMYALGIA

Substantial efforts have addressed the issue of sexual or physical abuse and its relationship with the psychiatric morbidity of patients with fibromyalgia. The first study was carried out by investigators from McGill University, Montreal, Quebec, Canada, who recruited 83 patients with fibromyalgia and 163 control subjects with other rheumatological disorders (Boisset-Pioro et al., 1995). The majority of control subjects (62 percent) had been diagnosed with inflammatory joint disease (i.e., rheumatoid arthritis, seronegative spondylarthritis, connective tissue diseases, or crystal arthropathies). The remaining control patients suffered from degenerative joint disease (19 percent) or localized soft-tissue rheumatism (19 percent). Fibromyalgia and control groups were similar with respect to age, annual income, ethnic group, and utilization of health services. Compared with control subjects, fewer fibromyalgia patients were employed at the time of entry in the study (51 versus 66 percent).

Data were collected with a seven-item questionnaire (Drossman et al., 1990). The questionnaire assessed past episodes of genital exposure, of being threatened with sexual intercourse, of having sex organs touched, of being sexually attacked, and of being beaten, hit, or kicked during childhood or adulthood.

Compared with well-matched control subjects with other rheumatic disorders, fibromyalgia patients reported significantly ($p < 0.01$) greater frequency of unwanted sexual contact (43 versus 30 percent), sexual abuse during childhood (37 versus 22 percent), sexual abuse during both childhood and adulthood (17 versus 6 percent), and physical abuse (18 versus 4 percent). A history of both sexual and physical abuse was identified in 17 percent of fibromyalgia patients, but in only 4 percent of control subjects ($p < 0.001$). The majority of these episodes had never been revealed to any agency or individual. The findings were interpreted to suggest that the psychological stress produced by sexual or physical abuse might contribute to the etiology of the pain symptoms of fibromyalgia.

A similar design was used by researchers from the Medical College of Wisconsin (Taylor et al., 1995). The authors obtained the participation of 82 female subjects; 40 had been diagnosed with fibromyalgia by the staff of the Rheumatology Division, and 42 were control subjects without major medical problems or evidence of connective tissue disorders. The fibromyalgia patients were somewhat older (46 versus 41 years) and more likely to be unemployed (42 versus 12 percent) than the control subjects. The groups were similar with regard to ethnic origin, marital status, and educational level.

Data regarding sexual abuse were collected with a five-item questionnaire adapted from the source (Drossman et al., 1990) used by Boisset-Pioro and her colleagues (1995). The frequency, duration, and degree of violence of sexual abuse were also recorded.

A history of sexual abuse was documented in 65 percent of patients with fibromyalgia and 52 percent of control subjects. The abuse consisted of sexual exposure (50 versus 36 percent), being forced to touch another's sex organs (50 versus 29 percent), having genitals touched by another (33 versus 17 percent), unwanted sexual intercourse (26 versus 14 percent), and being threatened with sexual intercourse (23 versus 19 percent). The frequency and severity of each type of abuse were similar in the two groups. A direct comparison of the fibromyalgia patients with ($N = 26$) and without ($N = 14$) a history of sexual abuse indicated that the abused patients were more likely to report feeling depressed (100 versus 57 percent), waking sluggish and tired (100 versus 79 percent), experiencing fatigue even with rest (100 versus 50 percent), suffering from abdominal cramping (88 versus 57 percent), complaining of numbness or tingling (88 versus 57 percent), having episodes of sudden weakness or faintness (77 versus 56 percent), and reporting unexplained weight changes (48 versus 7 percent). Overall, abused fibromyalgia patients reported significantly poorer health, more physical symptoms, greater severity of pain symptoms, and greater levels of recreational and social impairment. Although a causal link between sexual abuse and fibromyalgia could not be established, the authors felt that the main differences between abused and nonabused fibromyalgia patients reflected symptoms of depression (i.e., dysphoria, weight change, and fatigue).

A comprehensive evaluation of physical and emotional victimization of patients with fibromyalgia was conducted at the University of Washington, Seattle (Walker et al., 1997). The investigators sought to determine the prevalence of abuse and its relationship with other distressing interpersonal traumas and with the levels of dissociation and functional disability. The study compared consecutive series of 36 patients with fibromyalgia and 33 patients with rheumatoid arthritis. Patients with rheumatoid arthritis were older and more likely to be currently married than were patients with fibromyalgia. The main data collection instrument was the Child Maltreatment Interview (Briere, 1992a), which employs a semistructured format to detect abuse, neglect, parental unavailability, parental incapacitation by drugs or mental illness, and the subjects' reaction to maltreatment. A group of questions were added to assess unwanted physical or sexual experiences during adulthood. Dimensional trauma measurements were made with the Childhood Trauma Questionnaire (Bernstein et al., 1994). Self-report instruments with known reliability were used to measure dissociation (Carlson et al., 1993) and neuroticism (Costa and McCrae, 1980).

Patients with fibromyalgia had a higher prevalence of victimization by sexual and physical abuse (92 versus 67 percent, $p < 0.01$). The most striking difference between groups involved sexual assault with penetration, which was reported by 67 percent of patients with fibromyalgia, but only 23 percent of patients with rheumatoid arthritis ($p < 0.001$). Childhood sexual abuse involving penetration was also more common in the fibromyalgia group (33 versus 13 percent, $p < 0.06$). The prevalence of rape occurring both during childhood and adulthood was higher in the fibromyalgia group (25 versus 6 percent, $p < 0.05$). Compared with rheumatoid arthritis patients, the fibromyalgia patients were significantly more likely to report physical abuse during childhood (42 versus 17 percent, $p < 0.05$) and adulthood (47 versus 17 percent). Fibromyalgia patients reported more instances of emotional abuse, less parental psychological availability, more childhood unhappiness, and higher dissociation scores. The groups were similar with regard to neuroticism, coping, and illness appraisal. Further analyses pointed out the fact that physical abuse and rape occurring during adulthood had a specific and robust association with fibromyalgia, but not with rheumatoid arthritis. Moreover, the overall level of childhood abuse correlated highly with the physical disability perceived by fibromyalgia sufferers. The data were thought to indicate that childhood maltreatment leads to medically unexplained symptoms because "for many women this may be an acceptable method of indirectly obtaining care for their traumatic experiences" (Walker et al., 1997, p. 576). The victimization was also considered a contributing factor to a high level of self-assessed physical limitation and poorer response to treatment.

The fourth investigation exploring the link between sexual abuse and psychopathology in fibromyalgia was performed at the University of Alabama, Birmingham (Alexander et al., 1998). The authors recruited 75 women who had been diagnosed with fibromyalgia after being evaluated by the staff of the outpatient rheumatology clinic. Criteria for inclusion were age between 18 and 65 and the absence of other rheumatic disorders or chronic fatigue syndrome. The assessment of sexual and physical abuse relied on a seven-item interview similar to that used by Boisset-Pioro and colleagues (1995). Psychiatric disorders were identified with the computerized version of the Diagnostic Interview Schedule (Blouin et al., 1988). Self-administered questionnaires measured the severity of pain and fatigue, health-related quality of life, coping strategies, and daily environmental stress. Objective evaluations with a dolorimeter assessed the threshold for perceiving pain at 10 musculoskeletal sites.

Forty-three of the 75 fibromyalgia patients (57 percent) had a history of sexual or physical abuse. Of those abused, 31 (72 percent) had had their sexual organs touched against their will, 31 (72 percent) had been threatened with sex, 27 (63 percent) reported forced sexual relations, 15 (35 percent) had been the victim of exposure of sex organs during their childhood, 14 (33 percent) had been forced to touch the genitals of another person, 12 (28 percent) had been physically abused during childhood, and five (12 percent) had been physically abused after the age of 18. The abuse was exclusively physical in 7 percent of the 43 fibromyalgia patients. The abusive episodes occurred only during childhood in 47 percent and only during adulthood in 20 percent of patients.

The abused and nonabused fibromyalgia patient groups were similar with regard to age (45 versus 49 years), education (13 years in both groups), and duration of illness (7.7 versus 5.8 years). A number of psychiatric diagnoses were significantly more common among the abused fibromyalgia patients, including post-traumatic stress disorder (49 versus 9 percent, $p = 0.0003$), dysthymia (42 versus 9 percent, $p = 0.002$), somatization disorder (40 versus 6 percent, $p = 0.001$), agoraphobia (28 versus 3 percent, $p = 0.005$), alcohol abuse (19 versus 0 percent, $p = 0.02$), prescription drug abuse (16 versus 0 percent, $p = 0.02$), and bipolar disorder (16 versus 0 percent, $p = 0.02$). The psychiatric disorders with similar frequency in the two groups (abused and nonabused) were major depression (33 versus 22 percent), panic disorder (23 versus 13 percent), and bulimia nervosa (14 versus 16 percent). The average number of lifetime psychiatric diagnoses was much higher in the abused group (4 versus 1.4, $p = 0.001$).

Compared with nonabused subjects, fibromyalgia patients with a history of sexual or physical abuse reported significantly higher levels of daily stress ($p = 0.001$), fatigue ($p = 0.004$), and pain ($p = 0.02$). They also felt that the impact of their sickness had produced substantial psychosocial disability. In contrast, the perception of the severity of physical disability was similar in the two groups. Although pain thresholds were similar in the two groups, significant differences were noted with respect to pain perception. The abused group were much more likely to judge the experimental stimuli as painful regardless of the anatomical site (tender point versus control point) and dolorimetric pressure (mild versus moderate). Coping strategies (i.e., increasing pain behaviors, catastrophizing, and praying and hoping) and pain beliefs were similar in the two groups. The authors felt that "the willingness to consistently report pain is a modifiable behavior that is determined primarily by the large number of psychiatric disorders and high levels of stress" (Alexander et al., 1998, p. 112) associated with a history of sexual and physical abuse.

IRRITABLE BOWEL SYNDROME

The prevalence of physical and sexual victimization and its etiological relationship with irritable bowel syndrome has been the focus of a substantial body of clinical work, which was pioneered by researchers from the University of North Carolina School of Medicine at Chapel Hill (Drossman et al., 1990). The straightforward design of their work involved the administration of a brief questionnaire to a consecutive sample of patients seen in the gastroenterology outpatient unit of the North Carolina Memorial Hospital over a two-month period. Exclusion criteria were age outside the 18-to-70-year range and cognitive impairment rendering the patient unable to understand the questions.

Usable data were obtained from 206 of the 257 female patients seen in the clinic during the study period. The information collected on these patients evaluated demographic and socioeconomic dimensions; ascertained the presence of chronic abdominal or pelvic pain; recorded the presence of common nonabdominal symptoms (e.g., fatigue, headache, shortness of breath after light exertion, and joint pain or stiffness); and established the frequency of visits to health care providers. The history of victimization was investigated with a seven-item questionnaire. The phrasing of the questions was simple and direct: "During your childhood or adulthood has anyone ever exposed their sex organs of their body to you . . . threatened to have sex with you . . . touched the sex organs of your body . . . made you touch the sex organs of their body . . . tried forcefully or succeeded to have sex with you when you didn't want this?" (Drossman et al., 1990, p. 829). The questions assessing the history of physical abuse focused on instances during which the subject had been hit, kicked, or beaten.

The patient sample was divided according to the principal gastrointestinal diagnosis. Seventy-five patients (36 percent) received a functional diagnosis, i.e., irritable bowel syndrome, nonulcer dyspepsia, chronic abdominal pain, or constipation. More than half of these patients (53 percent) had been the victims of sexual abuse. The prevalence of any type of sexual abuse among patients with organic gastrointestinal disorders was 37 percent. Patients with functional disorders reported more episodes of sexual exposure (39 versus 23 percent), threat of sex (40 versus 23 percent), genital touching (37 versus 27 percent), and rape or incest (31 versus 18 percent) than did patients with organic disorders. Recurrent physical abuse was reported by 13 percent of patients with functional disorders, but by only 2 percent of those with organic conditions such as inflammatory bowel disease, acid peptic disease, or liver disorders. A close examination of the graphs included in the publication reveals that the overall lifetime frequency of abuse was at least 50 percent among patients with irritable bowel syndrome.

The evaluation of symptoms reported by the participants in this study indicated that individuals with a history of abuse were significantly more likely to have pelvic pain and a history of multiple medically unexplained complaints. These findings did not appear to be specific for patients with functional disorders. A history of abuse correlated with pelvic and upper abdominal pain only in patients with organic gastrointestinal disorders. The inference drawn from the data was appropriately modest as the authors felt that the higher rate of sexual and physical victimization of patients with functional disorders "raises questions about the role of psychosocial factors in the illness behaviors of these patients" (Drossman et al., 1990, p. 831).

The high prevalence of sexual victimization among patients with irritable bowel syndrome was also observed in a large study conducted among members of a California-based health maintenance organization (Longstreth and Wolde-Tsadik, 1993). The 1,956 subjects were asked to complete structured instruments assessing symptoms of irritable bowel syndrome, depression, anxiety, and childhood sexual and physical abuse. A total of 1,264 participants returned the questionnaires. The cohort had a mean age of 52 years and a slight female preponderance (54 percent).

The symptoms of irritable bowel syndrome were reported by 247 (19 percent) of the respondents. The syndrome was moderately severe in 202 and severe in 45 participants. The prevalence of childhood sexual abuse was significantly greater among subjects with symptoms indicating severe irritable bowel syndrome than among those with milder symptoms and subjects without functional gastrointestinal symptoms. For instance, the specific frequencies were 30 versus 15 versus 7 percent for sexual touching; 22 versus 10 versus 5 percent for sexual attack; and 22 versus 12 versus 5 percent for sexual exposure. At least one type of sexual abuse was reported by 36 percent of subjects with severe irritable bowel symptoms, 21 percent of those with moderate symptoms, and 10 percent of subjects without irritable bowel ($p < 0.01$). Overall, the presence of irritable bowel symptoms was strongly predicted by a history of childhood sexual abuse, history of alcohol abuse, number of nongastrointestinal symptoms, and number of visits to physicians. In contrast, the severity of depression and anxiety did not independently predict the presence of irritable bowel.

An attempt to confirm the association between self-reported physical or sexual abuse and the presence of symptoms suggestive of irritable bowel disorders was carried out by investigators from the University of Sydney, New South Wales, Australia, and the Mayo Clinic, Rochester, Minnesota (Talley et al., 1995). The study cohort was formed by a consecutive series of patients referred for evaluation to the gastroenterology outpatient unit at the Mayo Clinic. All patients were given a clinical assessment by a board-certified gastroenterologist and completed a 46-item questionnaire assessing the presence of gastrointestinal symptoms. The measurement of abuse was performed using the questionnaire pioneered by Drossman and his colleagues (1990) modified to include only items assessing emotional and verbal abuse. Levels of psychological distress were measured with the Brief Symptom Inventory (Derogatis and Melisaratos, 1983).

The clinical sample comprised 1,046 patients. Complete data sets were obtained from 997 individuals. Functional gastrointestinal disorders were identified in 440 patients; 203 had irritable bowel syndrome, 109 had functional dyspepsia, and 128 had other functional disorders. Compared with the group of patients with organic gastrointestinal disorders, the irritable bowel syndrome group was younger (55 versus 59 years) and had a preponderance of females (67 versus 48 percent). The two groups were similar with regard to marital status, educational level, main measures of psychological distress (i.e., anxiety, phobic anxiety, depression, and interpersonal sensitivity), and satisfaction with social support and health-related quality of life.

The prevalence of all forms of sexual and physical abuse was 22 percent among patients with functional gastrointestinal disorders and 16 percent for the group with organic diagnoses. The difference did not reach statistical significance. The distribution of types of abuse was similar in the two groups, i.e., 13 versus 9 percent for sexual/

physical abuse only, 2 versus 3 percent for emotional or verbal abuse only, and 6 versus 4 percent for both forms of abuse reported by the same person. Compared with all other participants, patients with symptoms of irritable bowel syndrome were twice as likely to have been the victims of some form of abuse (29 versus 15 percent, $p <$ 0.01). Detailed analyses indicated that 10 percent of patients with irritable bowel symptoms and 3 percent of the other subjects with gastrointestinal disorders ($p < 0.01$) had been the victims of both sexual and verbal abuse. Patients with irritable bowel symptoms were statistically more likely to have been victimized during both childhood and adulthood. The higher prevalence of abuse was identified in both men and women with symptoms of irritable bowel. The authors suggested that the increased prevalence of abuse leads to psychological distress, which in turn prompts clinical encounters during which patients endorse a large number of somatic symptoms.

The relationship between sexual victimization and psychiatric morbidity of patients was also carefully explored by investigators from the University of Washington, Seattle (Walker et al., 1995). The study represented a continuation of a pilot project involving 28 patients with irritable bowel syndrome and 19 with inflammatory bowel disease, which had demonstrated a significantly higher rate of lifetime sexual victimization (54 versus 5 percent) in the irritable bowel group (Walker et al., 1993). However, the size of the samples was too small to allow for the assessment of a relationship between sexual victimization and psychiatric morbidity. For their enlarged study, the authors recruited subjects from among all the patients seen during a six-month period in 1993 in the gastroenterology clinic of Virginia Mason Medical Center, a major tertiary care hospital in Seattle. The attending physicians staffing the clinic were asked to identify patients with irritable bowel syndrome, ulcerative colitis, and Crohn's disease. A nearly continuous sequential sample comprising 71 patients with irritable bowel syndrome (91 percent of those given this diagnosis) and 40 patients with inflammatory bowel disease (80 percent of patients with ulcerative colitis or Crohn's disease) was available for study. Data were collected no later than two weeks after the visit to the clinic. The instruments included a highly structured psychiatric interview (Robins et al., 1981), an inventory of functional gastrointestinal symptoms (Drossman et al., 1993), and a standardized maltreatment interview (Briere, 1992a). Self-report data assessed dissociative experiences (Bernstein and Putnam, 1986); three dimensions of personality, i.e., harm avoidance, reward dependence, and novelty seeking (Cloninger, 1987); and perceived health status and functional ability (Stewart et al., 1988).

The groups of patients with irritable bowel syndrome and inflammatory bowel disease were similar with regard to gender distribution, marital status, and socioeconomic class. Irritable bowel patients were significantly older than control subjects (51 versus 41 years). Health perceptions and self-perceived functional ability were similar in the two groups.

Patients with irritable bowel syndrome were significantly more likely to report a history of having been molested (43 versus 18 percent) or raped (24 versus 8 percent) during childhood. In contrast, the two groups were similar with respect to the frequencies of rape (32 versus 28 percent) and physical abuse (25 versus 20 percent) during adulthood. They also were more likely to have a history of major depression (76 versus 45 percent), somatization disorder (48 versus 3 percent), and generalized anxiety disorder (58 versus 35 percent). The striking difference in the proportion of patients diagnosed with somatization disorder retained its significance after the exclusion of gastrointestinal symptoms (17 versus 0 percent). Patients with irritable bowel syndrome also scored higher on the harm avoidance dimension of the personality construct. Regression analyses did not demonstrate a direct correlation between sexual victimization and the burden of psychopathology. Instead, the number of psychiatric diagnoses and degree of personality pathology was predicted by the number of medically unexplained symptoms.

Sexual abuse was also more frequently reported by irritable bowel syndrome patients than by patients with organic digestive diseases studied by the French Club of Digestive Motility (Delvaux et al., 1997). The participants were recruited sequentially from hospital-based academic gastroenterology units and private practices, and included 196 patients with irritable bowel syndrome and 135 individuals with organic digestive tract disorders exclusive of malignancies. Two additional control groups were recruited from among patients seen in ophthalmology clinics ($N = 200$) and healthy individuals ($N = 172$). The groups were similar with respect to age, but different with respect to gender distribution, which was predominantly female (86 percent) in the irritable bowel group and male (55 percent) in the organic digestive disorder group. The two other control groups had a majority of females. The data were collected with a questionnaire assessing a history of verbal aggression that included unsolicited sexual advances, exhibitionism, sexual harassment, sexual touch, rape, and physical abuse.

A history of sexual abuse was confirmed in 32 percent of patients with irritable bowel syndrome, but in only 14 percent of patients with organic digestive disorders, 13 percent of patients seen by ophthalmologists, and 8 percent of the healthy control group ($p < 0.001$). The frequency of rape with penetration was 9 percent in the irritable bowel group, 5 percent in the group with organic digestive tract disorders, 2 percent in the patients seen for eye ailments, and 0.5 percent among healthy subjects. Women and children whose parents were in an unstable marital relationship were much more likely than men to be the victims of sexual abuse. Nonetheless, gender differences in the composition of the groups did not fully explain the higher frequency of sexual abuse among patients with irritable bowel syndrome. For instance, the frequency of sexual abuse among male patients with irritable bowel syndrome was 19 percent, a much higher proportion than the 8 percent recorded for the patients with organic digestive disorders and 5 percent among healthy control subjects.

The association between abuse and irritable bowel syndrome was most recently explored in a population-based study carried out by researchers from the University of Sydney, New South Wales, Australia (Talley et al., 1998). The initial cohort comprised 1,500 individuals who had been randomly selected from the list of voters of the town of Penrith, Australia, a community quite representative of the country's population. The sample was mailed a questionnaire designed to identify the presence of irritable bowel syndrome; to detect sexual, physical, and emotional abuse; to screen for anxiety and depression; and to measure the personality trait neuroticism. Of the 1,177 subjects still living in the area at the time of the mailing, 730 returned the completed survey form. The assessment of sexual abuse was carried out with the instrument developed by Drossman et al. (1990).

Ninety participants (12 percent) fulfilled the standard diagnostic criteria for irritable bowel syndrome. The syndrome was more common among females and subjects with lower socioeconomic status. Subjects with irritable bowel syndrome reported significantly more frequent episodes of being threatened with sex (16 versus 8 percent), having genital organs touched by another (15 versus 8 percent), being forced to touch another's sex organs (13 versus 4 percent), and having been raped (15 versus 6 percent). The frequency of any adulthood sexual abuse was 23 percent in the irritable bowel syndrome group and 14 percent in the other subjects ($p < 0.05$). The frequency of sexual abuse during childhood was essentially similar in the two groups (27 versus 20 percent). Individuals with irritable bowel syndrome also reported a significantly higher frequency of physical and emotional/verbal abuse. Important differences were also noted for having been often bullied, threatened, or humiliated during childhood (13 versus 5 percent) or adulthood (11 versus 2 percent); for having been hit, kicked, or beaten often as a child (10 versus 5 percent) and during adulthood (7 versus 1 percent); and for having been subjected to verbal abuse during childhood (18 versus 7 percent) and as an adult (12 versus 6 percent). Overall, younger subjects more often reported all types of abuse, as did women and unmarried participants.

Psychological morbidity and neuroticism were statistically associated with episodes of abuse occurring at any point in life. The association was confirmed individually for each sexual abuse item and for the majority of the other types of abuse. As expected, subjects with irritable bowel syndrome reported higher psychological morbidity and neuroticism ($p < 0.001$). To test the previously established relationship between irritable bowel syndrome and abuse, the authors used logistic regression analyses that controlled for age, gender, neuroticism, and psychological morbidity. The output indicated that the association lost its significance when these factors were taken into account. Further mathematical modeling using path analysis showed that sexual abuse, particularly occurring during childhood, affected levels of neuroticism and psychological morbidity ($p < 0.001$). The severity of neuroticism was the factor that independently affected the prevalence of irritable bowel syndrome in women with this condition. The authors concluded that neuroticism, a personality trait leading to enhanced responsivity to physiological stimuli, might manifest itself in the form of unexplainable physical symptoms.

CHRONIC FATIGUE SYNDROME

A community-based study has explored the frequency of childhood sexual and physical abuse in patients with chronic fatigue syndrome and other chronic fatigue states (Taylor and Jason, 2001). Based at the University of Illinois and DePaul University in Chicago, the investigators used telephone screening to investigate the presence of chronic fatigue syndrome-like symptoms among 18,675 adults. A total of 780 individuals reported chronic fatigue and 408 of them also had at least four of the eight symptoms required by the definition of chronic fatigue syndrome (Fukuda et al., 1994). A control cohort ($N = 199$) was randomly selected from among the subjects without persistent tiredness. Forty-seven control subjects and 166 individuals with chronic fatigue syndrome-like symptoms agreed to undergo a comprehensive physical, laboratory, and psychiatric evaluation. Within the latter group, 32 subjects were diagnosed with chronic fatigue syndrome. The remaining individuals with fatigue were classified as having a psychiatric disorder ($N = 56$), a physical disorder ($N = 33$), or idiopathic chronic fatigue ($N = 45$). A past history of sexual and physical abuse was assessed with a standardized instrument (Drossman et al., 1995).

The frequencies of childhood sexual abuse were 16 percent in the chronic fatigue syndrome group and 2 percent in the control group. The highest prevalence of childhood sexual abuse was recorded in subjects with idiopathic chronic fatigue (34 percent). The frequency of childhood physical abuse was the highest among subjects with chronic fatigue syndrome (29 percent). The intergroup differences did not reach statistical significance.

The data presented in this chapter indicate that patients with fibromylagia and irritable bowel syndrome frequently report sexual and physical abuse. The prevalence of victimization among persons with these common functional illnesses is significantly higher than in healthy control subjects and in similarly disabled patients with organic disorders. Robust evidence points out that prior sexual abuse leads to perception of poor health, increased severity of pain, and multiple unexplained physical symptoms. Victims of abuse also score higher on measures of neuroticism, a personality trait thought to contribute to somatization. Data regarding the relationship between sexual or physical victimization and psychiatric morbidity are contradictory, but the majority of the evidence does not support abuse as a causal factor for depression and anxiety in these patients.

Chapter 14

Somatic Attributions in Functional Illness

Patients' interpretation of medically unexplained symptoms influences the illness presentation and the recognition of psychiatric morbidity in primary care (Bower et al., 2000). Symptom attribution styles and the severity of psychiatric distress have also been shown to be independent predictors of illnesses with unexplained physical symptoms, but not of those produced by well-defined organic disorders (Taylor et al., 2000). Among somatizers (i.e., individuals expressing psychoemotional distress with the language of bodily complaints), the attributional style is stable in middle-aged or older patients and in those with a chronic illness (Garcia-Campayo et al., 1997). In this chapter, we explore the attributional styles of patients with functional syndromes and their association with psychiatric morbidity and severity of illness.

CHRONIC FATIGUE SYNDROME

The first systematic exploration of attributional styles in chronic fatigue syndrome was performed in a controlled investigation carried out at the National Hospital for Nervous Diseases (Powell et al., 1990). The stimulus for this work was the authors' observation that 86 percent of patients with chronic fatigue syndrome, but only 14 percent of patients with depression, attributed their illness to a physical cause (Wessely and Powell, 1989). The investigators recruited 58 patients with chronic fatigue syndrome and 33 patients with depressive disorders. Patients with chronic fatigue syndrome were younger and had a longer duration of illness than the subjects from the depressed control group. A majority of patients in each group were female, and all subjects reported significant functional impairment. All patients underwent a structured psychiatric evaluation and completed questionnaires assessing attribution of symptoms, self-diagnosis, and satisfaction with medical care.

Most patients (80 percent) with chronic fatigue syndrome attributed their condition to a postviral illness or other somatic disorder. In contrast, only one patient (3 percent) with depression made this attribution. The analysis of the psychometric data indicated that 3 percent of the chronic fatigue syndrome patients and 63 percent of the depressed group had severely impaired self-esteem. Similar differences were noted for the prevalence of feelings of guilt (22 percent in the chronic fatigue syndrome group versus 81 percent in the major depression group) and overall severity of depressive symptomatology. The data were interpreted to indicate that the depressive syndrome identified in patients with chronic fatigue syndrome was qualitatively different than that exhibited by patients with major depression. The greater external (somatic) attribution in chronic fatigue syndrome was thought to lead to preservation of self-esteem and to minimize guilt. The authors felt that the somatic attributional style has some advantages, because it might protect the patients from the stigma associated with a psychiatric interpretation of their illness, decrease psychological distress, and avoid depression-related abnormalities in cognition. The negative consequences of this type of attribution include helplessness, decreased self-efficacy, and increased fatigue.

Illness attribution was next evaluated in a study of patients presenting with fatigue to an infectious disease clinic (Sharpe et al., 1992). The work was performed at Oxford University, Oxford, England. The study cohort comprised 200 patients evaluated for persistent tiredness. Usable follow-up questionnaires were returned by 144 subjects one year after their initial clinical assessment. The self-report data included current symptoms, beliefs about the cause of fatigue, coping behaviors, and severity of functional impairment.

Most patients attributed their illness to more than one cause. The common attributions were infection (94 percent), virus (83 percent), and stress (67 percent). The majority (65 percent) of patients was functionally impaired and only 13 percent of patients considered themselves to have fully recovered. The symptoms reported by the functionally impaired subgroup were emotional disorder (73 percent), sleep disturbance (69 percent), myalgia (58 percent), frequent headache (57 percent), and difficulty with concentration (43 percent). Univariate and logistic analyses identified the somatic attribution (viral infection) as a significant correlate of functional impairment at follow-up. Poorer outcomes were also predicted by current psychiatric disorders.

The relationship between attributions and outcome was also explored in a study conducted at the Prince Henry Hospital, Little Bay, New South Wales, Australia (Wilson et al., 1994). The authors had access to a large cohort of patients with chronic fatigue syndrome and invited 139 subjects to participate in a longitudinal study. Outcome data were obtained three years later from 103 subjects. Baseline measures included assessments of immune variables, psychiatric morbidity, neuroticism, and illness behavior. Illness behavior assessed disease conviction or the strength of the belief that the illness had a somatic rather than psychological origin. At follow-up, the subjects provided information regarding the outcome of their illness, psychological distress, and residual symptoms.

Three years after the onset of their fatigue illness, 6 percent of patients had completely recovered and 58 percent reported at least some improvement in their condition. The patients who did not improve were shown to have significantly higher scores for disease conviction. The somatic attributional bias correlated with the poor outcome, as reflected both in the investigators' assessments ($p < 0.004$) and in the patients' self-reports ($p = 0.01$). The presence of a previously undiagnosed psychiatric disorder was the only other strong predictor of lack of improvement. The data were interpreted to indicate that chronic fatigue syndrome patients who fare poorly are "subjects who deal with distress by somatization (presenting physical rather than psychological symptoms) and who discount the possible modulating effect of psychosocial factors" (Wilson et al., 1994, p. 758). The authors cautioned that although the somatic attribution contributed to higher levels of distress, a more severe course of illness during its initial phase may have shaped disease convictions and illness behavior.

The influence of a somatic attributional bias on the symptoms and clinical outcome of chronic fatigue patients was studied in primary care settings by investigators from the Hospital Nord, Saint-Etienne, France (Cathebras et al., 1995). The authors hypothesized that patients' belief about the etiology of their illness impacted on the course of illness, coping style, and emotional response to their health problems. The research was carried out on 231 patients with medically unexplained fatigue enrolled in the study by 65 general practitioners from three French regions. The subjects accepted into the study had no other acute or chronic medical disorders, no evidence of significant depressive symptomatology, and no current treatment with antibiotic or psychotropic drugs. Data were collected with self-administered instruments assessing the frequency of symptoms indicating subjective fatigue, depressive symptoms, and causal attributions of somatic symptoms. The specific causal attribution of fatigue was evaluated with a nine-item scale, which included three items each for somatic (i.e., infection or disease), psychological (i.e., stress or emotion), and normalizing (i.e., overwork or inadequate life rhythm) attributions. The scores on the somatic subscale were used to classify the top 33 percent of scores as patients with the strongest somatic attributions and the bottom 33 percent of the scores as patients with the weakest somatic attributions. The psychological and normalizing subscales were shown to have poor internal validity and were not used in further analyses of the data.

High ($N = 75$) and low ($N = 95$) scorers for somatic attribution of fatigue were similar with respect to age, gender distribution, severity of fatigue, and number of depressive symptoms. The high scorers endorsed significantly more symptoms and were more likely to have at least one other unexplainable somatic complaint. Symptoms such as memory loss, sleep problems, myalgias, headaches, anxiety, and irritability were significantly more common among subjects with a strong somatic attribution of their fatigue. The 42-day outcome of fatigue was similar in the two groups. The data were cautiously interpreted to indicate that in "primary care patients with fatigue not due to somatic illness or major depression, the tendency to attribute fatigue to somatic causes is not associated with a worse [short-term] outcome, but a higher number of reported symptoms" (Cathebras et al., 1995, p. 174).

Three years later, a large community study reexamined the attributional style of subjects with chronic fatigue (Chalder et al., 1996). The investigators were based at King's College School of Medicine, London, and carried out a survey of fatigue in the patient population ($N = 15,283$) of five general practices located in the southeast of England. The survey identified 38 individuals who attributed their chronic fatigue to myalgic encephalomyelitis, a construct that proposes that the symptom is due to an organic cause. The control groups were selected at random from among individuals who believed that their fatigue was caused either by social factors, e.g., family commitments ($N = 38$), or by a psychological problem, e.g., feeling depressed ($N = 40$). The groups were similar with regard to age, gender distribution, and level of professional training. Data were collected at baseline and 18 months later with instruments designed to measure fatigue, psychological distress, depression, anxiety, somatic symptoms, and functional impairment.

Chronic fatigue patients who attributed their condition to a somatic illness reported higher severity levels for their fatigue than the control groups. The difference was due to the perceived severity of physical fatigue. The severity of mental fatigue was similar in the three groups. The duration of fatigue was longer in the group with somatic attribution. Compared with the somatic attribution group, the patients with a psychological attribution indicated more anxiety, depression, and general psychological distress, but similar levels of fatigue and number of somatic symptoms. The subjects with a somatic attribution were significantly more likely than the other two groups to cope with their fatigue by curtailing their activities. The attributional style did not change during the follow-up period. The findings indicated that a somatic attributional bias is associated with more fatigue and more functional impairment, but less psychological distress than a psychological attribution. According to the authors of the study, these features "challenge the idea that psychiatric disturbance explains the symptom of fatigue in this setting" (Chalder et al., 1996, p. 799).

Another population-based study of the role of somatic attribution in chronic fatigue was carried out by researchers affiliated with Edinburgh University and Royal Edinburgh Hospital, Edinburgh, Scotland (Lawrie et al., 1997). The authors surveyed 695 adult subjects with a questionnaire recording demographic and care-seeking data; presence, duration, and severity of fatigue; and physical and psychiatric morbidity. The subjects' attributions for fatigue were categorized as physical, psychological, social, and occupational. Psychiatric interviews were conducted on subjects considered possible cases of chronic fatigue syndrome, as well as on a random sample of subjects classified as psychiatric cases or normal controls. All participants had participated in a survey of fatigue one year prior to the current study.

The study identified 41 new cases of chronic fatigue among the 542 subjects who returned the questionnaires. Major physical or psychiatric disorders had been diagnosed in 18 of the 41 chronic fatigue cases, leaving 23 with unexplained chronic fatigue. A somatic attributional bias was the most prominent risk factor for the development of chronic fatigue ($p < 0.06$). The other risk factors were the severity of fatigue and degree of psychological distress. However, multivariate analyses that controlled for the effect of psychological morbidity indicated that only the severity of fatigue was a significant risk factor for the development of an unexplained chronic fatigue illness. The authors were careful to point out that their findings did not support a somatic attributional bias in chronic fatigue, and suggested that such attribution is more common in patients seen in specialized settings than in primary care and that these explanatory models could be markers of symptom severity.

FIBROMYALGIA

The causal attributions of a large group of patients with fibromyalgia ($N = 56$) were compared with those endorsed by patients with chronic fatigue syndrome ($N = 95$) and control subjects with idiopathic pain or fatigue ($N = 41$) in a tertiary care setting by researchers from the Katholieke Universiteit, Leuven, Belgium (Neerinckx et al., 2000). The groups were well matched with regard to age, duration of symptoms, and occupational status. Patients with chronic fatigue syndrome were more likely to have had a premorbid episode of depression than patients with fibromyalgia and patients with idiopathic pain or fatigue (45 versus 32 versus 22 percent). Data were collected with a 71-item checklist of possible causes of illness. The attributions were categorized as physical or psychosocial.

Of the 192 patients entered in the study, 70 percent attributed their illness to a combination of physical and psychosocial causes, 25 percent believed that their condition had a physical cause, and 5 percent attributed it only to a psychosocial cause. Patients with fibromyalgia were more likely than chronic fatigue syndrome patients to indicate physical causes (changes of muscles or joints, high humidity, inflammation, and accidents), but less likely to attribute their condition to personal psychological problems. Air pollution and influence of weather were endorsed by a significant proportion of patients with fibromyalgia and chronic fatigue syndrome, but not by those with idiopathic symptoms. Patients with premorbid depression strongly endorsed psychosocial attributions such as personal psychological problems, lack of confidence, being upset, being unsatisfied or bored, stress, and traumatic experiences. Having been ill for longer than one year was clearly associated with unchangeable attributions, such as environmental pollution, terrestrial radiation, and problems in childhood. The findings suggested a prominent role of psychosocial attributions in patients with fatigue and pain. On the other hand, patients with a longer duration of these illnesses were considered to "show external, stable and global attributions that may compromise feelings of self-efficacy in dealing with illness" (Neerinchx et al., 2000, p. 1051).

The second study of somatic attribution in fibromyalgia was performed at the University of Leiden, the Netherlands (Brosschot and Aarsse, 2001). The all-female sample included 16 patients with fibromyalgia (mean age 49 years) and 17 healthy control subjects (mean age 35 years). Baseline data were collected with scales measuring symptom attribution, alexithymia, negative affectivity, anxiety, and emotional processing. The experiment consisted of showing three movie excerpts likely to induce sadness, anger, and fear. The subjects recorded their reaction to the material at intervals of 20 seconds during the 19-minute video projection. Before and after the experiment, the subjects completed a 12-item somatic symptom checklist and were asked to indicate whether they experienced the symptoms and to attribute a cause to them. The attributions were categorized as somatic, psychological, or external.

Fibromyalgia patients and healthy control subjects were similar with regard to somatic (24 versus 23 percent) and psychological (29 versus 32 percent) attributions for past physical symptoms. The baseline data also indicated that fibromyalgia patients were less likely to endorse external attributions for past symptoms (32 versus 36 percent, $p < 0.05$). As a group, patients with fibromyalgia had higher scores for trait anxiety, defensiveness, alexithymia, and negative affectivity than healthy control women. They endorsed more symptoms and a higher symptom severity before and after the experimental induction of negative emotions and were more likely than the control subjects to attribute them to a somatic rather than a psychological cause. The experiment did not produce a significant attributional shift after emotional stimulation. The authors felt that their fibromyalgia patients "clearly showed restrictive emotional processing and a predominance of somatic attribution at the expense of psychological attribution" and interpreted their observations to indicate "initial evidence for the existence of somatization in fibromyalgia" (Brosschot and Aarsse, 2001, p. 143).

PREMENSTRUAL SYNDROME

Researchers from the Manchester Royal Infirmary, Manchester, England, have evaluated the relationship between attributional patterns, moods, and menstrual cycle in a sample of 60 women obtaining care from a family planning clinic (Bains and Slade, 1988). The study's hypothesis stated that somatic attributions for negative premenstrual moods would be associated with more symptoms and debilitation. Data were collected with a personal perception questionnaire that presented four vignettes of women with negative or positive moods at two different times during their menstrual cycle. Additional scales assessed the presence, severity, and timing of 34 symptoms.

Somatic attributions were significantly related to the premenstrual phase and negative moods. In contrast, work and personality factors were often invoked as a justification for negative moods experienced during the intermenstrual phase. Positive moods were attributed to personality and external factors. The somatic attributional bias did not seem to affect the number and severity of physical, psychological, and behavioral symptoms reported by this group of subjects.

In conclusion, a somatic attributional bias is present in a majority of patients with chronic fatigue syndrome and fibromyalgia. This bias is associated with increased severity of illness and greater functional impairment. The attributional bias does not correlate with the severity of depressive symptomatology, but shows a relationship with the somatic manifestations of these syndromes and with disease conviction, worry, and irritability.

Chapter 15

Maladaptive Coping
in Functional Somatic Syndromes

Abnormal illness behavior is the central theme of a large body of research work in functional somatic syndromes. The working hypothesis suggests that patients with functional symptoms have a selection bias for illness-related stimuli, which leads to an overlap between three schemas: symptoms, illness, and self (Pincus and Morley, 2001). Such an enmeshment creates symptom amplification and illness maintenance, phenomena propelled by "the belief that one has a serious disease; the expectation that one's condition is likely to worsen; the 'sick role,' including the effect of litigation and compensation; and the alarming portrayal of the condition as catastrophic and disabling" (Barsky and Borus, 1999, p. 910). Abnormal illness behaviors produce nondeliberate distortions, but may also lead to intentional deception along "a continuum from unconscious symptom exaggeration to psychiatric disorders and malingering" (Ensalada, 2000, p. 739). This chapter reviews the evidence with the aim of assessing whether abnormal illness behavior correlates with psychopathology or is an independent feature of functional somatic syndromes.

CHRONIC FATIGUE SYNDROME

The psychosocial functioning of adolescent girls with chronic fatigue syndrome was studied in a controlled investigation by researchers from the North Shore University Hospital, Manhasset, New York (Pelcovitz et al., 1995). The authors hypothesized that the level of psychopathology correlates with family dysfunction such as enmeshment, rigidity, and overprotection. The ten patients with chronic fatigue syndrome had been referred for evaluation by their pediatricians and fulfilled standard criteria for this condition (Holmes et al., 1988). A control group of cancer patients who had completed initial treatment was recruited from the pediatric oncology unit of the same institution. These subjects were asymptomatic at the time of participation and had ended treatment for their malignancies at least six months prior to the study. A majority had been treated for Hodgkin's lymphoma or acute lymphoblastic leukemia and all were receiving follow-up evaluations from their oncologists. A second control group comprised healthy subjects. This group was recruited through a random digit-dialing procedure from the same community as patients with chronic fatigue syndrome and cancer in remission. The three groups were similar in age (range 15 to 6.5 years), socioeconomic status, and racial distribution.

The authors assessed the mothers' ratings of their children's behavioral abnormalities (Achenbach and Edelbrock, 1983) and the children's self-report of the same problems (Achenbach and Edelbrock, 1987). The format distinguished internalized behaviors (overcontrolled, fearful, or inhibited) from externalized behaviors (undercontrolled, aggressive, or antisocial). Depression, anxiety, and somatization were considered to be associated with internalized behaviors. In addition, the study investigated the subjects' perception of their families' flexibility and cohesiveness (Olson et al., 1985) and the care and protection dimensions of intrafamily bonding (Parker, 1983).

The most important differences between groups were noted on the youth self-reports. Patients with chronic fatigue syndrome showed a significantly higher degree of internalization than the adolescents included in the cancer and healthy control groups ($p = 0.007$). The magnitude of the difference between the chronic fatigue and the cancer groups was most marked for the somatization ($p = 0.004$) and depression ($p = 0.005$) subscales. The mothers' reports supported the somatizing tendency characteristic for chronic fatigue syndrome. The mothers did not perceive their chronically fatigued daughters as depressed. No intergroup differences were noted for the thought disorder component of the youth self-reports. The degree of child-parent bonding and family adaptability and cohesion were also similar in the three groups.

Factors influencing illness behavior in chronic fatigue syndrome in adolescents were the focus of an investigation performed at the

University of Washington in Seattle (Brace et al., 2000). Their hypothesis was similar to that formulated by Pelcovitz et al. (1995) and postulated that patients with chronic fatigue syndrome have families characterized by rigidity and enmeshment leading to parental reinforcement of abnormal illness behavior. A secondary hypothesis proposed that the subjects with abnormal illness behavior would be shown to have higher levels of psychosocial disability and depression than adolescents with other chronic diseases.

The initial cohort consisted of 18 patients (age range 11 to 17 years) diagnosed by adolescent medicine or rheumatology specialists to have chronic fatigue syndrome according to the U.S. definition for this condition (Fukuda et al., 1994). Fourteen subjects agreed to participate and ten completed all the requirements of the study. The control group of 16 patients with juvenile rheumatoid arthritis was recruited from among 58 patients who were invited to participate by their rheumatologists. All subjects had to have been symptomatic during the six months prior to entering the study, have no other chronic illnesses, and match the chronic fatigue patients for age, gender, and socioeconomic status. A matched healthy control group of 14 teenagers was recruited by pediatricians or volunteer workers affiliated with the children's hospital where this research was performed.

All subjects were white and 75 percent were female. Family reinforcement was measured with an instrument assessing adaptability/rigidity and family cohesion/enmeshment (Olson et al., 1982). Parental reinforcement of illness behavior was assessed with an inventory of activities such as telling other family members to be attentive with the patient or allowing her to stay home from school when feeling sick (Walker and Zeman, 1992). The presence and severity of depressive symptomatology was evaluated with an age-specific scale (Poznanski et al., 1984). The internalization of symptoms, reflecting evidence of anxiety, depression, somatization, and withdrawal, was measured with a validated child behavior checklist (Achenbach and Edelbrock, 1983). Finally, psychosocial and academic functioning were recorded with a structured instrument (Achenbach and Edelbrock, 1987).

Subjects with chronic fatigue syndrome were significantly more depressed than healthy subjects and teens with juvenile rheumatoid arthritis. As assessed by structured interviews, the difference remained highly significant ($p < 0.0001$) after the somatic symptoms were excluded from the calculation of the severity of depression. The illness behavior encouragement scores were significantly higher for patients with chronic fatigue syndrome. Other measures of the family contribution to illness behavior indicated no significant differences for family type, adaptability, and cohesion. Psychosocial functioning was the poorest among teenagers with chronic fatigue syndrome, as reflected by the fact that they had missed an average of 40 days of school during the previous six months, as compared with ten days for the juvenile arthritis group. The healthy control group subjects missed an average of three days of school. Similar differences were observed in the area of social competence. The authors' interpretation of the findings highlighted the fact that the families of teenagers with juvenile rheumatoid arthritis "expected symptoms to be a normal part of the teen's life and expected the teen to cope when symptoms occurred" (Brace et al., 2000, p. 336). In contrast, family members of teens with chronic fatigue syndrome appeared to be more concerned and encouraged maladaptive coping with illness.

An equally interesting line of inquiry was pursued by a group of investigators from the King's College Hospital, London (Cope et al., 1996). Their study focused on a cohort of 618 individuals given a diagnosis of viral illness in an outpatient general practice setting. All patients were assessed for psychiatric morbidity with a brief structured instrument (Hansen and Jacobsen, 1989) and had their illness attribution recorded with the Symptom Interpretation Questionnaire (Robbins and Kirmayer, 1991). Six months after their illness, they were sent a questionnaire assessing the presence and severity of fatigue. Eighty-eight of the 502 respondents were classified as having severe and persistent fatigue and were invited to participate in the study. Sixty-four chronic fatigue subjects accepted the offer and were then matched by gender and age with the next nonfatigued subject from the initial cohort. Twenty-three subjects (39 percent) with persistent tiredness fulfilled the British operational criteria for the diagnosis of chronic fatigue syndrome (Sharpe et al., 1991). The chronic fatigue and control subjects were assessed with instruments designed to quantify the duration, characteristics (mental versus physical), and impact of fatigue; psychiatric and somatic symptomatology; personal and family psychiatric history; and perception of stresses and supports. Data regarding beliefs in factors influencing health were collected with the Multidimensional Health Locus of Control (Wallston et al., 1978). The Ways of Coping Questionnaire (Folkman et al., 1986) was used to pinpoint strategies adopted in response to stressful conditions.

The chronic fatigue and nonfatigued control groups comprised 50 females and 14 males each. The mean age was 31 years in both groups. The groups were also similar with respect to socioeconomic status and level of education. Fifty-two of the chronic fatigue cases and 55 nonfatigued control subjects were employed. Fatigue was considered a problem by 95 percent of the cases, but only by 16 percent of the control subjects. Slightly more than half of the cases (53 percent) and 12 percent of the control group had recently consulted their general practitioner for fatigue.

The mental and physical fatigue experienced by chronic fatigue cases was significantly worse than that reported by the control subjects ($p < 0.001$). The onset of fatigue was described as gradual by 67 percent of the cases. At the time of the study, the symptom was getting better in 17 percent, getting worse in 6 percent, and staying at the same level in 77 percent of the subjects with postviral chronic fatigue. A substantial majority of the cases indicated that their fatigue had interfered with their work performance (75 percent), social functioning (86 percent), and sexual activity (52 percent). The subjects with chronic fatigue had experienced more physical symptoms, more painful conditions (e.g., dysmenorrhea, low back pain, migraine, and irritable bowel syndrome), and had visited their physician more often than the subjects from the control group ($p < 0.01$).

The structured psychiatric evaluation revealed that both depression and anxiety scores were clearly higher among the individuals with chronic fatigue ($p < 0.005$). Similar observations were made with regard to poor concentration and disordered sleep. In contrast, the frequency of irritability, worry, phobias and avoidance, compulsions, and obsessions were statistically similar in the two groups. Thirty-five subjects (65 percent) with chronic fatigue and nine control subjects (20 percent) met criteria for current psychiatric caseness ($p < 0.001$). The removal of fatigue from the symptom list produced only insignificant changes in these proportions (61 versus 13 percent). Fifty-five of the chronic fatigue subjects received a complete psychiatric evaluation and 42 (76 percent) were given a formal psychiatric diagnosis. The most common condition was depression, which was diagnosed in 30 cases. The groups also showed differences with regard to the prevalence of psychiatric treatments prior to the development of chronic fatigue (67 versus 48 percent). There were no differences in the number of subjects with a family history of psychiatric illnesses (50 versus 40 percent). A principal component analysis identified the past psychiatric history as the only predictor for current psychiatric caseness.

The fatigue was attributed to a purely psychological cause by 45 percent of subjects from the chronic fatigue group. A minority (20 percent) endorsed a purely or mainly physical attribution and 22 percent of the group felt that their fatigue was due to both physical and psychological causes. The overall interpretation of symptoms did not indicate the predominance of a psychologizing or somatizing pattern. Similarly negative results were obtained with regard to the health locus of control.

A comparison of the 23 cases of chronic fatigue syndrome revealed a couple of differences. First, the chronic fatigue syndrome cases were experiencing significantly more physical fatigue ($p < 0.05$), but similar levels of mental fatigue. Second, the proportion of psychiatric cases reached 75 percent among chronic fatigue syndrome patients and 50 percent in the other chronic fatigue subjects ($p < 0.07$). The results of principal component analysis showed that past psychiatric treatment or current psychiatric morbidity did not predict caseness for this group of patients. The strongest predictors of caseness were disability status (i.e., sick certification), a psychological attribution style, and the presence of fatigue at the onset of the viral illness. The analysis of the ways of coping demonstrated that subjects with chronic fatigue were more likely to adopt an escape-avoidant style ($p < 0.01$), especially among women. This coping style correlated strongly with all measures indicating the presence of a psychopathological state.

Investigators from the Karolinska Institute, Stockholm, Sweden, have studied the role of negative life events in shaping the illness behavior of patients with chronic fatigue syndrome (Theorell et al., 1999). The 46 participants with chronic fatigue syndrome were recruited from a university-based infectious disease clinic. These patients belonged to a 53-patient consecutive cohort who had been diagnosed according to standard criteria (Fukuda et al., 1994). The nonfatigued control group was recruited at two sites (a public insurance firm and a geriatric clinic). The control subjects matched the chronic fatigue patients with regard to age, gender, marital status, employment status, and type of job. A historical control group comprising 94 men and 89 women assembled six years prior to the study was used for some of the comparisons.

The researchers assessed the presence of 14 events with potential to lead to substantial life changes and the intensity of feverishness, pain, fatigue, sadness, and irritability experienced in the 12 months preceding the onset of chronic fatigue syndrome. Control subjects were asked to identify a difficult period in their lives at about the time of onset of chronic fatigue syndrome in the patient with whom they were matched.

The common life events (i.e., those with a prevalence of at least 10 percent per year) reported by chronic fatigue patients and healthy matched control subjects were increased responsibility at work (63 versus 54 percent), change of job (46 versus 38 percent), residential move (26 versus 17 percent), conflict at work (24 versus 15 percent), marital separation (24 versus 15 percent), conflict with spouse (22 versus 29 percent), deteriorated financial situation (17 versus 22 percent), conflict with close relative or friend (15 versus 15 percent), and new child (11 versus 4 percent). Compared with the sample of the general population, two of the 14 variables were found to be significantly higher in the chronic fatigue syndrome group, i.e., increased responsibility at work (63 versus 26 percent) and marital separation (24 versus 5 percent). The analysis of the temporal distribution of negative life events indicated a substantial difference between chronic fatigue syndrome patients and healthy control subjects. For the four-month period preceding the onset of chronic fatigue syndrome, the prevalence ratio for negative events was 90 percent greater in the chronic fatigue syndrome group.

Patients with chronic fatigue syndrome recalled experiencing fatigue, pain, and feverishness four to ten months prior to the onset of their illness. The self-scored severity of these symptoms was significantly greater than in the healthy control group. Both groups reported substantial worsening in the level of fatigue during the three months preceding the peak of crisis engendered by negative life events or the clinical onset of the syndrome. In the chronic fatigue syndrome group, the severity of fatigue abated only slightly during the following year. In contrast, in the healthy control group the level of energy returned to baseline after approximately six months. The same pattern was observed for the symptoms of pain and feverishness ($p <$ 0.001). The symptoms of sadness and irritability were equally prominent prior to the onset of chronic fatigue syndrome or the contemporary negative life event in the control group. The mood symptoms became significantly more severe at the onset of chronic fatigue syndrome and their severity remained high during the following year. In the control group, the crisis-related increase in the severity of sadness and irritability was not sustained, and the return to normal occurred over a period of eight to 12 months. The differences reached statistical significance for both symptoms ($p < 0.001$). Of great interest is the fact that patients with chronic fatigue syndrome did not experience more sadness or irritability after life crises.

Investigators from the University of Auckland, New Zealand (Moss-Morris and Petrie, 2001) have tested the hypothesis that patients with chronic fatigue syndrome have a "depressive" cognitive profile characterized by negative self-concepts and distorted thought processes (Beck, 1964). The construct postulated that cognitions in depression and chronic fatigue syndrome are organized around themes of defeat, loss, and abandonment. The associated distortions in thinking include catastrophizing, personalization (e.g., believing oneself responsible for unfavorable events), selective abstraction (i.e., focusing on negative aspects of events), and overgeneralization of negative experiences.

The authors compared 53 patients with chronic fatigue syndrome with 20 patients with major depression or dysthymia and 38 healthy control subjects. The diagnosis of chronic fatigue syndrome was established in accordance with standard criteria (Fukuda et al., 1994). A structured psychiatric interview identified current major depression in 12 and dysthymia in two of the 53 subjects. A past history of major depression or dysthymia was found in 58 percent of the chronic fatigue syndrome patients who were not currently depressed. The algorithm used for these diagnoses excluded from consideration somatic symptoms that may have been produced by physical illness. The subgroups of chronic fatigue patients with and without depression were similar with regard to age (43 versus 47 years), gender distribution (82 versus 86 percent female), duration of illness (9 versus 8 years), and rate of unemployment due to illness (59 versus 57 percent). The control group of patients with affective disorders (18 with major depression and two with dysthymia) did not have evidence of organic brain syndrome, psychosis, substance use disorder, or chronic physical illness. The demographic characteristics of this control group were statistically similar to the chronic fatigue syndrome patients. Finally, a group of healthy control subjects matched for age and gender with the other groups was recruited from the university and general community. These subjects had no clinical evidence or history of depression or chronic fatigue syndrome. The Beck Depression Inventory of depressive symptomatology (Beck, 1976) was used to confirm that the healthy control subjects were not depressed; the average score in this group was 4, as compared with 22 in the depressed group and 12 in the nondepressed chronic fatigue syndrome patients.

The main instruments used in this study measured negative self-esteem, self-perception as healthy or sick, somatic and affective components of distress, patients' beliefs about their illness, cognitive distortions, coping, and disability. These measures explored negative self-schemas, judgments about personal and interpersonal experiences, exposure to stress, and burden of illness as related to social interactions and home life. Follow-up data were obtained six months later from most of the patients enrolled in the study.

The severity of fatigue was similar in all three patient groups and significantly higher than in the control group. With or without a current depressive illness, patients with chronic fatigue syndrome rated themselves as physically sicker than the control groups. They were also significantly more likely than patients with a primary diagnosis of depression to attribute their illness to a somatic rather than psychological cause and to deal with illness by limiting physical activity. Stepwise regression indicated that the somatic attribution of illness was the strongest predictor of the severity of fatigue.

The cognitive errors questionnaire (Moss-Morris and Petrie, 1997) revealed a significant difference in the severity of distortions observed in the different groups of subjects included in this study. On the 12-item general category questionnaire, which tested the presence of thoughts leading to catastrophizing, selective abstraction, personalization, and overgeneralization, the patients with chronic fatigue syndrome (depressed or nondepressed) scored similarly to healthy control subjects, but much lower than patients with a primary diagnosis of depression. Contrasting results were obtained with the nine-item somatic scale of the same instrument, which assessed common symptoms experienced in the context of work, recreation, and family life. On this scale, the chronic fatigue syndrome and depression groups had similar scores, which in turn were much higher than those recorded for healthy subjects. These patterns were confirmed at the six-month follow-up evaluation. The severity of cognitive errors was unaffected by improvements in mood and level of disability. The somatic attribution of illness and the impact of somatic symptoms on interpersonal relationships were the best predictors of disability.

The negative schema characteristic for depression was not apparent in this group of patients with chronic fatigue syndrome, despite the fact that a majority had a past history or a current major affective disorder. Instead, chronic fatigue patients were characterized by an intense concern about their perceived poor health and by a strong conviction that their illness had a physical cause. In contrast with the general nature of disturbance observed in depressed patients, distorted thinking seemed to have a selective nature in chronic fatigue syndrome patients, because it became operational only when they felt that the situation might bring about or worsen their symptoms. This selectivity was not influenced by improvement in psychological well-being, a finding interpreted to suggest that these patterns of thinking are stable traits rather than illness-induced abnormalities.

FIBROMYALGIA

Investigators from the Harry S. Truman Memorial Veterans Center and the University of Missouri–Columbia School of Medicine have studied the psychological disturbances of patients with fibromyalgia and their relationship with the cardinal features of the syndrome, life stress, and illness behavior (Uveges et al., 1990). The authors recruited 35 patients diagnosed with primary fibromyalgia according to the Yunus criteria (Yunus et al., 1981) by rheumatologists practicing at two clinical sites. Twenty-five patients met the study's inclusion criteria, which required the absence of major psychiatric disorder, organic brain syndrome, secondary fibromyalgia, and unstable medical conditions. Forty-one patients with rheumatoid arthritis receiving care from the same rheumatologists were invited to participate as controls and 22 were found to be eligible for the study. The diagnosis of rheumatoid arthritis was established in accordance with the American Rheumatism Association's standard (Ropes et al., 1958). Psychological distress was assessed with the Symptom Checklist 90 (Derogatis and Melisaratos, 1983) and the Arthritis Impact Measurement Scales (Meenan et al., 1980); severity of pain with a visual analog scale and the McGill Pain Questionnaire (Melzack, 1975); life stress with the Hassles Scale (Kanner et al., 1981); and illness behavior with the Ways of Coping Scale (Folkman and Lazarus, 1980).

The fibromyalgia and rheumatoid arthritis groups were similar with regard to age (46 versus 50 years), educational level, and median income. The illness duration averaged eight years in the fibromyalgia group and ten years in the rheumatoid arthritis group. Three-quarters of patients in both groups were at least partially disabled. Patients with fibromyalgia reported significantly higher levels of pain and sleep disturbance. Compared with rheumatoid arthritis patients, the subjects from the fibromyalgia group were found to have similar physical function scores, but were significantly worse with respect to psychological status. Major differences were found for somatization, depression, anxiety, hostility, paranoid ideation, and psychoticism. The groups had similar scores on the measures of phobic anxiety, obsessive-compulsive behaviors, and interpersonal sensitivity. Fibromyalgia patients reported more hassles and considered their life stresses to have a higher severity than did patients with rheumatoid arthritis. The coping styles were similar in the two groups. The analysis of covariance indicated that life stress was a specific covariate for somatization, depression, psychoticism, and global severity in patients with fibromyalgia. In contrast, the severity of pain and sleep disturbance correlated only with the somatization scores.

Coping with illness, as reflected by the feelings, attitudes, and behaviors of patients with fibromyalgia, was also studied in a controlled investigation by researchers from the University of Gothenburg, Sweden (Gaston-Johansson et al., 1990). The authors recruited 31 female patients with fibromyalgia who had been referred for outpatient rehabilitation to Sahlgren's Hospital. The authors indicated that patients with psychiatric diagnoses were excluded. The control group comprised 30 women who had a definite diagnosis of rheumatoid arthritis, had been ill for three to 13 years, and had moderate functional impairment. In 12 of the 30 patients with rheumatoid arthritis, the erythrocyte sedimentation rate was abnormal, indicating active inflammatory changes. Data were collected with a questionnaire designed to explore feelings about self, preoccupation with pain, support from significant others, psychosomatic symptoms, activities of daily living, work situation, work environment, and expectations for the future. The instrument's reliability was ascertained by readministering the questionnaire after one month.

The fibromyalgia and rheumatoid arthritis groups were similar in age (mean 43 years), duration of illness (9.2 versus 7.6 years), marital status, level of education, occupation, and income. Patients with fibromyalgia reported significantly more sick days during the previous year (113 versus 52, $p < 0.05$). Compared with rheumatoid arthritis subjects, more of the fibromyalgia patients reported thinking often about their pain, experiencing pain, having difficulty sleeping, and needing more hours of diurnal rest ($p < 0.01$). Fibromyalgia patients were also more likely to indicate that pain, sleeplessness, fatigue, and headache were having a substantial impact on their daily living ($p < 0.01$). Fewer patients with fibromyalgia were experiencing their work environment as pleasant (68 versus 97 percent; $p < 0.001$) and more felt that their job was physically difficult (64 versus 27 percent, $p < 0.01$).

Compared with patients with rheumatoid arthritis, fibromyalgia patients stated that their pain symptoms had made them feel unsure of themselves (55 versus 13 percent; $p < 0.001$) and mistrusted by others (39 versus 3 percent; $p < 0.001$). Fibromyalgia patients were more negative with regard to their future, as fewer of them expected obtaining or maintaining employment ($p < 0.001$), relief from pain ($p < 0.01$), and better functional ability ($p < 0.01$). The data indicated that intense preoccupation with pain, low self-esteem, and pessimism are characteristics differentiating fibromyalgia from rheumatoid arthritis patients. The finding did not correlate with the presence of a psychiatric disorder.

The association between depression and illness behavior in fibromyalgia was the focus of a multicenter investigation coordinated by researchers from the University of Bologna, Italy (Ercolani et al., 1994). The 327 subjects were recruited from academic outpatient practices in Milan, Ancona, and Siena, Italy. The diagnosis of fibromyalgia was established in accordance with the Yunus criteria (Yunus et al., 1981). The mean age of the sample was 42 years, and 87 percent of the subjects were female. The presence and severity of depression were assessed with the Center for Epidemiologic Studies Depression Scale (CES-D), an extensively validated 20-item instrument designed for general populations (Radloff, 1977; Farmer et al., 1988). Illness behavior was assessed with a standard self-administered 62-item questionnaire (Pilowsky and Spence, 1975) measuring levels of hypochondriasis, disease conviction, somatic versus psychological focusing, affective inhibition, affective disturbance, denial, and irritability. The authors' assumption was that maladaptive coping is demonstrated by abnormal scores on three of these scales: disease conviction (i.e., an intense belief that a physical illness was present and rejection of a physician's reassuring statements to the contrary); somatic versus psychological focusing (i.e., the tendency to reject psychological factors as contributing to the illness); and denial of current life problems.

The CES-D classified 78 percent of patients as depressed (cutoff score 16), 49 percent as reaching a clinical level of depression (cutoff score 23), and 34 percent as severely depressed (cutoff score 28). The severity of depression correlated with age. The illness behavior questionnaire produced abnormal scores for disease conviction, somatic focusing, and denial. Of the seven dimensions of illness behavior, two (disease conviction and irritability) showed a positive correlation with age. The study identified a strong correlation between the severity of the depressive symptomatology and disease conviction, denial, and irritability. Disease conviction and denial were considered to contribute to the maladaptive coping of patients with fibromyalgia and were attributed by the authors to affective and cognitive disturbance. In the authors' words, depression should always be suspected when a patient with fibromyalgia "shows a hostile irritable behavior accompanied by focusing on somatic symptoms, and deep conviction to suffer from a severe organic disease" (Ercolani et al., 1994, p. 184).

The relationship between coping style and the severity of pain and depression experienced by women with fibromyalgia was carefully assessed in a study completed at the University of Medicine and Dentistry of New Jersey–Robert Wood Johnson Medical School, New Brunswick (Hassett et al., 2000). The authors hypothesized that patients with fibromyalgia have a tendency to perceive their illness as a catastrophe. This trait signifies psychological vulnerability and leads to inadequate coping strategies and higher levels of depression and pain. The participants were 64 women with fibromyalgia and 30 patients with rheumatoid arthritis. Eighty-two of the 94 subjects were recruited from a cohort of patients who had received or were currently receiving care from the university's rheumatology clinic. The other participants were recruited with the help of local support groups for patients with arthritis or through newspaper advertisements. The patients' diagnostic classifications were made in accordance with standard criteria for fibromyalgia (Wolfe et al., 1990) and rheumatoid arthritis (Arnett et al., 1988). The fibromyalgia and rheumatoid arthritis groups were similar with regard to age, years of education, marital status, and socioeconomic class. The duration of illness was significantly shorter in the fibromyalgia group (five versus ten years).

The pain-related coping strategies assessed in the study were diverting attention, reinterpreting pain sensations, coping self-statements, ignoring pain-sensations, praying or hoping, increasing activities, pain behaviors, and catastrophizing. The data were collected with an extensively validated 48-item checklist (Rosenstiel and Keefe, 1983; Keefe et al., 1989; Swartzman et al., 1994). The catastrophizing coping was identified by the subject's endorsements of statements indicating that the illness was awful and overwhelming; that she was worrying all the time about whether the suffering would get better or end; and that she could not go on. Pain was measured with scales assessing its severity and the magnitude of its sensory, affective, and evaluative dimensions (Melzack, 1975). Finally, depression was assessed with an improved version of an extensively used self-scored instrument (Beck et al., 1996). Statistical analyses considered catastrophizing and depression as predictor variables and pain as the principal dependent variable.

The severity of pain experienced by patients with fibromyalgia was similar to that reported by rheumatoid arthritis patients. The depression inventory indicated that fibromyalgia patients were significantly more depressed than patients with rheumatoid arthritis with comparable pain severity ($p < 0.02$). The difference was particularly obvious in the cognitive domain ($p < 0.01$). Close to 44 percent of subjects from the fibromyalgia group, but only 19 percent of the rheumatoid arthritis group, were classified as moderately to severely depressed. This difference was also reflected in the proportion of patients reporting suicidal ideation within two weeks prior to the assessment (34 versus 13 percent).

The analysis of coping strategies indicated that catastrophizing was significantly more prevalent among fibromyalgia patients ($p <$

0.02). Analyses of coping and pain showed that catastrophizing correlated with the severity of pain and depression in the fibromyalgia group. Catastrophizing patients with fibromyalgia relied on praying and hoping, while rheumatoid arthritis patients relied significantly more often on reinterpreting pain sensation.

The regression analysis indicated that depression explained 30 percent and catastrophizing 27 percent of the variance in the severity of pain ($p < 0.0001$ for both values). In contrast, duration of illness accounted for only 1 percent of the observed variance. The relationship between depression and maladaptive coping characterized by catastrophizing was significantly greater in the fibromyalgia group. The authors suggested that catastrophizing might be related to the illness experience of patients with fibromyalgia. The need to be taken seriously renders "adamant vocalization the only option for effective communication" (Hassett et al., 2000, p. 2498). Alternatively, a coping style dominated by catastrophic interpretations of events could be produced by negative cognition associated with the depressive syndrome often present in these patients.

A later investigation of the way in which patients with fibromyalgia cope with stressful events was conducted at Arizona State University (Davis et al., 2001). The work comprised a cross-sectional study of coping behaviors and an experimental manipulation of negative mood and stress.

The sample selected for the first study ($N = 50$) consisted of women who had received a clinical diagnosis of fibromyalgia. A control group ($N = 51$) included female patients with a diagnosis of osteoarthritis. Twenty-nine of these patients were scheduled to have total knee replacement surgery. Measurements included assessments of pain and functioning, social relationships, social support, affect, interpersonal sensitivity, and emotionality. Coping was tested with a modified version of the Vanderbilt Multidimensional Pain Coping Inventory (Smith et al., 1997). Based on previous work at their institution (Zautra et al., 1999), the authors used the instrument to identify three coping behaviors: active coping (e.g., positive reappraisal, problem solving, and stoicism), avoidant coping (e.g., catastrophizing, wishful thinking, mental disengagement, and self-isolation), and coping through social relationships (i.e., venting and social support).

For the study involving the experimental manipulation of stress and mood, the authors recruited 20 patients with fibromyalgia and 21 age-matched women with osteoarthritis. The subjects were randomly assigned to negative mood induction or to resting control. Reading a text describing a sad situation and then imagining oneself in that situation obtained the negative mood. The subjects were then asked to describe and discuss a recent conflict with a family member, friend, or physician. This portion of the experiment aimed to re-create the feelings experienced at the time of the conflict, and thus produce a stress stimulus. Physiological measures (i.e., heart rate and blood pressure) were performed throughout the experiment. Measures for pain, fatigue, and affect were carried out at baseline, at the end of the experiment, and after a ten-minute recovery period.

The fibromyalgia and osteoarthritis patients participating in the cross-sectional study were similar in age, educational level, marital status, and ethnic background. The proportion of subjects currently employed ranged from 22 percent in the fibromyalgia group to 31 percent in the surgical group. The fibromyalgia group rated their overall health status as poorer than the two osteoarthritis groups. The self-assessed severity of pain was similar in the fibromyalgia and the surgical osteoarthritis groups, and substantially greater than the pain experienced by the remaining osteoarthritis patients. A most important difference was the fact that patients with fibromyalgia had significantly lower levels of positive affect. They also indicated more emotional disturbance and were more likely to use avoidant coping than either of the osteoarthritis groups. Furthermore, fibromyalgia patients were more likely to use coping strategies involving social relationships, but reported more negative social ties and had fewer people in their social networks. Secondary analyses confirmed the link between conflictual social ties and decreased use of support networks in dealing with pain by patients with fibromyalgia.

The experimental induction of negative interpersonal stress helped clarify some of these issues. The groups participating in this phase of the research were similar with regard to baseline levels of fatigue and positive and negative affect. Objectively, the two groups had similar thresholds for pain, but the fibromyalgia patients perceived their pain symptoms as much more severe than those experienced by the subjects with osteoarthritis. The mood manipulations produced similar changes in both groups. The intensity of pain and fatigue experienced during the session correlated significantly with the negative mood condition in fibromyalgia and osteoarthritis patients. Patients with fibromyalgia suffered more pain during the recovery period, a finding interpreted to suggest a prolonged effect of the stressful stimuli. Stress and mood changes were associated with cardiovascular arousal in both groups. The data were interpreted to indicate that patients with fibromyalgia not only experience more interpersonal stress and are less able to maintain positive affect, but show maladaptive coping insofar as "elevations in negative mood may heighten their experience of pain during stress" (Davis et al., 2001, p. 224). The effect was restricted to pain perception and did not influence other cardinal features of illness, such as fatigue and pain threshold. The vulnerability identified by the authors in patients with fibromyalgia "may stem in part from an inability to maintain positive resources during times of pain and stress" (p. 225).

An important component of coping with illness is care-seeking behavior, a dimension well studied in work carried out at the University of Alabama School of Medicine, Birmingham (Kersh et al., 2001). The study used a self-regulatory model of health and illness behavior (Cameron et al., 1993) to investigate the role of personality traits, cognition, and environmental factors in the decision to seek care for the symptoms of fibromyalgia. The study cohort consisted of 118 patients who had been referred to the rheumatology clinic. Seventy-nine patients (74 women and five men) met criteria for the diagnosis of fibromyalgia (Wolfe at al., 1990); had no evidence of other rheumatologic disorders or chronic fatigue syndrome; were younger than 65 years of age; and completed all testing procedures. The control group was recruited through newspaper advertisements seeking individuals with myalgia who had not obtained medical care for their aches and pains during the previous decade. Of the 207 persons who responded, 46 were diagnosed with fibromyalgia and 39 (37 women and two men) met all of the criteria for inclusion in the study. A comprehensive battery of structured interviews and questionnaires was used to collect data from six separate domains: pain, psychiatric morbidity, personality variables, environmental stress, cognition, and overall state of health.

The groups of patients and nonpatients with fibromyalgia were similar in age (46 versus 49 years), ethnicity, level of education, and duration of pain (seven versus ten years). The patient group had a significantly higher number of lifetime psychiatric diagnoses (2.7 versus 1.3, $p < 0.001$). Fibromyalgia subjects had higher scores for neuroticism ($p < 0.001$), and lower scores for openness ($p = 0.001$) and extraversion ($p = 0.003$) as compared with the nonpatient group. Patients and nonpatients had similar scores for agreeableness and conscientiousness. Common stressful events had a greater negative impact on the patient group ($p = 0.001$). Fibromyalgia patients were also more likely to catastrophize and to believe themselves unable to manage the pain and other symptoms of their condition ($p < 0.001$). They had lower pain thresholds, higher pain severity ratings, more physical and psychosocial disability, and greater levels of anxiety and depression ($p < 0.001$).

The best independent predictors of whether a fibromyalgia sufferer will seek care for the condition were anxiety and depression ($p < 0.02$); decreased self-efficacy ($p < 0.02$); stressfulness of the environment ($p < 0.03$); and perceived severity of pain ($p < 0.04$). A longer duration of pain, maladaptive coping strategies, and psychiatric morbidity made a significant contribution to the decision to seek care. In contrast, personality variables and environmental stressors had only weak predictive power for this decision. Abnormal personality variables seemed to overlap with maladaptive coping and thus lost predictive power. The data were interpreted to indicate that "negative affect [trait anxiety and depression] and perceptions of stress are endogenous variables that may contribute to the development of abnormal pain sensitivity in some patients with fibromyalgia" (Kersh et al., 2001, p. 370).

IRRITABLE BOWEL SYNDROME

A collaborative effort of the Center for Functional Gastrointestinal and Motility Disorders, University of North Carolina, Chapel Hill, and the University of Toronto, Ontario (Drossman et al., 2000), attempted to determine whether physiological, psychosocial, or behavioral characteristics predict the severity of functional bowel disorder. The subjects recruited for the study were 211 female patients ages 18 through 65 who had experienced functional gastrointestinal symptoms for at least three months and were symptomatic at least two days each week. Irritable bowel syndrome was by far the most common diagnosis in this group (83 percent). Chronic functional abdominal pain was diagnosed in 7 percent of patients and painful functional constipation in 3 percent. Eligibility criteria required that the severity of illness be moderate or severe according to the Functional Bowel Disorder Severity Index (Drossman et al., 1995). The index verified the presence of the functional bowel disorder, assessed the severity of pain on a visual analog scale, and recorded the number of physician visits over the previous six months.

The illness dimensions measured were pain intensity, psychological distress, presence and severity of symptoms of depression, resiliency when confronted with stress, impact of sickness on daily activities, presence of dysfunctional attitudes, presence and self-perceived quality of social support, coping strategies, quality of life, and history of physical and sexual abuse. The measurements of behavior and health care utilization included the number of days in bed due to gastrointestinal symptoms, hospitalizations, surgical and endoscopic procedures, and visits and telephone contacts with physicians. Physiological data regarding rectal sensation were obtained in all subjects by quantitative assessments of the urge threshold, first pain report, and pain threshold.

The 211 patients had a mean age of 39 years and an average of 15 years in school. The severity of functional bowel disorder was moderate in 68 percent of the sample; the remaining patients were classified as having a severe disorder. The demographics of the two groups (moderate and severe) were similar. A history of physical or sexual abuse was slightly more common among patients with moderately severe illness (57 percent versus 40 percent).

The physiological parameters related to rectal sensation thresholds did not discriminate between patients with moderate and severe illness. Patients with severe disorders reported more physician contacts, more overnight hospitalizations, and more days in bed for gastrointestinal symptoms. The lifetime and current prevalence of surgeries and endoscopic procedures did not discriminate between the two groups. In contrast, substantial differences were noted with respect to psychosocial factors. Patients with severe functional bowel disorders were significantly more depressed, had a greater tendency to adopt a "catastrophic" coping style, and felt less able to control and decrease their symptoms. Impressive differences were also noted for the impact of illness on daily activities. For instance, the patients with severe illness were much more likely to report that the functional bowel disorder had affected their physical condition, eating patterns, and the ability to manage their home. On the other hand, the groups were similar with regard to the overall level of psychological distress, resiliency when confronted with stress, dysfunctional attitudes, and perceived social support. A multiple logistic regression analysis indicated that the best predictors of clinician-determined severity of illness were the physical and eating dysfunction attributed to the illness; the number of days spent in bed for gastrointestinal symptoms; and the number of times the patient had telephoned the physician to discuss gastrointestinal complaints. Thus, it appeared that illness severity was predicted by patient behaviors in response to pain, but not by visceral hypersensitivity or psychosocial factors.

The link between emotional abuse and the coping characteristics of patients with irritable bowel syndrome was examined through the prism of self-blame and self-silencing in a study conducted at the University of Toronto, Ontario, Canada (Ali et al., 2000). Self-silencing is a process that inhibits actions, feelings, and thoughts in order to create or maintain intimate and safe relationships with the downside of devaluation of one's own beliefs (Jack and Dill, 1992). The process correlates significantly with the presence of depressive symptomatology and may indicate a greater vulnerability to developing depression (Duarte and Thompson, 1999). The characterological self-blame is a reflection of low self-evaluation and excessive self-criticism and leads to the inappropriate assumption of responsibility or the feeling that one personally deserves negative life events (Janoff-Bulman, 1979). As is the case with self-silencing, the self-blame tendency is more marked among depressed individuals, in whom it is associated with decreased belief in personal control (Janoff-Bulman, 1979), dependency (Brewin and Furnham, 1987), and loneliness (Anderson et al., 1994).

The study group comprised 50 patients recruited over a period of six months by five gastroenterologists. Twenty-five patients had been diagnosed with irritable bowel syndrome according to standard criteria (Thompson et al., 1989). The control group included 25 patients with inflammatory bowel disease; 18 of these patients had Crohn's disease and seven suffered from ulcerative colitis.

The data were collected with a structured inventory of emotional abuse, which assessed public degradation, deliberate humiliation, verbal threats, being put down or insulted, and being denied economic or personal independence. Self-blame was measured with a random sequence of scenarios describing negative events. Self-silencing was assessed with a comprehensive instrument focusing on beliefs and behaviors related to interpersonal relationships. Other variables included the presence and severity of depressive symptomatology and a brief evaluation of past physical and sexual abuse.

The patients with irritable bowel syndrome and inflammatory bowel disease were similar with regard to age (mean 36 years), age at the onset of illness (mean 20 years), ethnic background, education, and socioeconomic status. A history of sexual abuse was more common among patients with irritable bowel than those with inflammatory bowel disease, especially in terms of having been sexually touched (44 versus 18 percent) and having been forced to have sexual intercourse (34 versus 14 percent). The frequency of physical abuse was statistically similar in the two groups (18 versus ten percent). Overall, the history of sexual and physical abuse had significant power for diagnostic discrimination. Differences were also noted with regard to the severity of depressive symptomatology, which was significantly higher among patients with irritable bowel syndrome. The authors further clarified this finding by noting that subjects with irritable bowel syndrome appeared mildly to moderately depressed, while those with inflammatory bowel disease scored in the range observed in nondepressed populations.

The main results indicated that the study's measures of emotional abuse, self-silencing, and self-blame were significantly interrelated in the two groups. Patients with irritable bowel syndrome reported more self-blame and self-silencing. The severity of depression was not significantly correlated with these features. The findings were interpreted to indicate that the patients with irritable bowel syndrome had been emotionally abused and had developed a tendency to blame themselves and take responsibility for negative events.

Work performed at the University of North Carolina at Chapel Hill has also contributed to the clarification of the cognitive schema of patients with irritable bowel syndrome (Gibbs-Gallagher et al., 2001). The authors hypothesized the existence of selective attention to gastrointestinal sensation in patients with this condition. The phenomenon was believed to be a component of hypervigilance and biased information processing necessary to support the subjects' belief that they suffer from an organic illness. The participants were 16 patients (13 women and three men; mean age 44 years) with irritable bowel syndrome recruited from a registry of individuals who attended lectures about the condition. The diagnosis was established in all cases according to standard criteria (Thompson et al., 1999). Nine patients (six women and three men; mean age 39 years) with bronchial asthma and eight healthy subjects (six women and two men; mean age 34 years) were recruited for the control group. A list of 20 gastrointestinal sensations, 20 respiratory sensations, and 20 personality traits (ten positive and ten negative) was used to create the word recall task. Each subject was shown 30 cards with words or short phrases describing ten items from each category. The cards were shown in random order for three seconds each. Following a 15-minute distraction task, the subjects were given five minutes to write down all the items they remembered. After completing the task, the subjects were asked to rate how often they had experienced gastrointestinal and respiratory sensations.

Patients with irritable bowel syndrome had experienced more gastrointestinal sensations and those with asthma more respiratory symptoms than the control group ($p < 0.05$). Patients with irritable bowel syndrome recalled more words describing gastrointestinal sensations (59 percent) than did patients with asthma and healthy control subjects (28 percent and 46 percent; $p < 0.001$). Similarly, patients with asthma were more likely to recall words designating respiratory sensations than did the other participants ($p < 0.001$). Previous symptomatic experiences were not predictive of the recalled words for either of the two patient groups. The three groups recalled similar proportions of the words describing personality traits. The observed selective recall was considered to indicate selective attention to symptoms characteristic for the illness experience of patients with irritable bowel and asthma. By analogy with similar research conducted in patients with depression (Segal, 1988), the authors interpreted the data as a demonstration of "the existence of organized belief systems influencing perception" and a tendency "to ignore or forget information that is inconsistent with these beliefs" (Gibbs-Gallagher et al., 2001, p. 1133).

In conclusion, the common denominator of the illness behavior in chronic fatigue syndrome, fibromyalgia, and irritable bowel syndrome is catastrophizing, a pattern of distorted thinking that exaggerates the significance of symptoms. This dimension of suffering correlates strongly with the number of functional somatic complaints, but only infrequently with the burden of depressive and anxiety symptoms. Other prominent features of this illness behavior are pessimism, low self-esteem, preoccupation with pain, and self-blame. These abnormalities have only a weak correlation with the burden of psychiatric morbidity associated with these syndromes. Internalized behaviors, including fearfulness and inhibition, and patterns of avoidant coping dominate the illness experience of some patients and correlate better with dimensions of somatization than with the depressive symptomatology.

References

Introduction

Barsky AJ, Borus JF. (1999). "Functional somatic syndromes," *Annals of Internal Medicine* 130(11): 910-921.

Hudson JI, Pope HG. (1990). "Affective spectrum disorder: Does antidepressant response identify a family of disorders with common pathophysiology?" *American Journal of Psychiatry* 147(5): 552-564.

Katon WJ, Walker EA. (1998). "Medically unexplained symptoms in primary care," *Journal of Clinical Psychiatry* 59(Suppl 20): 15-21.

Kellner R. (1994). "Psychosomatic syndromes, somatization and somatoform disorders," *Psychotherapy and Psychosomatics* 61(1-2): 4-24.

Lane TJ, Manu P, Matthews DA. (1991). "Depression and somatization in chronic fatigue syndrome," *American Journal of Medicine* 91(4): 335-344.

Manu P. (1998). "Definition and etiological theories" in Manu P (Ed.) *Functional Somatic Syndromes: Etiology, Diagnosis and Treatment.* New York: Cambridge University Press, 1-7.

Manu P, Affleck G, Tennen H, Morse PA, Escobar JI. (1996). "Hypochondriasis influences quality of life outcomes in patients with chronic fatigue," *Psychotherapy and Psychosomatics* 65(2): 76-81.

Manu P, Lane TJ, Matthews DA. (1989). "Somatization disorder in patients with a chief complaint of chronic fatigue," *Psychosomatics* 30(4): 388-395.

Manu P, Lane TJ, Matthews DA, Castriotta RJ, Watson RK, Abeles M. (1994). "Alpha-delta sleep in patients with a chief complaint of chronic fatigue," *Southern Medical Journal* 87(4): 465-470.

Manu P, Matthews DA, Lane TJ. (1991). "Panic disorder among patients with chronic fatigue," *Southern Medical Journal* 84(4): 451-456.

Manu P, Matthews DA, Lane TJ, Tennen H, Hesselbrock V, Mendola R, Affleck G. (1989). "Depression among patients with a chief complaint of chronic fatigue," *Journal of Affective Disorders* 12(2): 165-172.

Reid S, Whooley D, Crayford T, Hotopf M. (2001). "Medically unexplained symptoms—GP's attitude towards their cause and management," *Family Practice* 18(5): 519-523.

Sharpe M, Carson A. (2001). " 'Unexplained' somatic symptoms, functional syndromes, and somatization: Do we need a paradigm shift?" *Annals of Internal Medicine* 134(9 Part 2): 926-930.

Stern J, Murphy M, Bass C. (1993). "Personality disorders in patients with somatisation disorder," *British Journal of Psychiatry* 163(12): 785-789.

Stewart D. (1990). "The changing faces of somatization," *Psychosomatics* 31(2): 153-158.

Chapter 1

American Psychiatric Association. (1987). *Diagnostic and Statistical Manual of Mental Disorders* (Third Edition, Revised). Washington, DC: American Psychiatric Association.

American Psychiatric Association. (1994). *Diagnostic and Statistical Manual of Mental Disorders* (Fourth Edition). Washington, DC: American Psychiatric Association.

Bates DW, Buchwald D, Lee J, Kith P, Doolittle TH, Umali P, Komaroff AL. (1994). "A comparison of case definitions of chronic fatigue syndrome," *Clinical Infectious Diseases* 18(Suppl 1): S11-S15.

Bourdette DN, McCauley LA, Barkhuizen A, Johnston W, Wynn M, Joos SK, Storzbach D, Shuell T, Sticker D. (2001). "Symptom factor analysis, clinical findings, and functional status in a population-based control study of Gulf War unexplained illness," *Journal of Occupational and Environmental Medicine* 43(12): 1026-1040.

Croft P, Burt J, Schollum J, Thomas E, MacFarlane G, Silman A. (1996). "More pain, more tender points: Is fibromyalgia just one end of a continuous spectrum?" *Annals of Rheumatic Disease* 55(7): 482-485.

Croft P, Schollum J, Silman A. (1994). "Population study of tender point counts and pain as evidence of fibromyalgia," *British Medical Journal* 309(6956): 696-699.

Dubois RE, Seeley JK, Brus I, Sakamoto K, Ballow M, Harada S, Bechtold TA, Pearson G, Purtillo DT. (1984). "Chronic mononucleosis syndrome," *Southern Medical Journal* 77(11): 1376-1382.

Feinstein AR. (2001). "The Blame-X syndrome. Problems and lessons in nosology, spectrum, and etiology," *Journal of Clinical Epidemiology* 54(5): 433-439.

Fukuda K, Straus SE, Hickie I, Sharpe MC, Dobbins JG, Komaroff A. (1994). "The chronic fatigue syndrome: A comprehensive approach to its definition and study. International Chronic Fatigue Syndrome Study Group," *Annals of Internal Medicine* 121(12): 953-959.

Goldenberg DL, Felson DT, Dinerman H. (1986). "A randomized, controlled trial of amitriptyline and naproxen in the treatment of patients with fibromyalgia," *Arthritis and Rheumatism* 29(11): 1371-1377.

Haley RW, Kurt TL, Horn J. (1997). "Is there a Gulf War syndrome? Searching for syndromes by factor analysis of symptoms," *Journal of the American Medical Association* 277(3): 215-222.

Hammer J, Talley NJ. (1999). "Diagnostic criteria for the irritable bowel syndrome," *American Journal of Medicine* 107(5A): 5S-11S.

Hellinger WC, Smith TF, Van Scoy RE, Spitzer PG, Forgacs P, Edson RS. (1988). "Chronic fatigue syndrome and the diagnosis utility of antibody to Epstein-Barr virus early antigen," *Journal of American Medical Association* 260(7): 971-973.

Holmes GP, Kaplan JE, Gantz NM, Komaroff AL, Schonberger LB, Straus SE, Jones JF, Dubois RE, Cunningham-Rundles C, Tosato G, Brown NA, Pahwa S, Schooley RT. (1988). "Chronic fatigue syndrome: A working case definition," *Annals of Internal Medicine* 108(3): 387-389.

Holmes GP, Kaplan JE, Stewart JA, Hunt B, Pinsky PF, Schonberger LB. (1987). "A cluster of patients with a mononucleosis-like syndrome. Is Epstein-Barr virus the cause?" *Journal of American Medical Association* 257(17): 2297-2302.

Jones E, Hodgins-Vermaas R, McCartney H, Everitt B, Beech C, Poynter D, Palmer I, Hyams K, Wessely S. (2002). "Post-combat syndromes from the Boer War to the Gulf War: A cluster analysis of their nature and attribution," *British Medical Journal* 324(7333): 321-324.

Jones JF, Ray CG, Minnich LL, Hicks MJ, Kibler R, Lucas DO. (1985). "Evidence for active Epstein-Barr virus infection in patients with persistent, unexplained illnesses: Elevated anti-early antigen antibodies," *Annals of Internal Medicine* 102(1): 1-7.

Lloyd AR, Hickie I, Boughton CR, Spencer O, Wakefield D. (1990). "Prevalence of chronic fatigue syndrome in an Australian population," *Medical Journal of Australia* 153(9): 522-528.

Longstreth GF. (1998). "Irritable bowel syndrome," in Manu P (Ed.) *Functional Somatic Syndromes: Etiology, Diagnosis and Treatment.* New York: Cambridge University Press, 58-79.

Manning AP, Thompson WG, Heaton KW, Morris AF. (1978). "Towards positive diagnosis of the irritable bowel," *British Medical Journal* 2(6138): 653-654.

Mayou R, Farmer A. (2002). "Functional somatic symptoms and syndromes," *British Medical Journal* 325(7358): 265-268.

Moldofsky H, Scarisbrick P, England R, Smythe H. (1975). "Musculoskeletal symptoms and non-REM sleep disturbance in patients with 'fibrositis syndrome' and healthy subjects," *Psychosomatic Medicine* 37(4): 341-351.

Pawlikowska T, Chalder T, Hirsch SR, Wallace P, Wright DJ, Wessely SC. (1994). "A population-based study of fatigue and psychological distress," *British Medical Journal* 308(6931): 743-746.

Persian Gulf Veterans Coordinating Board. (1994). *Summary of the Issue Impacting upon the Health of Persian Gulf Veterans,* Version 2.2. Washington, DC: Persian Gulf Veterans Coordinating Board.

Sharpe M, Carson A. (2001). " 'Unexplained' somatic symptoms, functional syndromes, and somatization: Do we need a paradigm shift?" *Annals of Internal Medicine* 134(9 Part 2): 926-90.

Sharpe MC, Archard LC, Banatvala JE, Borysiewicz LK, Clare AW, David A, Edwards RH, Hawton KE, Lambert HP, Lane RJ. (1991). "A report—chronic fatigue syndrome: Guidelines for research," *Journal of the Royal Society of Medicine* 84(2): 118-121.

Smythe H. (1989). "Fibrositis syndrome: A historical perspective," *Journal of Rheumatology* 19(November): 2-6.

Smythe H, Moldofsky H. (1978). "Two contributions to understanding the 'fibrositis' syndrome," *Bulletin of Rheumatic Disease* 28(1): 928-931.

Straus SE, Dale JK, Tobi M, Lawley T, Preble O, Blaese RM, Hallahan C, Henle W. (1988). "Acyclovir treatment of the chronic fatigue syndrome. Lack of efficacy in a placebo-controlled trial," *New England Journal of Medicine* 319(26): 1692-1698.

Straus SE, Tosato G, Armstrong G, Lawley T, Preble O, Henle W, Davey R, Pearson G, Epstein J, Brus I, Blaese RM. (1985). "Persistent illness and fatigue in adults with evidence of Epstein-Barr virus infection," *Annals of Internal Medicine* 102(1): 7-16.

Thompson WG. (1999). "The road to Rome," *Gut* 45(Suppl 2): II80-II81.

Thompson WG, Creed F, Drossman DA, Heaton KW, Mazzacca G. (1992). "Functional bowel disorders and functional abdominal pain," *Gastroenterology International* 5(1): 75-91.

Thompson WG, Doterall G, Drossman DA, Keaton KW, Kruis W. (1989). "Irritable bowel syndrome: Guideline for the diagnosis (Working Team Report)," *Gastroenterology International* 2(1): 92-95.

Thompson WG, Longstreth GF, Drossman DA, Heaton KW, Irvine EJ, Muller-Lissner SA. (1999). "Functional bowel disorders and functional abdominal pain," *Gut* 45(Suppl 2): II43-II47.

Tobi M, Morag A, Ravid Z, Chowere I, Feldman-Weiss V, Michaeli Y, Ben-Chetrit E, Shalit M, Knobler H. (1982). "Prolonged atypical illness associated with serological evidence of persistent Epstein-Barr virus infection," *Lancet* 1(8263): 61-64.

Wessely S, Hotopf M. (1999). "Is fibromyalgia a distinct clinical entity? Historical and epidemiological evidence," *Bailliere's Clinical Rheumatology* 13(3): 427-436.

Wolfe F. (1997). "The relationship between tender points and fibromyalgia symptom variables: Evidence that fibromyalgia is not a discrete disorder in the clinic," *Annals of Rheumatic Disease* 56(4): 268-271.

Wolfe F, Hawley DJ, Cathey MA, Caro X, Russell IJ. (1985). "Fibrositis: Symptom frequency and criteria for diagnosis. An evaluation of 291 rheumatic disease patients and 58 normal individuals," *Journal of Rheumatology* 12(6): 1159-1153.

Wolfe F, Ross K, Anderson J, Russell IJ, Hebert L. (1995). "The prevalence and characteristics of fibromyalgia in the general population," *Arthritis and Rheumatism* 38(1): 19-38.

Wolfe F, Smythe HA, Yunus MB, Bennett RM, Bombardier C, Goldenberg DL, Tugwell P, Campbell SM, Abeles M, Clark P, Fam AG, Farber SJ, Fiechtner JJ, Franklin CM, Gatter RA, Hamaty D, Lessard J, Lichtbroun AS, Masi AT, McCain GA, Reynolds WJ, Romano TJ, Russell IJ, Sheon RP. (1990). "The American College of Rheumatology 1990 criteria for the classification of fibromyalgia: Report of the multicenter criteria committee," *Arthritis and Rheumatism* 33(2): 160-177.

Yunus M, Masi AT, Calabro JJ, Miller KA, Feigenbaum SL. (1981). "Primary fibromylagia (fibrositis): Clinical study of 50 patients with matched normal controls," *Seminars in Arthritis and Rheumatism* 11(1): 151-171.

Yunus MB, Masi AT, Aldag JC. (1989). "Preliminary criteria for primary fibromylagia syndrome (PFS): Multivariate analysis of a consecutive series of PFS, other pain patients, and normal subjects," *Clinical and Experimental Rheumatology* 7(1): 63-69.

Chapter 2

Aaron LA, Burke MM, Buchwald D. (2000). "Overlapping conditions among patients with chronic fatigue syndrome, fibromyalgia, and temporomandibular disorder," *Archives of Internal Medicine* 160(2): 221-227.

Aaron LA, Herrell R, Ashton S, Belcourt M, Schmaling K, Goldberg J, Buchwald D. (2001). "Comorbid clinical conditions in chronic fatigue: A co-twin control study," *Journal of General Internal Medicine* 16(1): 24-31.

Barsky AJ, Borus JF. (1999). "Functional somatic syndromes," *Annals of Internal Medicine* 130(11): 910-921.

Bourdette DN, McCauley LA, Barkhuizen A, Johnston W, Wynn M, Joos SK, Storzbach D, Shuell T, Sticker D. (2001). "Symptom factor analysis, clinical findings, and functional status in a population-based case control study of Gulf War unexplained illness," *Journal of Occupational and Environmental Medicine* 43(12): 1026-1040.

Deary IJ. (1999). "A taxonomy of medically unexplained symptoms," *Journal of Psychosomatic Research* 47(1): 51-59.

Fukuda K, Straus SE, Hickie I, Sharpe MC, Dobbins JG, Komaroff A. (1994). "The chronic fatigue syndrome: A comprehensive approach to its definition and study. International Chronic Fatigue Syndrome Study Group," *Annals of Internal Medicine* 121(12): 953-959.

Hudson JI, Pope HG Jr. (1990). "Affective spectrum disorder: Does antidepressant response identify a family of disorders with a common pathophysiology?" *American Journal of Psychiatry* 147: 552-564.

Mayer EA. (2000). "The neurobiology of stress and gastrointestinal disease," *Gut* 47: 861-869.

Moldofsky H, Scarisbrick P, England R, Smythe H. (1975). "Musculoskeletal symptoms and non-REM sleep disturbance in patients with 'fibrositis syndrome' and healthy subjects," *Psychosomatic Medicine* 37(4): 341-351.

Nimnuan C, Rabe-Hesketh S, Wessely S, Hotopf M. (2001). "How many functional somatic syndromes?" *Journal of Psychosomatic Research* 51(4): 549-557.

Robbins JM, Kirmayer LJ, Hemami S. (1997). "Latent variable models of functional somatic distress," *Journal of Nervous and Mental Disease* 185(10): 606-615.

Robins LN, Helzer JE. (1985). *Diagnostic Interview Schedule (DIS): Version III-A.* St. Louis, MO: Department of Psychiatry, Washington University School of Medicine.

Robins LN, Helzer JE, Croughan J, Ratcliff KS. (1981). "National Institute of Mental Health Diagnostic Interview Schedule: Its history, characteristics, and validity," *Archives of General Psychiatry* 38(4): 381-389.

Sharpe M, Carson A. (2001). " 'Unexplained' somatic symptoms, functional syndromes, and somatization: Do we need a paradigm shift?" *Annals of Internal Medicine* 134(9 Part 2): 926-930.

Tache Y, Martinez V, Million M, Rivier J. (1999). "Corticotropin-releasing factor and the brain-gut motor response to stress," *Canadian Journal of Gastroenterology* 13(Suppl A): 18A-25A.

Wessely S, Nimnuan C, Sharpe M. (1999). "Functional somatic syndromes: One or many?" *Lancet* 354: 936-939.

Whitehead WE, Palsson O, Jones KR. (2002). "Systematic review of the comorbidity of irritable bowel syndrome with other disorders: What are the causes and implications?" *Gastroenterology* 122(4): 1140-1156.

Chapter 3

American Psychiatric Association. (1987). *Diagnostic and Statistical Manual of Mental Disorders* (Third Edition, Revised). Washington, DC: American Psychiatric Association.

Farmer A, Jones I, Hillier J, Llewelyn M, Borysiewicz L, Smith A. (1995). "Neurasthenia revisited: ICD-10 and DSM-III-R psychiatric syndromes in chronic fatigue patients and comparison subjects," *British Journal of Psychiatry* 167(4): 503-506.

Fischler B, Cluydts R, De Gucht V, Kaufman L, De Meirleir K. (1997). "Generalized anxiety disorder in chronic fatigue syndrome," *Acta Psychiatrica Scandinavica* 95(5): 405-413.

Fukuda K, Straus SE, Hickie I, Sharpe MC, Dobbins JG, Komaroff A. (1994). "The chronic fatigue syndrome: A comprehensive approach to its definition and study. International Chronic Fatigue Syndrome Study Group," *Annals of Internal Medicine* 121 (12): 953-959.

Garralda ME, Rangel L. (2002). "Annotation: Chronic fatigue syndrome in children and adolescents," *Journal of Child Psychology and Psychiatry* 43(2): 169-176.

Gillespie NA, Zhu G, Heath AC, Hickie IB, Martin NG. (2000). "The genetic etiology of somatic distress," *Psychological Medicine* 30(5): 1051-1061.

Goldberg DP, Williams P. (1988). *The User's Guide to the General Health Questionnaire.* Slough, England: National Foundation for Educational Research.

Hickie I, Kirk K, Martin N. (1999). "Unique genetic and environmental determinants of prolonged fatigue: A twin study," *Psychological Medicine* 29(2): 259-268.

Holmes GP, Kaplan JE, Gantz NM, Komaroff AL, Schonberger LB, Straus SE, Jones JF, Dubois RE, Cunningham-Rundles C, Pahwa S, Brus I. (1988). "Chronic fatigue syndrome: A working case definition," *Annals of Internal Medicine* 108(3): 387-389.

Jason LA, Taylor RR, Kennedy CL, Jordan K, Huandy CF, Torres-Harding S, Song S, Johnson D. (2002). "A factor analysis of chronic fatigue symptoms in a community-based sample," *Social Psychiatry and Psychiatric Epidemiology* 37(4): 183-189.

Johnson SK, DeLuca J, Natelson BH. (1996). "Assessing somatization disorder in the chronic fatigue syndrome," *Psychosomatic Medicine* 58(1): 50-57.

Lane TJ, Manu P, Matthews DA. (1991). "Depression and somatization in the chronic fatigue syndrome," *American Journal of Medicine* 91(4): 335-344.

Lewis G, Pelosi A, Araya R, Dunn G. (1992). "Measuring psychiatric disorder in the community: A standardized assessment for use by lay interviewers," *Psychological Medicine* 22(2): 465-486.

Michiels V, Cluydts R. (2001). "Neuropsychological functioning in chronic fatigue syndrome: A review," *Acta Psychiatrica Scandinavica* 103(2): 84-93.

Morriss RK, Ahmed M, Wearden AJ, Mullis R, Strickland P, Appleby L, Campbell IT, Pearson D. (1999). "The role of depression in pain, psychophysiological syndromes and medically unexplained symptoms associated with chronic fatigue syndrome," *Journal of Affective Disorders* 55(2-3): 143-148.

Robins L, Cottler L, Keating S. (1991). *Diagnostic Interview Schedule (DIS): Version III-Revised.* St. Louis, MO: Washington University School of Medicine.

Robins LN, Helzer JE. (1985). *Diagnostic Interview Schedule (DIS): Version III-A.* St. Louis, MO: Department of Psychiatry, Washington University School of Medicine.

Roy-Byrne P, Afari N, Ashton S, Fischer M, Goldberg J, Buchwald D. (2002). "Chronic fatigue and anxiety/depression: A twin study," *British Journal of Psychiatry* 180(1): 29-34.

Sharpe MC, Archard LC, Banatvala JE, Borysiewicz LK, Clare AW, David A, Edwards RH, Hawton KE, Lambert HP, Lane RJ. (1991). "A report—chronic fatigue syndrome: Guidelines for research," *Journal of the Royal Society of Medicine* 84(2): 118-121.

Spitzer R, Endicott J. (1978). *Schedule for Affective Disorders and Schizophrenia.* New York: New York State Psychiatric Institute.

Spitzer RL, Williams JBW, Gibbon M, First MB. (1990). *Structured Clinical Interview for DSM-III-R—Patient Edition (with Psychotic Screen)—SCID-P (w/ Psychotic Screen)—Version 1.0.* Washington, DC: American Psychiatric Press.

Valentine AD, Meyers CA. (2001). "Cognitive and mood disturbance as causes and symptoms of fatigue in cancer patients," *Cancer* 92(6 Suppl): 1694-1698.

Wessely S, Chalder T, Hirsch S, Wallace P, Wright D. (1996). "Psychological symptoms, somatic symptoms, and psychiatric disorder in chronic fatigue and chronic fatigue syndrome: A prospective study in the primary care setting," *American Journal of Psychiatry* 153(8): 1050-1059.

Wessely S, Powell R. (1989). " 'Fatigue syndromes' a comparison of chronic 'postviral' fatigue with neuromuscular and affective disorders," *Journal of Neurology, Neurosurgery and Psychiatry* 52(8): 940-948.

Wing JK, Babor T, Brugha T, Burke J, Cooper JE, Giel R, Jablenski A, Regier D, Sartorius N. (1990). "SCAN. Schedules for Clinical Assessment in Neuropsychiatry," *Archives of General Psychiatry* 47(6): 589-593.

Zigmond AS, Snaith RP. (1983). "The Hospital Anxiety and Depression Scale," *Acta Psychiatrica Scandinavica* 67(6): 361-370.

Chapter 4

Ahles TA, Khan SA, Yunus MB, Spiegel DA, Masi AT. (1991). "Psychiatric status of patients with primary fibromyalgia, patients with rheumatoid arthritis, and subjects without pain: A blind comparison of *DSM-III* diagnoses," *American Journal of Psychiatry* 148(12): 1721-1726.

American Psychiatric Association. (1987). *Diagnostic and Statistical Manual of Mental Disorders* (Third Edition, Revised). Washington, DC: American Psychiatric Association.

American Psychiatric Association, Committee on Nomenclature and Statistics. (1980). *Diagnostic and Statistical Manual of Mental Disorders* (Third Edition). Washington, DC: American Psychiatric Association.

Arata CM, Saunders BE, Kilpatrick DO. (1991). "Concurrent validity of a crime-related post-traumatic stress disorder scale for women within the Symptom Checklist-90-Revised," *Violence and Victims* 6(3): 191-199.

Bech P, Rafaelsen OJ. (1980). "The use of rating scales exemplified by a comparison of the Hamilton and the Bech-Rafaelsen Melancholia Scale," *Acta Psychiatrica Scandinavica* 62(2): 128-131.

Carney MWP, Roth M, Garside RF. (1965). "The diagnosis of depressive syndromes and prediction of ECT response," *British Journal of Psychiatry* 111(7): 659-674.

Cathebras P, Lauwers A, Rousset H. (1998). "[Fibromyalgia. A critical review]," *Annales de Medicine Interne* 149(7): 406-414.

Croft P, Schollum J, Silman A. (1994). "Population study of tender point counts and pain as evidence of fibromyalgia," *British Medical Journal* 309(6956): 696-699.

Derogatis L. (1983). *The SCL-90-R Manual-II: Administration, Scoring and Procedures.* Towson, MD: Clinical Psychometric Research.

Epstein SA, Kay G, Clauw D, Heaton R, Klein D, Krupp L, Kuck J, Leslie V, Masur D, Wagner M, Waid R, Zisook S. (1999). "Psychiatric disorders in patients with fibromyalgia," *Psychosomatics* 40(1): 57-63.

Fassbender K, Samborsky W, Kellner M, Muller W, Lautenbacher S. (1997). "Tender points, depressive and functional symptoms: Comparison between fibromyalgia and major depression," *Clinical Rheumatology* 16(1): 76-79.

Goldberg D, Williams P. (1988). *A User's Guide to the General Health Question-naire.* Windsor, Great Britain: Nelson.

Hamilton M. (1959). "Assessment of anxiety states by rating," *British Journal of Medical Psychology* 32(1): 50-55.

Hudson JI, Hudson MS, Pliner LF, Goldenberg DL, Pope HG Jr. (1985). "Fibro-myalgia and major affective disorder: A controlled phenomenology and family history study," *American Journal of Psychiatry* 142(4): 441-446.

Johnson SK, DeLuca J, Natelson BH. (1996). "Assessing somatization disorder in the chronic fatigue syndrome," *Psychosomatic Medicine* 58(1): 50-57.

Kerns RD, Turk DC, Rudy TE. (1985). "The West Haven-Yale Multidimensional Pain Inventory (WHYMPI)," *Pain* 23(4): 345-356.

Kessler RC, McGonagle KA, Zhao S, Nelson CB, Hughes M, Eshleman S, Wittchen HU, Kendler KS. (1994). "Lifetime and 12-month prevalence of DSM-III-R psychi-atric disorders in the United States. Results from the national Comorbidity Survey," *Archives of General Psychiatry* 51(1): 8-19.

Kirmayer LJ, Robbins JM, Kapusta MA. (1988). "Somatization and depression in fibromyalgia syndrome," *American Journal of Psychiatry* 145(8): 950-954.

Krag NJ, Norregaard J, Larsen JK, Danneskiold-Samsoe B. (1994). "A blinded, controlled evaluation of anxiety and depressive symptoms in patients with fibromyalgia, as measured by standardized psychometric interview scales," *Acta Psychiatrica Scandinavica* 89(6): 370-375.

Larsen JK, Gjerris A, Holm P, Anderson J, Bille A, Christensen EM, Hoyer E, Jensen H, Mejlhede A, Langargergaard A. (1991). "Moclobemide in depression: A randomized, multicenter trial against isocarboxazide and clomipramine, em-phasizing atypical depression," *Acta Psychiatric Scandinavica* 84(6): 564-570.

McBeth J, Silman AJ. (2001). "The role of psychiatric disorders in fibromyalgia," *Current Rheumatology Reports* 3(2): 157-164.

Meenan RF, Gertman PM, Mason JH. (1980). "Measuring health status in arthritis: The arthritis impact measurement scales," *Arthritis and Rheumatism* 23(2): 146-152.

Neeck G. (2002). "Pathogenic mechanisms of fibromyalgia," *Ageing Research Re-views* 1(2): 243-255.

Othmer E, Penick EC, Powell BJ. (1983). *Psychiatric Diagnostic Interview (PDI) Manual.* Los Angeles: Western Psychological Services.

Powell BJ, Penick EC, Othmer E. (1985). "The discriminate validity of the Psychi-atric Diagnostic Interview," *Journal of Clinical Psychiatry* 46(8): 320-322.

Robins LN, Helzer JE, Croughan J. (1980). *NIMH Diagnostic Interview Schedule Version II.* Rockville, MD: National Institute for Mental Health.

Ropes MW, Bennett GA, Cobb S, Jacox R, Jessar RA. (1958). "1958 revision of di-agnostic criteria for rheumatoid arthritis," *Bulletin on the Rheumatic Diseases* 9(2): 175-176.

Sherman JJ, Turk DC, Okifuji A. (2000). "Prevalence and impact of posttraumatic stress disorder-like symptoms on patients with fibromyalgia syndrome," *Clini-cal Journal of Pain* 16(2): 127-134.

Spitzer RL, Williams JBW, Gibbon M. (1990). *Structured Clinical Interview for DSM-III-R*. Washington, DC: American Psychiatric Press, Inc.

Walker EA, Keegan D, Gardner G, Sullivan M, Katon WJ, Bernstein D. (1997). "Psychosocial factors in fibromyalgia compared with rheumatoid arthritis: I. Psychiatric diagnoses and functional disability," *Psychosomatic Medicine* 59(6): 565-571.

Weller RA, Penick EC, Powel BJ, Othmer E, Rice AS, Kent TA. (1985). "Agreement between two structured psychiatric interviews: DIS and the PDI," *Comprehensive Psychiatry* 26(2): 157-163.

Wolfe F, Ross K, Anderson J, Russell IJ. (1995). "Aspects of fibromyalgia in the general population: Sex, pain threshold and fibromyalgia symptoms," *Journal of Rheumatology* 22(1): 151-156.

Wolfe F, Ross K, Anderson J, Russell IJ, Herbert L. (1995). "The prevalence and characteristics of fibromyalgia in the general population," *Arthritis and Rheumatism* 38(1): 19-28.

Wolfe F, Smythe HA, Yunus MB, Bennett RM, Bombardier C, Goldenberg DL, Tugwell P, Campbell SM, Abeles M, Clark P, Fam AG, Farber SJ, Fiechtner JJ, Franklin C, Gatter RA, Hamaty D, Lessard J, Lichtbroun AS, Masi AT, McCain GA, Reynolds WJ, Romano TJ, Russell IJ, Sheon RP. (1990). "The American College of Rheumatology 1990 criteria for the classification of fibromyalgia. Report of the Multicenter Criteria Committee," *Arthritis and Rheumatism* 33(2): 160-172.

Yunus M, Masi AT, Calabro JJ, Miller KA, Feigenbaum SL. (1981). "Primary fibromyalgia (fibrositis): Clinical study of 50 patients with matched normal controls," *Seminars in Arthritis and Rheumatism* 11(1): 151-171.

Yunus MB. (2001). "The role of gender in fibromyalgia syndrome," *Current Rheumatology Reports* 3(2): 128-134.

Zung WW. (1965). "A self-rating depression scale," *Archives of General Psychiatry* 12(1): 63-70.

Chapter 5

American Psychiatric Association. (1987). *Diagnostic and Statistical Manual of Mental Disorders* (Third Edition, Revised).Washington, DC: American Psychiatric Association.

American Psychiatric Association. (1994). *Diagnostic and Statistical Manual of Mental Disorders* (Fourth Edition). Washington, DC: American Psychiatric Association.

Bailey JW, Cohen LS. (1999). "Prevalence of mood and anxiety disorders in women who seek treatment for premenstrual syndrome," *Journal of Women's Health & Gender-Based Medicine* 8(9): 1181-1184.

Brewerton TD, Berrettini WH, Nurnberger JI Jr., Linnoila M. (1988). "Analysis of seasonal fluctuations of CSF monoamine metabolites and neuropeptides in normal controls: Findings with 5HIAA and HVA," *Psychiatry Research* 23(3): 257-265.

Burt VK, Stein K. (2002). "Epidemiology of depression throughout the female life cycle," *Journal of Clinical Psychiatry* 63(Suppl 7): 9-15.

Endicott J, Spitzer RL. (1978). "A diagnostic interview: The Schedule for Affective Disorders and Schizophrenia," *Archives of General Psychiatry* 35(7): 837-844.

Eriksson E, Andersch B, Ho HP, Landen M, Sundblad C. (2002). "Diagnosis and treatment of premenstrual dysphoria," *Journal of Clinical Psychiatry* 63(Suppl 7): 16-23.

Graze KK, Nee J, Endicott J. (1990). "Premenstrual depression predicts future major depressive disorder," *Acta Psychiatrica Scandinavica* 81(2): 201-205.

Harrison WM, Endicott J, Nee J, Glick H, Rabkin JG. (1989). "Characteristics of women seeking treatment for premenstrual syndrome," *Psychosomatics* 30(4): 405-411.

Hartlage SA, Arduino KE, Gehlert S. (2001). "Premenstrual dysphoric disorder and risk for major depressive disorder: A preliminary study," *Journal of Clinical Psychology* 57(12): 1571-1578.

Kasper S, Wehr TA, Bartko JJ, Grant PA, Rosenthal NE. (1989). "Epidemiological findings of seasonal changes in mood and behavior: A telephone survey in Montgomery County, Maryland," *Archives of General Psychiatry* 46(9): 823-833.

Lesch KP, Bengel D, Heils A, Sabol SZ, Greenberg BD, Petri S, Benjamin J, Muller CR, Hamer DH, Murphy DL. (1996). "Association of anxiety-related traits with a polymorphism in the serotonin transporter gene regulatory region," *Science* 274(5292): 1527-1531.

Limosin F, Ades J. (2001). "[Psychiatric and psychological aspects of premenstrual syndrome]," *Encephale* 27(6): 501-508.

Maskall DD, Lam RW, Misri S, Carter D, Kuan AJ, Yatham LN, Zis AP. (1997). "Seasonality of symptoms in women with late luteal phase dysphoric disorder," *American Journal of Psychiatry* 154(10): 1436-1441.

Pearlstein TB, Frank E, Rivera-Tovar A, Thoft JS, Jacobs E, Miczkowski TA. (1990). "Prevalence of axis I and axis II disorders in women with late luteal phase dysphoric disorder," *Journal of Affective Disorders* 20(2): 129-134.

Praschak-Rieder N, Willeit M, Neumeister A, Hilger E, Stastny J, Thierry N, Lenzinger E, Kasper S. (2001). "Prevalence of premenstrual dysphoric disorder in female patients with seasonal affective disorder," *Journal of Affective Disorders* 63(1-3): 239-242.

Praschak-Rieder N, Willeit M, Winkler D, Neumeister A, Hilger E, Zill P, Hornik K, Stastny J, Thierry N, Ackenheil M, Bondy B, Kasper S. (2002). "Role of family history and 5-HTTLPR polymorphism in female seasonal affective disorder patients with and without premenstrual dysphoric disorder," *European Neuro-psychopharmacology* 12(2): 129-134.

Rosenthal NE, Bradt GH, Wehr TA. (1987). *Seasonal Pattern Assessment Questionnaire*. Washington, DC: National Institute of Mental Health.

Rosenthal NE, Mazzanti CM, Barnett RL, Hardin TA, Turner EH, Lam GK, Ozaki N, Goldman D. (1998). "Role of serotonin transporter promoter repeat length polymorphism (5-HTTLPR) in seasonality and seasonal affective disorder," *Molecular Psychiatry* 3(2): 175-177.

Sarrias MJ, Artigas F, Martinez E, Gelpi E. (1989). "Seasonal change in plasma serotonin and related parameters: Correlations with environmental measures," *Biological Psychiatry* 26(7): 695-706.

Chapter 6

American Psychiatric Association. (1987). *Diagnostic and Statistical Manual of Mental Disorders* (Third Edition, Revised). Washington, DC: American Psychiatric Press.

American Psychiatric Association. (1994). *Diagnostic and Statistical Manual of Mental Disorders* (Fourth Edition). Washington, DC: American Psychiatric Press.

Beck AT. (1978). *Beck Depression Inventory*. Philadelphia: Center for Cognitive Therapy.

Creed F. (1999). "The relationship between psychosocial parameters and outcome in irritable bowel syndrome," *American Journal of Medicine* 107(5A): 74S-80S.

Derogatis LR, Lipman RS, Covi L. (1973). "SCL-90: An outpatient psychiatric rating scale—preliminary report," *Psychopharmacology Bulletin* 9(1): 13-28.

Derogatis LR, Melisaratos N. (1983). "Brief symptom inventory: An introductory report," *Psychological Medicine* 13(3): 595-605.

Lydiard RB. (2001). "Irritable bowel syndrome, anxiety, and depression: What are the links?" *Journal of Clinical Psychiatry* 62(Suppl 8): 38-45; discussion 46-47.

Lydiard RB, Fossey MD, Marsh W, Ballenger JC. (1993). "Prevalence of psychiatric disorders in patients with irritable bowel syndrome," *Psychosomatics* 34(3): 229-234.

Main CJ. (1983). "The Modified Somatic Perception Questionnaire (MSPQ)," *Journal of Psychosomatic Research* 27(6): 503-514.

Manning AP, Thompson WG, Heaton KW, Morris AF. (1978). "Towards positive diagnosis of the irritable bowel," *British Medical Journal* 2(6138): 653-654.

Miller AR, North CS, Clouse RE, Wetzel RD, Spitznagel EL, Alpers DH. (2001). "The association of irritable bowel syndrome and somatization disorder," *Annals of Clinical Psychiatry* 13(1): 25-30.

Pilowski I. (1967). "Dimensions of hypochondriasis," *British Journal of Psychiatry* 131(1): 89-93.

Robins L, Cottler L, Bucholz K, Compton W, North CS, Rourke K. (1995). *Diagnostic Interview Schedule for DSM-IV (DIS-IV)*. St. Louis, MO: Washington University.

Robins LN, Helzer JE, Croughan J, Ratcliff KS. (1981). "National Institute of Mental Health Diagnostic Interview Schedule: Its history, characteristics and validity," *Archives of General Psychiatry* 38(4): 381-389.

Spitzer RL, Williams JBW, Gibbon M. (1990). *Structured Clinical Interview for DSM-III-R.* Washington, DC: American Psychiatric Press.

Talley NJ, Howell S, Poulton R. (2001). "The irritable bowel syndrome and psychiatric disorders in the community: Is there a link?" *American Journal of Gastroenterology* 96(4): 943-945.

Thompson WG, Dotevall G, Drossman DA, Heaton KW, Kruis W. (1989). "Irritable bowel syndrome: Guidelines for the diagnosis," *Gastroenterology International* 2(2): 92-95.

Thompson WG, Longstreth GF, Drossman DA, Heaton KW, Irvine EJ, Muller-Lissner SA. (1999). "Functional bowel disorders and functional abdominal pain," *Gut* 45(suppl II): II43-II47.

Walker EA, Roy-Byrne PP, Katon WJ, Li L, Amos D, Jiranek G. (1990). "Psychiatric illness and irritable bowel syndrome: A comparison with inflammatory bowel disease," *American Journal of Psychiatry* 147(12): 1656-1661.

Whitehead WE, Palsson O, Jones KR. (2002). "Systematic review of the comorbidity of irritable bowel syndrome with other disorders: What are the causes and implications?" *Gastroenterology* 122(4): 1140-1156.

Woodman CL, Breen K, Noyes R Jr, Moss C, Fagerholm R, Yagla SJ, Summers R. (1998). "The relationship between irritable bowel syndrome and psychiatric illness. A family study," *Psychosomatics* 39(1): 45-54.

Chapter 7

Blake DD, Weathers FW, Nagy LM, Kaloupek DG, Gusman FD, Charney DS, Keane TM. (1995). "The development of a clinician administered PTSD scale." *Journal of Traumatic Stress* 8(1): 75-90.

Derogatis LR, Lipman RS, Rickels K, Uhlenhuth EH, Covi L. (1974). "The Hopkins Symptom Checklist (HSCL): A self-report symptom inventory," *Behavioral Sciences* 19(1): 1-15.

De Vries M, Soetekouw PM, van Bergen LF, van der Meer JW, Bleijenberg G. (1999). "[Somatic and psychological symptoms in soldiers after military clashes and peace-keeping missions]," *Nederlands Tijdschrift voor Geneeskunde* 143(51): 2557-2562.

Doebbeling BN, Clarke WR, Watson D, Torner JC, Woolson RF, Voelker MD, Barrett DH, Schwartz DA. (2000). "Is there a Persian Gulf War syndrome? Evidence from a large population-based survey of veterans and nondeployed controls," *American Journal of Medicine* 108(9): 695-704.

Ford JD, Campbell KA, Storzbach D, Binder LM, Anger WK, Rohlman DS. (2001). "Posttraumatic stress symptomatology is associated with unexplained illness attributed to Persian Gulf War military service," *Psychosomatic Medicine* 63(5): 842-849.

Fukuda K, Straus SE, Hickie I, Sharpe MC, Dobbins JG, Komaroff A. (1994). "The chronic fatigue syndrome: A comprehensive approach to its definition and study. International Chronic Fatigue Syndrome Study Group," *Annals of Internal Medicine* 121(12): 953-959.

Keane TM, Caddell JM, Taylor KL. (1988). "Mississippi Scale for Combat-Related Posttraumatic Stress Disorder: Three studies in reliability and validity," *Journal of Consulting and Clinical Psychology* 56(1): 85-90.

Knoke JD, Smith TC, Gray GC, Kaiser KS, Hawksworth AW. (2000). "Factor analysis of self-reported symptoms: Does it identify a Gulf War syndrome?" *American Journal of Epidemiology* 152(4): 379-388.

Labbate LA, Cardena E, Dimitreva J, Roy M, Engel CC. (1998). "Psychiatric syndromes in Persian Gulf War veterans: An association of handling dead bodies with somatoform disorders," *Psychotherapy and Psychosomatics* 67(4): 275-279.

Marcus S, Robins LN, Bucholz K. (1990). *Quick Diagnostic Interview Schedule 3R Version.* St. Louis, MO: Washington University School of Medicine.

Natelson BH, Tiersky L, Nelson J. (2001). "The diagnosis of posttraumatic stress disorder in Gulf veterans with medically unexplained fatiguing illness," *Journal of Nervous and Mental Disease* 189(11): 795-796.

Sartin JS. (2000). "Gulf war illnesses: Causes and controversies," *Mayo Clinic Proceedings* 75(8): 811-819.

Spitzer RL, Williams JBW, Gibbon M, First MB. (1990). *User's Guide for the Structured Clinical Interview: SCID.* Washington, DC: American Psychiatric Association.

Tournier JN, Drouet E, Jouan A. (2002). "[The Gulf war syndrome]," *Presse Medicale* 31(1 Pt 1): 3-9.

White RF, Proctor SP, Heeren T, Wolfe J, Krengel M, Vasterling J, Lindem K, Heaton KJ, Sutker P, Ozonoff DM. (2001). "Neuropsychological function in Gulf War veterans: Relationship to self-reported toxicant exposures," *American Journal of Industrial Medicine* 40(1): 42-54.

Chapter 8

American Psychiatric Association. (1987). *Diagnostic and Statistical Manual of Mental Disorders* (Third Edition, Revised). Washington, DC: American Psychiatric Association.

Buchwald D, Cheney PR, Peterson DL, Henry B, Wormsley SB, Geiger A, Ablashi DV, Salahuddin Z, Saxinger Z, Biddle R, Kikinis R, Jolesz FA, Folks T, Balachandran N, Peter JB, Gallo RC, Komaroff AL. (1992). "Chronic illness characterized by fatigue, neurologic and immunologic disorders, and active human herpesvirus type 6 infection," *Annals of Internal Medicine* 116(2): 103-113.

Contreras D, Steriade M. (1995). "Cellular basis of EEG slow rhythms: A study of dynamic corticothalamic relationships," *Journal of Neuroscience* 15(1 Part 2): 604-622.

Cook DB, Lange G, DeLuca J, Natelson BH. (2001). "Relationship of brain MRI abnormalities and physical functional status in chronic fatigue syndrome," *International Journal of Neuroscience* 107(1): 1-6.

Costa DC, Tannock C, Brostoff J. (1995). "Brainstem perfusion is impaired in chronic fatigue syndrome," *Quarterly Journal of Medicine* 88(11): 767-773.

Davidson RJ, Abercrombie H, Nitschke JB, Purnam K. (1999). "Regional brain function, emotion and disorders of emotion," *Current Opinions in Neurobiology* 9(2): 228-234.

Davis KD, Kiss ZH, Tasker RR, Dostrovsky JO. (1996). "Thalamic stimulation-evoked sensations in chronic pain patients and in nonpain (movement disorder) patients," *Journal of Neurophysiology* 75(3): 1026-1037.

Fischler B, D'Haenen H, Cluydts R, Michiels V, Demets K, Bossuyt A, Kaufman L, De Meirleir K. (1996). "Comparison of 99m Tc HMPAO SPECT scan between chronic fatigue syndrome, major depression and healthy controls: An exploratory study of clinical correlates of regional blood flow," *Neuropsychobiology* 34(4): 175-183.

Fukuda K, Straus SE, Hickie I, Sharpe MC, Dobbins JG, Komaroff A, International Chronic Fatigue Syndrome Study Group. (1994). "The chronic fatigue syndrome: A comprehensive approach to its definition and study," *Annals of Internal Medicine* 121(12): 953-959.

Grant R, Condon B, Lawrence A, Hadley A, Patterson J, Bone I, Teasdale GM. (1988). "Is cranial CSF volume under hormonal influence? An MR study," *Journal of Computer Assisted Tomography* 12(1): 36-39.

Greco A, Tannock C, Brostoff J, Costa DC. (1997). "Brain MR in chronic fatigue syndrome," *American Journal of Neuroradiology* 18(8): 1265-1269.

Haley RW, Hom J, Roland PS, Bryan WW, Van Ness PC, Bonte FJ, Devous MD Sr, Mathews D, Fleckenstein JL, Wians FH Jr, Wolfe GI, Kurt TL. (1997). "Evaluation of neurologic function in Gulf War veterans. A blinded case-control study," *Journal of the American Medical Association* 277(3): 223-230.

Haley RW, Kurt TM, Hom J. (1997). "Is there a Gulf War syndrome? Searching for syndromes by factor analysis of symptoms," *Journal of the American Medical Association* 277(3): 215-222.

Holmes GP, Kaplan JE, Gantz NM, Komaroff AL, Schonberger LB, Straus SE, Jones JF, Dubois RE, Cunningham-Rundles C, Pahwa S, Brus I. (1988). "Chronic fatigue syndrome: A working case definition," *Annals of Internal Medicine* 108(3): 387-389.

Janssen RS, Cornblath DR, Epstein LG, McArthur J, Price RW. (1989). "Human immunodeficiency virus (HIV) infection and the nervous system: Report from the American Academy of Neurology AIDS task Force," *Neurology* 39(1): 119-122.

Johansson G, Risberg J, Rosenhall U, Orndahl G, Svennerholm L, Nystrom S. (1995). "Cerebral dysfunction in fibromyalgia: Evidence from regional blood flow measurements, otoneurological tests and cerebrospinal fluid analysis," *Acta Psychiatrica Scandinavica* 95(2): 86-94.

Ketter TA, Wang PW. (2002). "Predictors of treatment response in bipolar disorders: Evidence from clinical and brain imaging studies," *Journal of Clinical Psychiatry* 63(Suppl 3): 21-25.

Kinomura S, Larsson J, Gulyas B, Roland PE. (1996). "Activation by attention of the human reticular formation and thalamic intralaminar nuclei," *Science* 271(5248): 512-515.

Kiss ZH, Tsoukatos J, Tasker RR, Davis KD, Dostrovsky JO. (1995). "Sleeping cells in the human thalamus," *Stereotactic and Functional Neurosurgery* 65(1-4): 125-129.

Kwiatek R, Barnden L, Tedman R, Jarrett R, Chew J, Rowe C, Pile K. (2000). "Regional cerebral blood flow in fibromyalgia. Single-photon-emission computed tomography evidence of reduction in the pontine tegmentum and thalami," *Arthritis and Rheumatism* 43(12): 2823-2833.

Lange G, DeLuca J, Maldjian JA, Lee HJ, Tiersky LA, Natelson BH. (1999). "Brain MRI abnormalities exist in a subset of patients with chronic fatigue syndrome," *Journal of the Neurological Sciences* 171(1): 3-7.

Lange G, Holodny AI, DeLuca J, Lee HJ, Yan XM, Steffener J, Natelson BH. (2001). "Quantitative assessment of cerebral ventricular volumes in chronic fatigue syndrome," *Applied Neurophysiology* 8(1): 23-30.

Lenz FA, Gracely RH, Baker FH, Richardson RT, Dougherty PM. (1998). "Reorganization of sensory modalities evoked by microstimulation in region of the thalamic principal sensory nucleus in patients with pain due to nervous system injury," *Journal of Comparative Neurology* 399(1): 125-138.

MacHale SM, Lawrie SM, Cavanagh JTO, Glabus MF, Murray CL, Goodwin GM, Ebmeier K. (2000). "Cerebral perfusion in chronic fatigue syndrome and depression," *British Journal of Psychiatry* 176(June): 550-556.

Markus S, Robins LN, Bucholz, K. (1991). *Quick Diagnostic Interview Schedule 3R Version I.* St. Louis, MO: Washington University School of Medicine.

Mertz H, Morgan V, Tanner G, Pickens D, Price R, Shyr Y, Kessler R. (2000). "Regional cerebral activation in irritable bowel syndrome and control subjects with painful and nonpainful rectal distention," *Gastroenterology* 118(5): 842-848.

Mountz JM, Bradley LA, Modell JG, Alexander RW, Triana-Alexander M, Aaron LA, Stewart KE, Alarcon GS, Mountz JD. (1995). "Fibromyalgia in women: Abnormalities of regional cerebral blood flow in the thalamus and the caudate nucleus are associated with low pain threshold levels," *Arthritis and Rheumatism* 38(7): 926-938.

Mowbray RM. (1972). "The Hamilton rating scale for depression: A factor analysis," *Psychological Medicine* 2(3): 272-280.

Natelson BH, Cohen JM, Brassloff I, Lee HJ. (1993). "A controlled study of brain magnetic resonance imaging in patients with the chronic fatigue syndrome," *Journal of the Neurological Sciences* 120(2): 213-217.

Schmidt R, Roob G, Kapeller P, Schmidt H, Berghold A, Lechner A, Fazekas F. (2000). "Longitudinal change of white matter abnormalities," *Journal of Neural Transmission* 59(Suppl): 9-14.

Schwartz RB, Garada BM, Komaroff AL, Tice HM, Gleit M, Jolesz FA, Holman BL. (1994). "Detection of intracranial abnormalities in patients with chronic fatigue syndrome: Comparison of MR imaging and SPECT," *American Journal of Roentgenology* 162(4): 935-941.

Schwartz RB, Komaroff AL, Garada BM, Gleit M, Doolittle TH, Bates DW, Vasile RG, Holman BL. (1994). "SPECT imaging of the brain: Comparison of findings in patients with chronic fatigue syndrome, AIDS dementia complex, and major unipolar depression," *American Journal of Roentgenology* 162(4): 943-951.

Soares JC, Mann JJ. (1997). "The anatomy of mood disorders—review of structural neuroimaging studies," *Biological Psychiatry* 41(1): 86-106.

Steriade M, Contreras D. (1995). "Relations between cortical and thalamic cellular events during transition from sleep patterns to paroxysmal activity," *Journal of Neuroscience* 15(1 Part 2): 623-642.

Stewart AL, Hays RD, Ware JE Jr. (1988). "The MOS short-form general health survey: Reliability and validity in a patient population," *Medical Care* 26(7): 724-735.

Tupler LA, Coffey CE, Logue PE, Djang WT, Fagan SM. (1992). "Neuropsychological importance of subcortical white matter hyperintensity," *Archives of Neurology* 49(12): 1248-1252.

Weese GD, Phillips JM, Brown VJ. (1999). "Attentional orienting is impaired by unilateral lesions of the thalamic reticular nucleus in the rat," *Journal of Neuroscience* 19(22): 10135-10139.

Wolfe F, Smythe HA, Yunus MB, Bennett RM, Bombardier C, Goldenberg DL, Tugwell P, Campbell SM, Abeles M, Clark P, Fam AG, Farber SJ, Fiechtner JJ, Franklin C, Gatter RA, Hamaty D, Lessard J, Lichtbroun AS, Masi AT, McCain GA, Reynolds WJ, Romano TJ, Russell IJ, Sheon RP. (1990). "The American College of Rheumatology 1990 criteria for the classification of fibromyalgia. Report of the Multicenter Criteria Committee," *Arthritis and Rheumatism* 33(2): 160-172.

Zigmond AS, Snaith RP. (1983). "The hospital anxiety and depression scale," *Acta Psychiatrica Scandinavica* 67(6): 361-370.

Chapter 9

Adams RL, Trenton SL. (1981). "Development of a paper- and pen-form of the Halstead Category test," *Journal of Consulting and Clinical Psychology* 49(2): 298-299.

Anger WK. (1990). "Worksite behavioral research: Results, sensitive methods, test batteries and the transition from laboratory data to human health," *Neurotoxicology* 11(4): 627-717.

Austin MP, Mitchell P, Goodwin GM. (2001). "Cognitive deficits in depression: Possible implications for functional neuropathology," *British Journal of Psychiatry* 178(March): 200-206.

Bates ME, Tracy JL. (1990). "Cognitive functioning in young 'social drinkers.' Is there impairment to detect?" *Journal of Abnormal Psychology* 99: 242-249.

Beck AT, Ward CH, Mendelson M. (1961). "An inventory for measuring depression," *Archives of General Psychiatry* 4(6): 561-571.

Benton AL. (1974). *Revised Visual Retention Test* (Fourth Edition). San Antonio, TX: Psychological Corporation.

Benton AL, Hamsher K. (1983). *Multilingual Aphasia Examination.* Iowa City, IA: AJA Associates.

Binder LM, Storzbach D, Campbell KA, Rohlman DS, Anger WK. (2001). "Neurobehavioral deficits associated with chronic fatigue syndrome in veterans with Gulf War unexplained illness," *Journal of International Neuropsychological Society* 7(7): 835-839.

Bornstein RA. (1986). "Normative data on intermanual differences on three tests of motor performance," *Journal of Clinical and Experimental Neuropsychology* 8(1): 12-20.

Buschke H. (1973). "Selective reminding for analysis of memory and learning," *Journal of Verbal Learning and Verbal Behavior* 12(5): 543-550.

Buschke H, Fuld PA. (1974). "Evaluating storage, retention, and retrieval in disordered memory and learning," *Neurology* 24(11): 1019-1025.

College Entrance Examination Board. (1993). *Scholastic Aptitude Test Administered May 1993.* Princeton, NJ: Educational Testing Services.

Cornblatt BA, Risch NJ, Faris G, Friedman G, Erlenmeyer-Kimling. (1988). "The continuous performance test, identical-pairs version: I. New findings about sustained attention in normal families," *Psychiatry Research* 26(2): 223-238.

Derogatis LR. (1992). *SCL-90-R Administration, Scoring & Procedures Manual II* (Second Edition). Towson, MD: Clinical Psychometric Research.

Derogatis LR, Melisaratos N. (1983). "The Brief Symptom Inventory: An introductory report," *Psychological Medicine* 13(3): 593-605.

DiClementi JD, Schmaling KB, Jones JF. (2001). "Information processing in chronic fatigue syndrome. A preliminary investigation of suggestibility," *Journal of Psychosomatic Research* 51(5): 679-686.

Fiedler N, Kipen HM, DeLuca J, Delly-McNeil K, Natelson BH. (1996). "A controlled comparison of multiple chemical sensitivities and chronic fatigue syndrome," *Psychosomatic Medicine* 58(1): 38-49.

Fossati P, Ergis AM, Allilaire JF. (2002). "[Executive functioning in unipolar depression: A review]," *Encephale* 28(2): 97-107.

Fukuda K, Straus SE, Hickie I, Sharpe MC, Dobbins JG, Komaroff A. (1994). "The chronic fatigue syndrome: A comprehensive approach to its definition and study. International Chronic Fatigue Syndrome Study Group," *Annals of Internal Medicine* 121(12): 953-959.

Golden JC. (1978). *Stroop Color and Word Test*. Chicago: Stoelting.

Holmes GP, Kaplan JE, Gantz NM, Komaroff AL, Schonberger LB, Straus SE, Jones JF, Dubois RE, Cunningham-Rundles C, Pahwa S, Brus I. (1988). "Chronic fatigue syndrome: A working case definition," *Annals of Internal Medicine* 108(3): 387-389.

Jastak JF, Wilkinson G. (1984). *The Wide Range Achievement Test—Revised: Administration Manual*. Wilmington, DE: Jastak Associates.

Jensen AR. (1987). "Individual differences in the Hick paradigm." In Vernon P (Ed.), *Speed of Information Processing and Intelligence*. Norwood, NJ: Ablex Publishing, pp. 101-175.

Kovera CA, Anger WK, Campbell KA, Binder LM, Storzbach D, Davis KL, Rohlman DS. (1996). "Computer-administration of questionnaires: A health screening system (HHS) developed for veterans," *Neurotoxicology and Teratology* 18(4): 511-518.

Krupp LB, Sliwinski M, Masur DM, Friedberg F, Coyle PK. (1994). "Cognitive functioning and depression in patients with chronic fatigue syndrome and depression," *Archives of Neurology* 51(7): 705-710.

Lange G, Tiersky LA, Scharer JB, Policastro T, Fiedler N, Morgan TE, Natelson BH. (2001). "Cognitive functioning in Gulf War Illness," *Journal of Clinical and Experimental Neuropsychology* 23(2): 240-249.

Liotti M, Mayberg HS. (2001). "The role of functional neuroimaging in the neuropsychology of depression," *Journal of Clinical and Experimental Neuropsychology* 23(1): 121-136.

Loftus EF, Donders K, Hoffman HG, Schooler JW. (1989). "Creating new memories that are quickly accessed and confidently held," *Memory and Cognition* 17(5): 607-617.

Marcus S, Robins LN, Bucholz K. (1990). *Quick Diagnostic Interview Schedule 3R Version*. St. Louis, MO: Washington University School of Medicine.

Marshall PS, Forstot M, Callies A, Peterson PK, Schenk CH. (1997). "Cognitive slowing and working memory difficulties in chronic fatigue syndrome," *Psychosomatic Medicine* 59(1): 58-66.

Mialet JP, Pope HG, Yurgelun-Todd D. (1996). Impaired attention in depressive states: A non-specific deficit? *Psychological Medicine* 26(5): 1009-1020.

Poser CM, Paty DW, Scheinberg C, McDonald WI, Davis FA, Ebers GC, Johnson KP, Sibley WA, Silberberg DH, Tourtelotte WW. (1983). "New diagnostic criteria for multiple sclerosis: Guidelines for research protocols," *Annals of Neurology* 13(3): 227-231.

Radloff LS, Locke BZ. (1986). "The community mental health assessment survey and the CES-D scale." In Weismann MM, Meyers JK, Ross CE (Eds.), *Commu-*

nity Survey of Psychiatric Disorders. New Brunswick, NJ: Rutgers University Press, pp. 177-187.

Reitan SM, Wolfson D. (1985). *The Halstead-Reitan Neuropsychological Test Battery: Theory and Interpretation.* Tucson, AZ: Neuropsychology Press.

Roman DD, Edwall GE, Buchanan RJ. (1991). "Extended norms for the Paced Auditory Serial Addition Task," *Clinical Neuropsychologist* 5(1): 33-40.

Salthouse TA. (1994). "The aging of working memory," *Neuropsychology* 8(4): 535-543.

Schagen S, Schmand B, deSterke S, Lindeboom J. (1997). "Amsterdam Short-Term Memory test: A new procedure for the detection of feigned memory deficits," *Journal of Clinical and Experimental Neuropsychology* 19(1): 43-51.

Schmand B, Lindeboom J, Schagen S, Heijt R, Koene T, Hamburger HL. (1998). "Cognitive complaints in patients after whiplash injury: The impact of malingering," *Journal of Neurology Neurosurgery and Psychiatry* 64(3): 339-343.

Sillanpaa MC, Agar LM, Milner IB, Podany EC, Axelrod BN, Brown G. (1997). "Gulf War veterans: A neuropsychological explanation," *Journal of Clinical and Experimental Neuropsychology* 19(2): 211-219.

Smith A. (1973). *Symbol Digit Modalities Test.* Los Angeles, CA: Western Psychological Services.

Spiegel H, Spiegel D. (1978). *Trance and Treatment: Clinical Uses of Hypnosis.* Washington, DC: American Psychiatric Press.

Stinissen J, Willems PJ, Coetsier L, Hulsman WLL. (1970). *[Manual of the Dutch Edition of WAIS].* Amsterdam: Swets and Zeitlinger.

Storzbach D, Rohlman DS, Anger WK, Binder LM, Campbell KA. (2001). "Neurobehavioral deficits in Persian Gulf veterans: Additional evidence from a population-based study," *Environmental Research Section A* 85(1): 1-13.

Trenerry MR, Crossen B, DeBoe J, Leber WR. (1989). *Stroop Neuropsychological Screening Test Manual.* Odessa, FL: Psychological Assessment Resources.

Van der Werf SP, de Vree B, Van der Meer JW, Bleijenberg G. (2002). "The relations among body consciousness, somatic symptom report, and information processing speed in chronic fatigue syndrome," *Neuropsychiatry, Neuropsychology and Behavioral Neurology* 15(1): 2-9.

Van der Werf SP, Prins JB, Jongen PJH, Van der Meer JWM, Bleijenberg G. (2000). "Abnormal neuropsychological findings are not necessarily a sign of cerebral impairment: A matched comparison between chronic fatigue syndrome and multiple sclerosis," *Neuropsychiatry, Neuropsychology and Behavioral Neurology* 13(3): 199-203.

Wechsler D. (1981). *Wechsler Adult Intelligence Scale—Revised Manual.* New York: Psychological Corporation.

Wechsler D. (1987). *Memory Scale—Revised.* San Antonio, TX: Psychological Corporation.

White RF, Proctor SP, Heeren T, Wolfe J, Krengel M, Vasterling J, Lindem K, Heaton KJ, Sutker P, Ozonoff DM. (2001). "Neuropsychological function in

Gulf War veterans: Relationship to self-reported toxicant exposures," *American Journal of Industrial Medicine* 40(1): 42-54.

Chapter 10

Altemus M, Dale JK, Michelson D, Demitrack MA, Gold PW, Straus SE. (2001). "Abnormalities in response to vasopressin infusion in chronic fatigue syndrome," *Psychoneuroendocrinology* 26(2): 175-188.

American Psychiatric Association. (1987). *Diagnostic and Statistical Manual of Mental Disorders* (Third Edition, Revised). Washington, DC: American Psychiatric Association.

American Psychiatric Association. (1994). *Diagnostic and Statistical Manual of Mental Disorders* (Fourth Edition). Washington, DC: American Psychiatric Association.

Birmaher B, Heydl P. (2001). "Biological studies in depressed children and adolescents," *International Journal of Neuropsychopharmacology* 4(2): 149-157.

Blackburn-Munro G, Blackburn-Munro RE. (2001). "Chronic pain, chronic stress and depression: Coincidence or consequence?" *Journal of Neuroendocrinology* 13(12): 1009-1023.

Burke PM, Reichler RJ, Smith E, Dugaw K, McCauley E, Mitchell J. (1985). "Correlation between serum and salivary cortisol levels in depressed and non-depressed children and adolescents," *American Journal of Psychiatry* 142(9): 1065-1967.

Catley D, Kaell AT, Kirschbaum C, Stone AA. (2000). "A naturalistic evaluation of cortisol secretion in persons with fibromyalgia and rheumatoid arthritis," *Arthritis Care and Research* 13(1): 51-61.

Crofford LJ, Pillemer SR, Kalogeras KT, Cash LM, Michelson D, Kling MA, Sternberg EM, Gold PW, Chrousos GP, Wilder RL. (1994). "Hypothalamic-pituitary-adrenal axis perturbations in patients with fibromyalgia," *Arthritis and Rheumatism* 37(11): 1583-1592.

Demitrack MA, Dale JK, Straus SE, Laue L, Listwak SJ, Kruesi MJP, Chrousos GP, Gold PW. (1991). "Evidence for impaired activation of the hypothalamic-pituitary-adrenal axis in patients with chronic fatigue syndrome," *Journal of Clinical Endocrinology and Metabolism* 73(6): 1224-1234.

Elsenbruch S, Lovallo WR, Orr WC. (2001). "Psychological and physiological responses to postprandial mental stress in women with the irritable bowel syndrome," *Psychosomatic Medicine* 63(5): 805-813.

Fukuda K, Straus SE, Hickie I, Sharpe MC, Dobbins JG, Komaroff A. (1994). "The chronic fatigue syndrome: A comprehensive approach to its definition and study. International Chronic Fatigue Syndrome Study Group," *Annals of Internal Medicine* 121(12): 953-959.

Gold PW, Chrousos GP. (2002). "Organization of the stress system and its dys-regulation in melancholic and atypical depression: High vs low CRH/NE states," *Molecular Psychiatry* 7(3): 254-275.

Gold PW, Gwirtsman H, Avgerinos PC, Nieman CK, Gallucci WT, Kaye W, Jimerson D, Ebert M, Rittmeister R, Loriaux DL. (1986). "Abnormal hypotha-lamic-pituitary-adrenal function in anorexia nervosa: Pathophysiologic mecha-nisms in underweight and weight-corrected patients," *New England Journal of Medicine* 314(21): 1335-1342.

Gold PW, Loriaux DL, Roy A, Kling MA, Calabrese JR, Kellner CH, Nieman LK, Post RM, Pickar D, Gallucci W, Paul S, Oldfield EH, Cutler GR Jr, Chrousos GP. (1986). "Response to CRH in the hypercortisolism of depression and Cush-ing's disease: Pathophysiologic and diagnostic implications," *New England Journal of Medicine* 314(21): 1329-1334.

Goodyer IM, Herbert J, Altham PM, Pearson J, Secher SM, Shiers HM. (1996). "Adrenal secretion during major depression in 8- to 16-year-olds. I. Altered diur-nal rhythms in salivary cortisol and dehydroepiandrosterone (DHEA) at presen-tation," *Psychological Medicine* 26(2): 245-256.

Griep EN, Boersma JW, de Kloet ER. (1993). "Altered reactivity of the hypotha-lamic-pituitary-adrenal axis in the primary fibromyalgia syndrome," *Journal of Rheumatology* 20(3): 469-474.

Griep EN, Boersma JW, Lentjes EG, Prins AP, van der Koorst JK, de Kloet ER. (1998). "Function of the hypothalamic-pituitary-adrenal axis in patients with fibromyalgia and low back pain," *Journal of Rheumatology* 25(7): 1374-1381.

Holmes GP, Kaplan JE, Gantz NM, Komaroff AL, Schonberger LB, Straus SE, Jones JF, Dubois RE, Cunningham-Rundles C, Pahwa S, Brus I. (1988). "Chronic fa-tigue syndrome: A working case definition," *Annals of Internal Medicine* 108(3): 387-389.

Joseph-Vanderpool JR, Rosenthal NE, Chrousos GP, Wehr TA, Skwerer R, Kasper S, Gold PW. (1991). "Abnormal pituitary-adrenal responses to corticotropin-releasing hormone in patients with seasonal affective disorder: Clinical and pathophysiological implications," *Journal of Clinical Endocrinology and Me-tabolism* 72(6): 1382-1387.

Kathol RG, Anton R, Noyes R, Gehris T. (1989). "Direct comparison of urinary free cortisol excretion in patients with depression and panic disorder," *Biological Psychiatry* 25(7): 873-878.

Luger A, Deuster PA, Kyle SB, Galucci WT, Montgomery LC, Gold PW, Loriaux DL, Chrousos GP. (1987). "Acute hypothalamic-pituitary-adrenal responses to the stress of treadmill exercise. Physiologic adaptations to physical training," *New England Journal of Medicine* 316(21): 1309-1315.

Maes M, Lin A, Bonaccorso S, van Hunsel F, Van Gastel A, Delmeire L, Biondi M, Bosmans E, Kenis G, Scharpe S. (1998). "Increased 24-hour urinary cortisol ex-cretion in patients with post-traumatic stress disorder and patients with major depression, but not in patients with fibromyalgia," *Acta Psychiatric Scandinavica* 98(4): 328-335.

Ockenfels MC, Porter LS, Smyth J, Kirschbaum C, Hellhammer DH, Stone AA. (1995). "Effect of chronic stress associated with unemployment on cortisol: Overall cortisol levels, diurnal rhythm, and acute stress reactivity," *Psychosomatic Medicine* 57(5): 460-467.

Odber J, Cawood EHH, Bancroft J. (1998). "Salivary cortisol in women with and without perimenstrual mood changes," *Journal of Psychosomatic Research* 45(6): 557-568.

Patacchioli FR, Angelucci L, Dell'Erba G, Monnazzi P, Leri O. (2001). "Actual stress, psychopathology and salivary cortisol levels in irritable bowel syndrome," *Journal of Endocrinological Investigation* 24(3): 173-177.

Purba JS, Hoogendjijk WJ, Hofman MA, Swaab DF. (1996). "Increased numbers of vasopressin and oxytocin-expressing neurons in the paraventricular nucleus of the hypothalamus in depression," *Archives of General Psychiatry* 53(2): 137-143.

Raadsheer FC, Hoogendijk WJ, Stam FC, Tilders FJ, Swaab DF. (1994). "Increased numbers of corticotropin-releasing hormone expressing neurons in the hypothalamic paraventricular nucleus of depressed patients," *Neuroendocrinology* 60(4): 436-444.

Rabin DS, Schmidt PJ, Campbell G, Gold PW, Jensvold M, Rubinow DR, Chrousos GP. (1990). "Hypothalamic-pituitary-adrenal function in patients with the premenstrual syndrome," *Journal of Clinical Endocrinology and Metabolism* 71(5): 1158-1162.

Rosenbaum AH, Maruta T, Schatzberg AF, Orsulak PJ, Jiang NS, Cole JO, Schildkraut JJ. (1983). "Toward a biochemical classification of depressive disorders, VII: Urinary free cortisol and urinary MHPG in depressions," *American Journal of Psychiatry* 140(3): 314-318.

Scott LV, Dinan TG. (1998). "Urinary free cortisol in chronic fatigue syndrome, major depression and in healthy volunteers," *Journal of Affective Disorders* 47(1-3): 49-54.

Scott LV, Medbak S, Dinan TG. (1999). "Desmopressin augments pituitary-adrenal responsivity to corticotropin-releasing hormone in subjects with chronic fatigue syndrome and in healthy volunteers," *Biological Psychiatry* 45(11): 1447-1454.

Scott LV, Salahuddin F, Cooney J, Svec F, Dinan TG. (1999). "Differences in adrenal steroid profile in chronic fatigue syndrome, in depression and in health," *Journal of Affective Disorders* 54(1-2): 129-137.

Sharpe MC, Archard LC, Banatvala JE, Borysiewicz LK, Clare AW, David A, Edwards RH, Hawton KE, Lambert HP, Lane RJ. (1991). "A report—chronic fatigue syndrome guidelines for research," *Journal of the Royal Society of Medicine* 84(2): 118-121.

Strickland P, Morriss R, Wearden A, Deakin B. (1998). "A comparison of salivary cortisol in chronic fatigue syndrome, community depression and healthy controls," *Journal of Affective Disorders* 47(1-3): 191-194.

Thalen BE, Kjellman BF, Ljunggren JG, Akner G, Kagedal B, Wahlund B, Wetterberg L. (1993). "Release of corticotropin after administration of corticotropin-releasing hormone in depressed patients in relation to the dexamethasone suppression test," *Acta Psychiatrica Scandanavica* 87(2): 133-140.

Thase ME, Dube S, Bowler K, Howland RH, Myers JE, Friedman E, Jarrett DB. (1996). "Hypothalamic-pituitary-adrenocortical activity and response to cognitive behavior therapy in unmedicated, hospitalized depressed patients," *American Journal of Psychiatry* 153(7): 886-891.

Thompson WG, Dotevall G, Drossman DA, Heaton KW, Kruis W. (1989). "Irritable bowel syndrome: Guidelines for the diagnosis," *Gastroenterology International* 2(2): 92-95.

Wolfe F, Smythe HA, Yunus MB, Bennett RM, Bombardier C, Goldenberg DL, Tugwell P, Campbell SM, Abeles M, Clark P, Fam AG, Farber SJ, Fiechtner JJ, Franklin CM, Gatter RA, Hamaty D, Lessard J, Lichtbroun AS, Masi AT, McCain GA, Reynolds WJ, Romano TJ, Russell IJ, Sheon RP. (1990). "The American College of Rheumatology 1990 criteria for the classification of fibromyalgia: Report of the multicenter criteria committee," *Arthritis and Rheumatism* 33(2): 160-177.

Young AH, Sharpe M, Clements A, Dowling B, Hawton KE, Cowen PJ. (1998). "Basal activity of the hypothalamic-pituitary-adrenal axis in patients with the chronic fatigue syndrome (neurasthenia)," *Biological Psychiatry* 43(3): 236-237.

Young EA, Aggen SH, Prescott CA, Kendler KS. (2000). "Similarity in saliva cortisol measures in monozygotic twins and the influence of past major depression," *Biological Psychiatry* 48(1): 70-74.

Chapter 11

American Psychiatric Association. (1987). *Diagnostic and Statistical Manual of Mental Disorders* (Third Edition, Revised). Washington, DC: American Psychiatric Association.

American Psychiatric Association. (1994). *Diagnostic and Statistical Manual of Mental Disorders* (Fourth Edition). Washington, DC: American Psychiatric Association.

Ashby CR Jr, Carr LA, Cook CL, Steptoe MM, Franks DD. (1988). "Alteration of platelet serotonergic mechanisms and monoamine oxidase activity in premenstrual syndrome," *Biological Psychiatry* 24(2): 225-233.

Bancroft J, Cook A. (1995). "The neuroendocrine response to d-fenfluramine in women with premenstrual depression," *Journal of Affective Disorders* 36(1-12): 57-64.

Cleare AJ, Bearn J, Allain T, McGregor A, Wessely S, Murray RM, O'Keane V. (1995). "Contrasting neuroendocrine responses in depression and chronic fatigue syndrome," *Journal of Affective Disorders* 34(4): 283-289.

Cleare AJ, Bond AJ. (1997). "Does central serotonergic function correlate inversely with aggression? A study using D-fenfluramine in healthy subjects," *Psychiatry Research* 69(2-3): 89-95.

Cowen PJ, Charig EM. (1987). "Neuroendocrine responses to intravenous tryptophan in major depression," *Archives of General Psychiatry* 44(11): 958-966.

Demitrack MA, Gold PW, Dale JK, Krahn DD, Kling MA, Straus SE. (1992). "Plasma and cerebrospinal fluid monoamine metabolism in patients with chronic fatigue syndrome: Preliminary findings," *Biological Psychiatry* 32(10): 1065-1077.

Dinan TG, Majeed T, Lavelle E, Scott LV, Berti C, Behan P. (1997). "Blunted serotonin-mediated activation of the hypothalamic-pituitary-adrenal axis in chronic fatigue syndrome," *Psychoneuroendocrinology* 22(4): 261-267.

Feeney S, Goodall E, Silverstone T. (1993). "The prolactin response to *d*- and *l*-fenfluramine and to *d*-amphetamine in human subjects," *International Clinical Psychopharmacology* 8(1): 49-54.

FitzGerald M, Malone KM, Li S, Harrison WM, McBride PA, Endicott J, Cooper T, Mann JJ. (1997). "Blunted serotonin response to fenfluramine challenge in premenstrual dysphoric disorder," *American Journal of Psychiatry* 154: 556-558.

Flory JD, Mann JJ, Manuck SB, Muldoon MF. (1998). "Recovery from major depression is not associated with normalization of serotonergic function," *Biological Psychiatry* 43(5): 320-326.

Freeman EW, Rickels K, Arredondo F, Kao LC, Pollack SE, Sondheimer SJ. (1999). "Full- or half-cycle treatment of severe premenstrual syndrome with a serotonergic antidepressant," *Journal of Clinical Psychopharmacology* 19(1): 3-8.

Girdler SS, Straneva PA, Light KC, Pedersen CA, Morrow AL. (2001). "Allopregnanolone levels and reactivity to mental stress in premenstrual dysphoric disorder," *Biological Psychiatry* 49(9): 788-797.

Goldenberg DL, Mayskiy M, Mossey C, Ruthazer R, Schmid, C. (1996). "A randomized, double-blind crossover trial of fluoxetine and amitriptyline in the treatment of fibromyalgia," *Arthritis and Rheumatism* 39(11): 1852-1859.

Gorard DA, Taylor TM, Medbak SH, Perry LA, Libby GW, Farthing MJ. (1993). "Plasma prolactin, adrenocorticotropic hormone and cortisol after administration of d-fenfluramine or placebo to healthy subjects," *International Clinical Psychopharmacology* 8(2): 123-128.

Heninger GR, Charney DS, Sternberg DE. (1984). "Serotonergic function in depression: Prolactin response to intravenous tryptophan in depressed patients and healthy subjects," *Archives of General Psychiatry* 41(4): 398-402.

Hirschfeld RM. (2000). "History and evolution of the monoamine hypothesis of depression," *Journal of Clinical Psychiatry* 61 (Suppl 6): 4-6.

Holmes GP, Kaplan JE, Gantz NM, Komaroff AL, Schonberger LB, Straus SE, Jones JF, Dubois RE, Cunningham-Rundles C, Pahwa S, Brus I. (1988). "Chronic fatigue syndrome: A working case definition," *Annals of Internal Medicine* 108(3): 387-389.

Kravitz HM, Katz R, Kot E, Helmke N, Fawcett J. (1992). "Biochemical clues to a fibromyalgia-depression link: Imipramine binding in patients with fibromyalgia or depression and in healthy controls," *Journal of Rheumatology* 19(9): 1428-1432.

Leonard BE. (2000). "Evidence for a biochemical lesion in depression," *Journal of Clinical Psychiatry* 61(Suppl 6): 12-17.

Lichtenberg P, Shapira B, Gillon D, Kindler S, Cooper TB, Newman ME, Lerer B. (1992). "Hormone responses to fenfluramine and placebo challenge in endogenous depression," *Psychiatry Research* 43(2): 137-146.

Magni G, Andreoli F, Arduino C, Arie D, Ceccherelli F, Ambrosio F, Dodi G, Eandi M. (1987). "Modifications of 3H-imipramine binding sites in patients of chronic pain patients treated with mianserin," *Pain* 30(3): 311-320.

Mann JJ. (1999). "Role of the serotonergic system in the pathogenesis of major depression and suicidal behavior," *Neuropsychopharmacology* 21(2 Suppl): 99S-105S.

Marazziti D, Perugi G, Deltito J, Lenzi A, Maremmani I, Placidi GF, Cassano GB. (1988). "High-affinity 3H-imipramine binding sites: A possible state-dependent marker for major depression," *Psychiatry Research* 23(2): 229-237.

Mellerup ET, Bech P, Hansen HJ, Langemark M, Loldrup D, Plenge P. (1988). "Platelet 3H-imipramine binding in psychogenic pain patients," *Psychiatry Research* 26(2): 149-156.

Mitchell P, Smythe G. (1990). "Hormonal responses to fenfluramine in depressed and control subjects," *Journal of Affective Disorders* 19(1): 43-51.

O'Keane V, Dinan TG. (1991). "Prolactin and cortisol responses to d-fenfluramine in major depression: Evidence for diminished responsivity of central serotonergic function," *American Journal of Psychiatry* 148(8): 1009-1015.

O'Keane V, McLoughlin D, Dinan TG. (1992). "D-fenfluramine-induced prolactin and cortisol release in major depression: Response to treatment," *Journal of Affective Disorders* 26(3): 143-150.

O'Keane V, O'Hanlon M, Webb M, Dinan TG. (1991). "D-fenfluramine/prolactin response throughout the menstrual cycle: Evidence for an oestrogen-induced alteration," *Clinical Endocrinology* Oxford 34(4): 289-292.

Paul SM, Rehavi M, Skolnick P, Ballenger JC, Goodwin FK. (1981). "Depressed patients have decreased binding of tritiated imipramine to platelet serotonin 'transporter,'" *Archives of General Psychiatry* 38(12): 1315-1317.

Raisman R, Briley MS, Bouchami F, Sechter D, Zarifian E, Langer SZ. (1982). "3H-imipramine binding and serotonin uptake in platelets from untreated depressed patients and control volunteers," *Psychopharmacology* (Berlin) 77(4): 332-335.

Rapkin AJ, Morgan M, Goldman L, Brann DW, Simone D, Mahesh VB. (1997). "Progesterone metabolite allopregnanolone in women with premenstrual syndrome," *Obstetrics Gynecology* 90: 709-714.

Rasgon N, McGuire M, Tanavoli S, Fairbanks L, Rapkin A. (2000). "Neuro-endocrine response to an intravenous L-tryptophan challenge in women with premenstrual syndrome," *Fertility and Sterility* 73(1): 144-149.

Rasgon N, Serra M, Biggio G, Pisu MG, Fairbanks L, Tanavoli S, Rapkin A. (2001). "Neuroactive steroid-serotonergic interaction: Responses to an intravenous L-tryptophan challenge in women with premenstrual syndrome," *European Journal of Endocrinology* 45(1): 25-33.

Rojansky N, Halbreich U, Zander K, Barkai A, Goldstein S. (1991). "Imipramine receptor binding and serotonin uptake in platelets of women with premenstrual changes," *Gynecologic and Obstetric Investigation* 31(3): 146-152.

Russell IJ, Michalek JE, Vipraio GA, Fletcher EM, Javors MA, Bowden CA. (1992). Platelet 3H-imipramine uptake receptor density and serum serotonin levels in patients with fibromyalgia/fibrositis syndrome," *Journal of Rheumatology* 19(1): 104-109.

Russell IJ, Vaeroy H, Javors M, Nyberg F. (1992). "Cerebrospinal fluid biogenic amine metabolites in fibromyalgia/fibrositis syndrome and rheumatoid arthritis," *Arthritis and Rheumatism* 35(5): 550-556.

Shapira B, Cohen J, Newman ME, Lerer B. (1993). "Prolactin response to fen-fluramine and placebo challenge following maintenance pharmacotherapy withdrawal in remitted depressed patients," *Biological Psychiatry* 33(7): 531-535.

Steege JF, Stout AL, Knight DL, Nemeroff CB. (1992). "Reduced platelet tritium-labeled imipramine binding sites in women with premenstrual syndrome," *American Journal of Obstetrics and Gynecology* 167(1): 168-172.

Steiner M, Steinberg S, Stewart D, Carter D, Berger C, Reid R, Grover D, Streiner D and the Canadian Fluoxetine/Premenstrual Dysphoria Collaborative Study Group. (1995). "Fluoxetine in the treatment of premenstrual syndrome," *New England Journal of Medicine* 332(23): 1529-1534.

Steiner M, Yatham LN, Coote M, Wilkins A, Lepage P. (1999). "Serotonergic dysfunction in women with pure premenstrual dysphoric disorder: Is the fenfluramine challenge test still relevant?" *Psychiatry Research* 87(2-3): 107-115.

Suranyi-Cadotte B, Quirion R, McQuade P, Nair NP, Schwartz G, Mosticyan S, Wood PL. (1984). "Platelet 3H-imipramine binding: A state-dependent marker in depression," *Progress in Neuropsychopharmacology and Biological Psychiatry* 8(4-6): 368-371.

Vassallo CM, Felman E, Peto T, Castell L, Sharpley AL, Cowen PJ. (2001). "Decreased tryptophan availability but normal post-synaptic 5-HT2c receptor sensitivity in chronic fatigue syndrome," *Psychological Medicine* 31(4): 585-591.

Vercoulen JHMM, Swanink CMA, Zitman FG, Vreden SGS, Hoofs MPE, Fennis JFM, Galama JMD, van der Meer JWM, Bleinjenberg G. (1996). "Randomized, double-blind, placebo-controlled study of fluoxetine in chronic fatigue syndrome," *Lancet* 347(9005): 858-861.

Wang M, Seippel L, Purdy RH, Backstrom T. (1996). "Relationship between symptom severity and steroid variation in women with premenstrual syndrome," *Journal of Clinical Endocrinology and Metabolism* 81: 1076-1082.

Wearden AJ, Morriss RK, Mullis R, Strickland PL, Pearson DJ, Appleby L, Campbell IT, Morris JA. (1998). "Randomized, double-blind, placebo-controlled treatment trial of fluoxetine and graded exercise for chronic fatigue syndrome," *British Journal of Psychiatry* 172(6): 485-490.

Wolfe F, Russell IJ, Vipraio GA, Ross K, Anderson J. (1997). "Serotonin levels, pain threshold, and fibromyalgia symptoms in the general population," *Journal of Rheumatology* 24(3): 555-559.

Yatham LN, Morehouse RL, Chisholm BT, Haase DA, MacDonald DD, Marrie TJ. (1995). "Neuroendocrine assessment of serotonin (5-HT) function in chronic fatigue syndrome," *Canadian Journal of Psychiatry* 41(2): 129-131.

Yonkers KA, Halbreich U, Freeman E, Brown C, Endicott J, Frank E, Parry B, Pearlstein T, Severino S, Stout A, Stone A, Harrison W, for the Sertraline Premenstrual Dysphoric Collaborative Study Group. (1997). "Symptomatic improvement of premenstrual dysphoric disorder with sertraline treatment. A randomized controlled trial," *Journal of the American Medical Association* 278(12): 983-988.

Zarifian E, Sechter D, Bouchami F, Cuche H, Olie JP, Susini JR, Briley M, Raisman R, Langer SZ. (1982). "[3H-imipramine binding to human platelets. A peripheral index in depressive syndromes]," *Nouvelle Presse Medicale* 11(18): 1385-1387.

Chapter 12

Achenbach TM, Verhulst FC, Baron GD, Althaus M. (1987). "A comparison of syndromes derived from the Child Behavior Checklist for American and Dutch boys aged 6-11 and 12-16," *Journal of Child Psychology and Psychiatry* 28(3): 437-453.

Ahles TA, Yunus MB, Riley SD, Bradley JM, Masi AT. (1984). "Psychological factors associated with primary fibromyalgia syndrome," *Arthritis and Rheumatism* 27(10): 1101-1106.

American Psychiatric Association. (1987). *Diagnostic and Statistical Manual of Mental Disorders* (Third Edition, Revised). Washington, DC: American Psychiatric Association,

Bakker CB, Bakker-Rabdau MK, Breit S. (1978). "The measurement of assertiveness and aggressiveness," *Journal of Personality Assessment* 42(3): 277-284.

Benjamin J, Osher Y, Lichtenberg P, Bachner-Melman R, Gritsenko I, Kotler M, Belmaker RH, Valsky V, Drendel M, Ebstein RP. (2000). "An interaction between the catechol-*O*-methyltransferase and the serotonin transporter promoter region polymorphism contributes to tridimensional personality questionnaire persistence scores in normal subjects," *Neuropsychobiology* 41(1): 48-53.

Berlin RE, Raju JD, Schmidt PJ, Adams LF, Rubinow DR. (2001). "Effects of the menstrual cycle on measures of personality in women with premenstrual syndrome: A preliminary study," *Journal of Clinical Psychiatry* 62(5): 337-342.

Binder LM, Storzbach D, Campbell KA, Rohlman DS, Anger WK, Salinsky MC, Campbell BR, Mueller R. (2000). "Comparison of MMPI-2 profiles of Gulf War veterans with epileptic and nonepileptic seizure patients," *Assessment* 7(1): 73-78.

Blakely AA, Howard RC, Sosich RM, Murdoch JC, Menkes DB, Spears GFS. (1991). "Psychiatric symptoms, personality and ways of coping in chronic fatigue syndrome," *Psychological Medicine* 21(2): 347-362.

Blanchard EB, Keefer L, Galovski TE, Taylor AE, Turner SM. (2001). "Gender differences in psychological distress among patients with irritable bowel syndrome," *Journal of Psychosomatic Research* 50(5): 271-275.

Bradley LA, Prokop CK, Margolis R, Gentry WD. (1978). "Multivariate analysis of MMPI profiles of low back pain patients," *Journal of Behavioral Medicine* 1(3): 253-272.

Buckley L, MacHale SM, Cavanagh JTO, Sharpe M, Deary IJ, Lawrie SM. (1998). "Personality dimensions in chronic fatigue syndrome and depression," *Journal of Psychosomatic Research* 46(4): 395-400.

Buss AH, Darkee A. (1957). "An inventory for assessing different kinds of hostility," *Journal of Consulting Psychology* 21(4): 343-348.

Christodoulou C, DeLuca J, Johnson SK, Lange G, Gaudino EA, Natelson BH. (1999). "Examination of Cloninger's dimensions of personality in fatiguing illness: Chronic fatigue syndrome and multiple sclerosis," *Journal of Psychosomatic Research* 47(6): 597-607.

Cloninger CR. (1987a). "A systematic method for clinical description and classification of personality variants," *Archives of General Psychiatry* 44(6): 573-588.

Cloninger CR. (1987b). *The Tridimensional Personality Questionnaire, Version IV.* St. Louis, MO: Department of Psychiatry, Washington University School of Medicine.

Costa PT, McCrae T. (1985). *The NEO Personality Inventory Manual.* Odessa, FL: Psychological Assessment Resources.

Critchlow DG, Bond AJ, Wingrove J. (2001). "Mood disorder history and personality assessment in premenstrual dysphoric disorder," *Journal of Clinical Psychiatry* 62(9): 688-693.

Crowne DP, Marlowe D. (1960). "A new scale of social desirability independent of psychopathology," *Journal of Consulting Psychology* 24(3): 394-354.

Dahlstrom WG, Welsh GS, Dahlstrom LE. (1972). *MMPI Handbook,* Volume 1. Minneapolis: University of Minnesota Press.

De Ronchi D, Muro A, Marziani A, Rucci P. (2000). "Personality disorders and depressive symptoms in late luteal phase dysphoric disorder," *Psychotherapy and Psychosomatics* 69(1): 27-34.

Enns MW, Cox BJ. (1997). "Personality dimensions and depression: Review and commentary," *Canadian Journal of Psychiatry* 42(3): 249-250.

Eysenck HJ, Eysenck SBG. (1968). *Personality Structure and Measurement.* Baltimore, MD: Edits Publishers.

Eysenck HJ, Eysenck SBG. (1975). *Manual of the Eysenck Personality Questionnaire.* London: Hodder and Stoughton.

Fiedler N, Lange G, Tiersk L, DeLuca J, Policastro T, Kelly-McNeil K, McWilliams R, Korn L, Natelson B. (2000). "Stressors, personality traits, and coping of Gulf War veterans with chronic fatigue," *Journal of Psychosomatic Research* 48(6): 525-535.

First MB, Spitzer RL, Gibbon M. (1997). *Structured Clinical Interview for DSM-IV Axis I Disorders: Clinician Version (SCID-CV).* Washington, DC: American Psychiatric Press.

Fock KM, Chew CN, Tay LK, Peh LH, Chan S, Pang EP. (2001). "Psychiatric illness, personality traits and the irritable bowel syndrome," *Annals of the Academy of Medicine, Singapore* 30(6): 61-64.

Frost RO, Marten P, Lahart C, Rosenblate R. (1990). "The dimensions of perfectionism," *Cognitive Therapy Research* 14(6): 449-468.

Fukuda K, Straus SE, Hickie I, Sharpe MC, Dobbins JG, Komaroff A. (1994). "The chronic fatigue syndrome: A comprehensive approach to its definition and study. International Chronic Fatigue Syndrome Study Group," *Annals of Internal Medicine* 121(12): 953-959.

Goldberg D, Williams P. (1988). *A User's Guide to the General Health Questionnaire.* Windsor, Great Britain: Nelson.

Gray D, Parker-Cohen NY, White T, Clark ST, Seiner SH, Achilles J, McMahon WM. (2001). "A comparison of individual and family psychology of adolescents with chronic fatigue syndrome, rheumatoid arthritis, and mood disorders," *Developmental and Behavioral Pediatrics* 22(4): 234-242.

Hollander E, DeCaria CM, Nitescu A, Gully R, Suckow RF, Cooper TB, Gorman JM, Klein DF, Liebowitz MR. (1992). "Serotonergic function in obsessive-compulsive disorder: Behavioral and endocrine responses to oral *m*-chlorophenylpiperazine and fenfluramine in patients and healthy volunteers," *Archives of General Psychiatry* 49(1): 21-28.

Holmes GP, Kaplan JE, Gantz NM, Komaroff AL, Schonberger LB, Straus SE, Jones JF, Dubois RE, Cunningham-Rundles C, Pahwa S, Brus I. (1988). "Chronic fatigue syndrome: A working case definition," *Annals of Internal Medicine* 108(3): 387-389.

Holmes TH, Rahe RH. (1967). "The social readjustment rating scale," *Journal of Psychosomatic Research* 11(2): 213-218.

Hyler SE, Rieder RO. (1986). *Personality Diagnostic Questionnaire—Revised.* New York: New York State Psychiatric Institute.

Hyler SE, Rieder RO. (1987). *PDQ-R: Personality Disorders Questionnaire—Revised.* New York: New York State Psychiatric Institute.

Johnson SK, DeLuca J, Natelson BH. (1996). "Personality dimensions in the chronic fatigue syndrome: A comparison with multiple sclerosis and depression," *Journal of Psychiatric Research* 30(1): 9-20.

Katon WJ, Walker EA. (1998). "Medically unexplained symptoms in primary care," *Journal of Clinical Psychiatry* 59(Suppl 20): 15-21.

Kirmayer LJ, Robbins JM, Paris J. (1994). "Somatoform disorders personality and the social matrix of somatic distress," *Journal of Abnormal Psychology* 103(1): 125-136.

Kovera CA, Anger WK, Campbell KA, Binder LM, Storzbach D, Davis KL, Rohlman DS. (1996). "Computer-administration of questionnaires: A health screening system (HHS) developed for veterans," *Neurotoxicology and Teratology* 18(4): 511-518.

Lloyd AR, Hickie I, Boughton CR, Spencer O, Wakefield D. (1990). "Prevalence of chronic fatigue syndrome in an Australian population," *Medical Journal of Australia* 153(9): 522-528.

Loranger AW, Janca A, Sartorius N. (1997). *Assessment and Diagnosis of Personality Disorders. The ICD-10 International Personality Disorder Examination (ICDE)*. New York: Cambridge University Press.

Marcus S, Robins LN, Bucholz, K. (1990). *Quick Diagnostic Interview Schedule 3R Version I*. St Louis, MO: Washington University School of Medicine.

Millon T. (1987). *Manual for the MMCI-II* (Second Edition). Minneapolis, MN: National Computer Systems.

Moldofsky H, Scarisbrick P, England R, Smythe H. (1975). "Musculoskeletal symptoms and non-REM sleep disturbance in patients with 'fibrositis syndrome' and healthy subjects," *Psychosomatic Medicine* 37(4): 341-351.

Montgomery SA, Asberg M. (1979). "A new depression scale designed to be sensitive to change," *British Journal of Psychiatry* 134(4): 382-389.

Parry BL, Ehlers CL, Mostofi N, Phillips E. (1996). "Personality traits in LLPDD and normal controls during follicular and late menstrual-cycle phases," *Psychological Medicine* 26(1): 197-202.

Payne TC, Leavitt F, Garron DC, Katz RS, Golden HE, Glickman PB, Vanderplate C. (1982). "Fibrositis and psychological disturbance," *Arthritis and Rheumatism* 25(2): 213-217.

Pepper CM, Krupp LB, Friedberg F, Doscher C, Coyle PK. (1993). A comparison of neuropsychiatric characteristics in chronic fatigue syndrome, multiple sclerosis, and major depression. *Journal of Neuropsychiatry and Clinical Neurosciences* 5(2): 200-205.

Poser CM, Paty DW, Scheinberg L, McDonald WI, Davis FA, Ebers OC, Johnson KP, Sibley WA, Silberberg DH, Tourtellotte WW. (1983). "New diagnostic criteria for multiple sclerosis: Guidelines for research protocols," *Annals of Neurology* 13(3): 227-231.

Rey JM, Starling J, Wever C, Dossetor DR, Plapp JM. (1995). "Inter-rater reliability of global assessment of functioning in a clinical setting," *Journal of Child Psychology and Psychiatry* 36(5): 787-792.

Reynolds WM. (1982). "Development of reliable and valid short forms of the Marlowe-Crowne social desirability scale," *Journal of Clinical Psychology* 38(2): 119-125.

Robins L, Cottler L, Keating S. (1991). *Diagnostic Interview Schedule (DIS): Version III-Revised.* St. Louis, MO: Washington University School of Medicine.

Ropes MW, Bennett GA, Cobb S, Jacox R, Jessar RA. (1958). "1958 revision of diagnostic criteria for rheumatoid arthritis," *Bulletin on the Rheumatic Diseases* 9(2): 175-176.

Rosenberg M. (1965). *Society and the Adolescent Self-Image.* Princeton, NJ: Princeton University Press.

Shaffer D, Fisher P, Dulcan MK, Davies M, Piacentini J, Schwab-Stone ME, Lahey BB, Bourdon K, Jensen PS, Bird HR, Canino G, Regier DA. (1996). "The NIMH Diagnostic Interview Schedule for Children Version 2.3 (DISC-2.3): Description, acceptability, prevalence rates, and performance in the Methods for the Epidemiology of Child and Adolescent Mental Disorders Study," *Journal of the American Academy of Child and Adolescent Psychiatry* 35: 865-877.

Shapurian R, Hojat M, Nayerahmadi H. (1987). "Psychometric characteristics and dimensionality of a Persian version of Rosenberg Self-Esteem Scale," *Perceptual and Motor Skills* 65(1): 27-34.

Sharpe MC, Archard LC, Banatvala JE, Borysiewicz LK, Clare AW, David A, Edwards RH, Hawton KE, Lambert HP, Lane RJ. (1991). "A report—chronic fatigue syndrome guidelines for research," *Journal of the Royal Society of Medicine* 84(2): 118-121.

Spitzer RL, Williams JBW, Gibbon M. (1987). *Structured Clinical Interview for the DSM-III-R Personality Disorders (SCID-II).* Washington, DC: American Psychiatric Association.

Spitzer RL, Williams JB, Gibbon M, First MB. (1992). "The Structured Clinical Interview for DSM-III-R (SCID). I. History, rationale, and description," *Archives of General Psychiatry* 49(8): 624-629.

Taylor GJ. (2000). "Recent developments in alexithymia theory and research," *Canadian Journal of Psychiatry* 45(2): 134-142.

Taylor GJ, Bagby RM, Ryan DP, Parker JD, Doody KF, Keefe P. (1988). "Criterion validity of the Toronto Alexythymia Scale," *Psychosomatic Medicine* 50(5): 500-509.

Thompson WG, Dotevall G, Drossman DA, Heaton KW, Kruis W. (1989). "Irritable bowel syndrome: Guidelines for the diagnosis," *Gastroenterology International* 2(2): 92-95.

Watson M, Greer S. (1983). "Development of a questionnaire measure of emotional control," *Journal of Psychosomatic Research* 27(4): 299-305.

White C, Schweitzer R. (2000). "The role of personality in the development and perpetuation of chronic fatigue syndrome," *Journal of Psychosomatic Research* 48(6): 515-524.

Widiger TA, Rogers JH. (1989). "Prevalence and comorbidity of personality disorders," *Psychiatric Annals* 19(2): 132-136.

Williams JB, Gibbon M, First MB, Spitzer RL, Davies M, Borus J, Howes MJ, Kane J, Pope HO Jr., Rounsaville B. (1992). "The Structured Clinical Interview for DSM-III-R (SCID). II. Multisite test-retest reliability," *Archives of General Psychiatry* 49(8): 630-636.

Wolfe F, Smythe HA, Yunus MB, Bennett RM, Bombardier C, Goldenberg DL, Tugwell P, Campbell SM, Abeles M, Clark P, Fam AG, Farber SJ, Fiechtner JJ, Franklin C, Gatter RA, Hamaty D, Lessard J, Lichtbroun AS, Masi AT, McCain GA, Reynolds WJ, Romano TJ, Russell IJ, Sheon RP. (1990). "The American College of Rheumatology 1990 criteria for the classification of fibromyalgia. Report of the Multicenter Criteria Committee," *Arthritis and Rheumatism* 33(2): 160-172.

Wood B, Wessely S. (1999). "Personality and social attitudes in chronic fatigue syndrome," *Journal of Psychosomatic Research* 47(4): 385-397.

Yunus M, Masi AT, Calabro JJ, Miller KA, Feigenbaum SL. (1981). "Primary fibromyalgia (fibrositis): Clinical study of 50 patients with matched normal controls," *Seminars in Arthritis and Rheumatism* 11(1): 151-171.

Chapter 13

Alexander RW, Bradley LA, Alarcon GS, Triana-Alexander M, Aaron LA, Alberts KR, Martin MY, Stewart KE. (1998). "Sexual and physical abuse in women with fibromyalgia: Association with outpatient health care utilization and pain medication usage," *Arthritis Care and Research* 11(2): 102-115.

Bernstein D, Fink L, Handelsman L, Foote J, Lovejoy M, Wenzel K, Sapareto E, Ruggiero J. (1994). "Initial reliability and validity of a new retrospective measure of child abuse and neglect," *American Journal of Psychiatry* 151(8): 1132-1136.

Bernstein EM, Putnam FW. (1986). "Development, reliability and validity of a dissociation scale," *Journal of Nervous and Mental Disease* 174(12): 727-735.

Blouin AG, Perez EL, Blouin JH. (1988). "Computerized administration of the Diagnostic Interview Schedule," *Psychiatry Research* 23(3): 335-344.

Boisset-Pioro MH, Esdaile JM, Fitzcharles MA. (1995). "Sexual and physical abuse in women with fibromyalgia syndrome," *Arthritis and Rheumatism* 38(2): 235-241.

Briere J. (1992a). *Child Abuse Trauma.* Newbury Park, NJ: Sage Publications.

Briere J. (1992b). "Methodological issues in the study of sexual abuse effects," *Journal of Clinical and Consulting Psychology* 60(2): 196-203.

Carlson EB, Putnam FW, Ross CA, Torem M, Coons P, Dill DL, Lowenstein RJ, Braun BG. (1993). "Validity of the Dissociative Experiences Scale in screening for multiple personality disorder: A multicenter study," *American Journal of Psychiatry* 150(7): 1030-1036.

Cloninger CR. (1987). "A systematic method for clinical description and classification of personality variants: A proposal," *Archives of General Psychiatry* 44(6): 573-588.

Costa PT, McCrae RR. (1980). "Influence of extroversion and neuroticism on subjective well-being: Happy and unhappy people," *Journal of Personality and Social Psychology* 38: 668-678.

Delvaux M, Denis P, Allemand H. (1997). "Sexual abuse is more frequently reported by IBS patients than by patients with organic digestive diseases or controls. Results of a multicentre inquiry, French Club of Digestive Motility," *European Journal of Gastroenterology and Hepatology* 9(4): 345-352.

Derogatis LR, Melisaratos N. (1983). "The Brief Symptom Inventory: An introductory report," *Psychological Medicine* 13(3): 595-605.

Drossman DA, Leserman J, Nachman G, Li Z, Gluck H, Toomey TC, Mitchell CM. (1990). "Sexual and physical abuse in women with functional and organic gastrointestinal disorders," *Annals of Internal Medicine* 113(11): 828-833.

Drossman DA, Li Z, Andruzzi E, Temple RD, Talley NJ, Thompson WG, Whitehead WE, Janssen J, Funch-Jensen P, Corazziari E, Richter JE, Kock GG. (1993). "US householder survey of functional gastrointestinal disorders: Prevalence, sociodemography and health impact," *Digestive Diseases and Sciences* 9: 1569-1580.

Drossman DA, Talley NJ, Leserman J, Olden KW, Barreiro MA. (1995). "Sexual and physical abuse and gastrointestinal illness: Review and recommendations," *Annals of Internal Medicine* 123: 782-794.

Frayne SM, Skinner KM, Sullivan LM, Tripp TJ, Hankin CS, Kressin NR, Miller DR. (1999). "Medical profile of women Veterans Administration outpatients who report a history of sexual assault occurring while in the military," *Journal of Womens' Health and Gender Based Medicine* 8(6): 835-845.

Fukuda K, Straus SE, Hickie I, Sharpe MC, Dobbins JG, Komaroff A. (1994). "The chronic fatigue syndrome: A comprehensive approach to its definition and study. International Chronic Fatigue Syndrome Study Group," *Annals of Internal Medicine* 121(12): 953-959.

Golding JM, Cooper ML, George LK. (1997). "Sexual assault history and health perceptions: Seven general population studies," *Health Psychology* 16(5): 417-425.

Holmes MM, Resnick HS, Frampton D. (1998). "Follow-up of sexual assault victims," *American Journal of Obstetrics and Gynecology* 179(2): 336-342.

Longstreth GF, Wolde-Tsadik G. (1993). "Irritable bowel-type symptoms in HMO examinees. Prevalence, demographic, and clinical correlates," *Digestive Diseases and Science* 38(9): 1581-1589.

Robins LN, Helzer JE, Croughan J, Ratcliff KS. (1981). "National Institute of Mental Health Diagnostic Interview Schedule: Its history, characteristics, and validity," *Archives of General Psychiatry* 38(4): 381-389.

Stewart AL, Hays RD, Ware JE Jr. (1988). "The MOS short-form general health survey: Reliability and validity in a patient population," *Medical Care* 26(7): 724-735.

Talley NJ, Boyce PM, Jones M. (1998). "Is the association between irritable bowel syndrome and abuse explained by neuroticism? A population based study," *Gut* 41(1): 47-53.

Talley NJ, Fett SL, Zinsmeister AR. (1995). "Self-reported abuse and gastrointestinal disease in outpatients: Association with irritable bowel-type symptoms," *American Journal of Gastroenterology* 90(3): 335-337.

Taylor ML, Trotter DR, Csuka ME. (1995). "The prevalence of sexual abuse in women with fibromyalgia," *Arthritis and Rheumatism* 38(2): 229-234.

Taylor RR, Jason LA. (2001). "Sexual abuse, physical abuse, chronic fatigue, and chronic fatigue syndrome: A community-based study," *Journal of Nervous and Mental Disease* 189(10): 709-715.

Walker EA, Gelfand AN, Gelfand MD, Katon WJ. (1995). "Psychiatric diagnoses, sexual and physical victimization, and disability in patients with irritable bowel syndrome or inflammatory bowel disease," *Psychological Medicine* 25(6): 1259-1267.

Walker EA, Katon WJ, Roy-Byrne PP, Jemelka RP, Russo J. (1993). "Histories of sexual victimization in patients with irritable bowel syndrome or inflammatory bowel disease," *American Journal of Psychiatry* 150(10): 1502-1506.

Walker EA, Keegan D, Gardner G, Sullivan M, Bernstein D, Katon WJ. (1997). "Psychosocial factors in fibromyalgia compared with rheumatoid arthritis. II. Sexual, physical, and emotional abuse and neglect," *Psychosomatic Medicine* 59(6): 572-577.

Chapter 14

Bains GK, Slade P. (1988). "Attributional patterns, moods, and the menstrual cycle," *Psychosomatic Medicine* 50(5): 469-476.

Bower P, West R, Taylee A, Hann M. (2000). "Symptom attribution and the recognition of psychiatric morbidity," *Journal of Psychosomatic Research* 48(2): 157-160.

Brosschot JF, Aarsse HR. (2001). "Restricted emotional processing and somatic attribution in fibromyalgia," *International Journal of Psychiatry in Medicine* 31(2): 127-146.

Cathebras P, Jacquin L, Le Gal M, Fayol C, Bouchou K, Rousset H. (1995). "Correlates of somatic causal attributions in primary care patients with fatigue," *Psychotherapy and Psychosomatics* 63(6-4): 174-180.

Chalder T, Power MJ, Wessely S. (1996). "Chronic fatigue in the community: 'A question of attribution,' " *Psychological Medicine* 26(4): 791-800.

Garcia-Campayo J, Larrubia J, Lobo A, Perez-Echeverria MJ, Campos R. (1997). "Attribution in somatizers: Stability and relationship to outcome at 1-year follow-up," *Acta Psychiatrica Scandinavica* 95(5): 433-438.

Lawrie SM, Manders DN, Geddes JR, Pelosi AJ. (1997). "A population-based incidence study of chronic fatigue," *Psychological Medicine* 27(2): 343-353.

Neerinckx E, Van Houdenhove B, Lysens R, Vertommen H, Onghena P. (2000). "Attributions in chronic fatigue syndrome and fibromyalgia syndrome in tertiary care," *Journal of Rheumatology* 27(4): 1051-1055.

Powell R, Dolan R, Wesselly S. (1990). "Attributions and self-esteem in depression and chronic fatigue syndromes," *Journal of Psychosomatic Research* 34(6): 665-673.

Sharpe M, Hawton K, Seagrott V, Pasvol G. (1992). "Follow up of patients presenting with fatigue to an infectious disease clinic," *British Medical Journal* 305(6846): 147-152.

Taylor RE, Mann AH, White NJ, Goldberg DP. (2000). "Attachment style in patients with unexplained physical complaints," *Psychological Medicine* 30(4): 931-941.

Wessely S, Powell R. (1989). "Fatigue syndromes: A comparison of chronic 'postviral' fatigue with neuromuscular and affective disorders," *Journal of Neurology, Neurosurgery and Psychiatry* 52: 940-948.

Wilson A, Hickie I, Lloyd A, Hadzi-Pavlovic D, Boughton C, Dwyer J, Wakefield D. (1994). "Longitudinal study of outcome in chronic fatigue syndrome," *British Medical Journal* 308(6931): 756-759.

Chapter 15

Achenbach T, Edelbrock C. (1983). *Manual for the Child Behavior Checklist, Revised Child Behavior Profile.* Burlington, VT: University of Vermont, Department of Psychiatry.

Achenbach T, Edelbrock C. (1987). *Manual for the Youth Self-Report, Revised Youth Self-Report Profile.* Burlington, VT: University of Vermont, Department of Psychiatry.

Ali A, Toner BB, Stuckless N, Gallop R, Diamant NE, Gould MI, Vidins EI. (2000). "Emotional abuse, self-blame, and self-silencing in women with irritable bowel syndrome," *Psychosomatic Medicine* 62(1): 76-82.

Anderson CA, Miller RS, Riger AL, Dill JC, Sedikides C. (1994). "Behavioral and characterological attributional styles as predictors of depression and loneliness: Review, refinement, and test," *Journal of Personality and Social Psychology* 66(3): 549-558.

Arnett FC, Edworthy SM, Bloch DA, McShane DJ, Fries JF, Cooper NS, Healey LA, Kaplan SR, Liang MH, Luthra HS. (1988). "The American Rheumatism Association 1987 revised criteria for the classification of rheumatoid arthritis," *Arthritis and Rheumatism* 31(3): 315-324.

Barsky AJ, Borus JF. (1999). "Functional somatic syndromes," *Annals of Internal Medicine* 130(11): 910-921.

Beck AT. (1964). "Thinking and depression. II. Theory and therapy," *Archives of General Psychiatry* 10: 561-571.

Beck AT. (1976). *Beck Depression Inventory.* Philadelphia: Center for Cognitive Therapy.

Beck AT, Steer RA, Brown GK. (1996). *Manual for Beck Depression Inventory—II.* San Antonio, TX: Psychological Corporation.

Brace MJ, Scott Smith M, McCauley E, Sherry DD. (2000). "Family reinforcement of illness behavior: A comparison of adolescents with chronic fatigue syndrome, juvenile arthritis, and healthy controls," *Journal of Developmental and Behavioral Pediatrics* 21(5): 332-339.

Brewin CR, Furnham A. (1987). "Dependency, self-criticism and depressive attributional style," *British Journal of Clinical Psychology* 26(Pt 3): 225-226.

Cameron L, Leventhal EA, Leventhal H. (1993). "Symptom representation and affect as determinants of care seeking in a community dwelling, adult sample population," *Health Psychology* 12: 171-179.

Cope H, Mann A, Pelosi A, David A. (1996). "Psychosocial risk factors for chronic fatigue and chronic fatigue syndrome following a presumed viral illness: A case-control study," *Psychological Medicine* 26(6): 1197-1209.

Davis MC, Zautra AJ, Reich JW. (2001). "Vulnerability to stress among women in chronic pain from fibromyalgia and osteoarthritis," *Annals of Behavioral Medicine* 25(3): 215-226.

Derogatis LR, Melisaratos N. (1983). "Brief symptom inventory: An introductory report," *Psychological Medicine* 13(3): 595-605.

Drossman DA, Li Z, Toner BB, Diamant NE, Creed FH, Thompson D, Read NW, Babbs C, Barreiro M, Bank L. (1995). "Functional bowel disorders. A multicenter comparison of health status and development of illness severity index," *Digestive Diseases and Science* 40(5): 986-995.

Drossman DA, Whitehead WE, Toner BB, Diamant N, Hu YJ, Bangdiwala SI, Jia H. (2000). "What determines severity among patients with functional bowel disorders?" *American Journal of Gastroenterology* 95(4): 974-980.

Duarte LM, Thompson JM. (1999). "Sex differences in self-silencing," *Psychological Reports* 85(1): 145-161.

Ensalada LH. (2000). "The importance of illness behavior in disability management," *Occupational Medicine* 15(4): 739-754.

Ercolani M, Trombini G, Chattat R, Cervini C, Piergiacomi G, Salaffi F, Zeni S, Marcolongo R. (1994). "Fibromyalgic syndrome: Depression and abnormal illness behavior," *Psychotherapeutics and Psychosomatics* 61(3-4): 178-186.

Farmer ME, Locker BZ, Moscicki EK, Dannenberg AL, Larson DB, Radloff LS. (1988). "Physical activity and depressive symptoms: The NHANES I Epidemiologic Follow-Up Study," *American Journal of Epidemiology* 128(6): 1340-1351.

Folkman F, Lazarus RF. (1980). "An analysis of coping in a middle-aged community sample," *Journal of Health and Social Behavior* 21(3): 219-239.

Folkman S, Lazarus RS, Dunkel-Schetter C, DeLongis A, Gruen RJ. (1986). "Dynamics of a stressful encounter: Cognitive appraisal, coping and encounter outcomes," *Journal of Personality and Social Psychology* 50(5): 992-1003.

Fukuda K, Straus SE, Hickie I, Sharpe MC, Dobbins JG, Komaroff A. (1994). "The chronic fatigue syndrome: A comprehensive approach to its definition and study. International Chronic Fatigue Syndrome Study Group," *Annals of Internal Medicine* 121(12): 953-959.

Gaston-Johansson F, Gustafsson M, Felldin R, Sanne H. (1990). "A comparative study of feelings, attitudes and behaviors of patients with fibromyalgia and rheumatoid arthritis," *Social Science and Medicine* 31(8): 941-947.

Gibbs-Gallagher N, Palsson OS, Levy RL, Meyer K, Drossman DA, Whitehead WE. (2001). "Selective recall of gastrointestinal-sensation words: Evidence for a cognitive-behavioral contribution to irritable bowel syndrome," *American Journal of Gastroenterology* 96(4): 1133-1138.

Hansen V, Jacobsen BK. (1989). "Mental distress and social conditions and lifestyle in northern Norway," *British Medical Journal* 299(6691): 85-88.

Hassett AL, Cone JD, Patella SJ, Sigal LH. (2000). "The role of catastrophizing in the pain and depression of women with fibromyalgia syndrome," *Arthritis and Rheumatism* 43(11): 2493-2500.

Holmes GP, Kaplan JE, Gantz NM, Komaroff AL, Schonberger LB, Straus SE, Jones JF, Dubois RE, Cunningham-Rundles C, Pahwa S, Brus I. (1988). "Chronic fatigue syndrome: A working case definition," *Annals of Internal Medicine* 108(3): 387-389.

Jack DC, Dill D. (1992). "Silencing the Self Scale: Schemas of intimacy associated with depression in women," *Psychology of Women Quarterly* 19(3): 337-353.

Janoff-Bulman R. (1979). "Characterological versus behavioral self-blame: Inquiries into depression and rape," *Journal of Personality and Social Psychology* 37(10): 1798-1809.

Kanner A, Coyne J, Schaefer C, Lazarus R. (1981). "Comparison of two modes of stress measurement: Daily hassles and uplifts versus major life events," *Journal of Behavioral Medicine* 4(1): 1-39.

Keefe FJ, Brown GK, Wallston KA, Caldwell DS. (1989). "Coping with rheumatoid arthritis pain: Catastrophizing as a maladaptive strategy," *Pain* 37(1): 51-56.

Kersh BC, Bradley LA, Alarcon GS, Alberts KR, Sotolongo A, Martin MY, Aaron LA, Dewaal DF, Domino ML, Chaplin WF, Palardy NR, Cianfrini LR, Triana-Alexander M. (2001). "Psychosocial and health status variables independently predict health care seeking in fibromyalgia," *Arthritis Care and Research* 45(4): 362-371.

Meenan RF, Gertman PM, Mason JH. (1980). "Measuring health status in arthritis: The arthritis impact measurement scales," *Arthritis and Rheumatism* 23(2): 146-152.

Melzack R. (1975). "The McGill Pain Questionnaire: Major properties and scoring methods," *Pain* 1(3): 277-299.

Moss-Morris R, Petrie KJ. (1997). "Cognitive distortions of somatic experiences—revision and validation of a measure," *Journal of Psychosomatic Research* 43: 293-306.

Moss-Morris R, Petrie KJ. (2001). "Discriminating between chronic fatigue syndrome and depression: A cognitive analysis," *Psychological Medicine* 31(3): 469-479.

Olson D, Porter J, Bell R. (1982). *FACES II: Family Adaptability and Cohesion Evaluation Scales*. St. Paul, MN: University of Minnesota, Family Social Sciences.

Olson D, Porter J, Lavee Y. (1985). *FACES III*. St. Paul, MN: University of Minnesota, Family Social Sciences.

Parker G. (1983). *Parental Overprotection: A Risk Factor for Psychosocial Development*. New York: Grune and Stratton.

Pelcovitz D, Friedman A, Krilov LR, Mandel F, Kaplan S. (1995). "Psychosocial correlates of chronic fatigue syndrome in adolescent girls," *Developmental and Behavioral Pediatrics* 16(5): 333-338.

Pilowsky I, Spence ND. (1975). "Patterns of illness behaviour in patients with intractable pain," *Journal of Psychosomatic Research* 19(4): 279-287.

Pincus T, Morley S. (2001). "Cognitive-processing bias in chronic pain: A review and integration," *Psychological Bulletin* 127(5): 599-617.

Poznanski EO, Grossman JA, Buchsbaum Y, Banegas M, Freeman L, Gibbons R. (1984). "Preliminary studies of the reliability and validity of the Children's Depression Rating Scale," *Journal of the American Academy of Child Psychiatry* 23(2): 191-197.

Radloff LS. (1977). "The CES-D scale," *Applied Psychological Measures* 1(5): 385-401.

Robbins JM, Kirmayer LJ. (1991). "Attribution of common somatic symptoms," *Psychological Medicine* 21(4): 1029-1045.

Robins LN, Helzer JE, Croughan J, Ratcliff KS. (1981). "National Institute of Mental Health diagnostic interview schedule: Its history, characteristics and validity," *Archives of General Psychiatry* 38(4): 381-389.

Ropes MW, Bennett GA, Cobb S, Jacox R, Jessar RA. (1958). "1958 revision of diagnostic criteria for rheumatoid arthritis," Bulletin of the Rheumatic Diseases 9(2): 175-176.

Rosenstiel AK, Keefe FJ. (1983). "The use of coping strategies in low back pain: Relationship to patient characteristics and current adjustment," *Pain* 17(1): 32-44.

Segal ZV. (1988). "Appraisal of the self schema construct in cognitive models of depression," *Psychological Bulletin* 103(2): 147-162.

Sharpe MC, Archard LC, Banatvala JE, Borysiewicz LK, Clare AW, David A, Edwards RH, Hawton KE, Lambert HP, Lane RJ. (1991). "A report—chronic fatigue syndrome guidelines for research," *Journal of the Royal Society of Medicine* 84(2): 118-121.

Smith CA, Wallston KA, Dwyer KA, Dowdy SW. (1997). "Beyond good and bad," *Annals of Behavioral Medicine* 19(1): 11-21.

Swartzman LC, Gwadry FG, Shapiro AP, Teasell RW. (1994). "The factor structure of the Coping Strategies Questionnaire," *Pain* 57(3): 311-316.

Theorell T, Blomkvist V, Lindh G, Evengard B. (1999). "Critical life events, infections, and symptoms during the year preceding chronic fatigue syndrome (CFS):

An examination of CFS patients and subjects with a nonspecific life crisis," *Psychosomatic Medicine* 61(3): 304-310.

Thompson WG, Dotevall G, Drossman DA, Heaton KW, Kruis W. (1989). "Irritable bowel syndrome: Guidelines for the diagnosis," *Gastroenterology International* 2(2): 92-95.

Thompson WG, Longstreth GF, Drossman DA, Heaton KW, Irvine EJ, Muller-Lissner SA. (1999). "Functional bowel disorder and functional abdominal pain," *Gut* 45(suppl II): 1143-1147.

Uveges JM, Parker JC, Smarr KL, McGowan JF, Lyon MG, Irvin WS, Meyer AA, Buckelew SP, Morgan RK, Delmonico RL, Hewett JE, Kay DR. (1990). "Psychological symptoms in primary fibromyalgia syndrome: Relationship to pain, life stress, and sleep disturbance," *Arthritis and Rheumatism* 33(8): 1279-1283.

Walker LS, Zeman JL. (1992). "Parental response to child illness behavior," *Journal of Pediatric Psychology* 17(1): 49-71.

Wallston KA, Wallston BS, DeVellis R. (1978). "Development of the Multidimensional Health Locus of Control Scale," *Health Education Monograph* 6: 160-170.

Wolfe F, Smythe HA, Yunus MB, Bennett RM, Bombardier C, Goldenberg DL, Tugwell P, Campbell SM, Abeles M, Clark P, Fam AG, Farber SJ, Fiechtner JJ, Franklin CM, Gatter RA, Hamaty D, Lessard J, Lichtbroun AS, Masi AT, McCain GA, Reynolds WJ, Romano TJ, Russell IJ, Sheon RP. (1990). "The American College of Rheumatology 1990 criteria for the classification of fibromyalgia: Report of the multicenter criteria committee," *Arthritis and Rheumatism* 33(2): 160-177.

Yunus M, Masi AT, Calabro JJ, Miller KA, Feigenbaum SL. (1981). "Primary fibromyalgia (fibrositis): Clinical study of 50 patients with matched normal controls," *Seminars in Arthritis and Rheumatism* 11(1): 151-171.

Zautra AJ, Hamilton NA, Burke HM. (1999). "Comparison of stress responses in women with two types of chronic pain: Fibromyalgia and osteoarthritis," *Cognitive Therapy and Research* 23(2): 209-230.

Index

THE PSYCHOPATHOLOGY OF FUNCTIONAL SOMATIC SYNDROMES

Neurobiology and Illness Behavior in Chronic Fatigue Syndrome, Fibromyalgia, Gulf War Illness, Irritable Bowel, and Premenstrual Dysphoria

_____ in hardbound at $59.96 (regularly $79.95) (ISBN: 0-7890-1259-6)

_____ in softbound at $26.21 (regularly $34.95) (ISBN: 0-7890-1260-X)

Or order online and use special offer code HEC25 in the shopping cart.

COST OF BOOKS_____

OUTSIDE US/CANADA/
MEXICO: ADD 20%_____

POSTAGE & HANDLING_____
*(US: $5.00 for first book & $2.00
for each additional book)*
*(Outside US: $6.00 for first book
& $2.00 for each additional book)*

SUBTOTAL_____

IN CANADA: ADD 7% GST_____

STATE TAX_____
*(NY, OH, MN, CA, IN, & SD residents,
add appropriate local sales tax)*

FINAL TOTAL_____
*(If paying in Canadian funds,
convert using the current
exchange rate, UNESCO
coupons welcome)*

☐ **BILL ME LATER:** ($5 service charge will be added)

(Bill-me option is good on US/Canada/Mexico orders only;
not good to jobbers, wholesalers, or subscription agencies.)

☐ Check here if billing address is different from
shipping address and attach purchase order and
billing address information.

Signature_____

☐ **PAYMENT ENCLOSED:** $_____

☐ **PLEASE CHARGE TO MY CREDIT CARD.**

☐ Visa   ☐ MasterCard   ☐ AmEx   ☐ Discover
☐ Diner's Club   ☐ Eurocard   ☐ JCB

Account # _____

Exp. Date_____

Signature_____

Prices in US dollars and subject to change without notice.

NAME_____

INSTITUTION_____

ADDRESS_____

CITY_____

STATE/ZIP_____

COUNTRY_____ COUNTY (NY residents only)_____

TEL_____ FAX_____

E-MAIL_____

May we use your e-mail address for confirmations and other types of information? ☐ Yes ☐ No
We appreciate receiving your e-mail address and fax number. Haworth would like to e-mail or fax special discount offers to you, as a preferred customer. **We will never share, rent, or exchange your e-mail address or fax number.** We regard such actions as an invasion of your privacy.

Order From Your Local Bookstore or Directly From

The Haworth Press, Inc.

10 Alice Street, Binghamton, New York 13904-1580 • USA
TELEPHONE: 1-800-HAWORTH (1-800-429-6784) / Outside US/Canada: (607) 722-5857
FAX: 1-800-895-0582 / Outside US/Canada: (607) 771-0012
E-mailto: orders@haworthpress.com

PLEASE PHOTOCOPY THIS FORM FOR YOUR PERSONAL USE.
http://www.HaworthPress.com   BOF03